MENTAL HEALTH NURSING

Mental Health Nursing

Competencies for Practice

Edited by

Stephan D. Kirby,
Denis A. Hart, Dennis Cross &
Gordon Mitchell

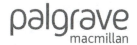

First published 2004 by
PALGRAVE MACMILLAN
Houndmills, Basingstoke, Hampshire RG21 6XS and
175 Fifth Avenue, New York, N.Y. 10010
Companies and representatives throughout the world

PALGRAVE MACMILLAN is the global academic imprint of the Palgrave
Macmillan division of St. Martin's Press, LLC and of Palgrave Macmillan Ltd.
Macmillan® is a registered trademark in the United States, United Kingdom
and other countries. Palgrave is a registered trademark in the European
Union and other countries.

ISBN 1–4039–0262–3 paperback

This book is printed on paper suitable for recycling and made from fully
managed and sustained forest sources.

A catalogue record for this book is available from the British Library.

10   9   8   7   6   5   4   3   2   1
13   12   11   10   09   08   07   06   05   04

Printed and bound in Great Britain by
J. W. Arrowsmith Ltd, Bristol

Contents

Overview **464**
Stephan D. Kirby, Denis A. Hart, Dennis Cross, and Gordon Mitchell

List of Figures

List of Tables

List of Boxes

Foreword

STEPHAN D. KIRBY AND GORDON MITCHELL

At a meeting of mental health educators in November 1999 a recommendation was made that it would be extremely helpful to develop a subset of the UKCC competencies specifically for mental health nurses. The project to develop these competencies was instigated by The Northern Centre for Mental Health.

So, not long after that meeting a group of leading clinicians, academics, service providers and service users from the North East of England met to discuss and plant the seeds of what was to become the 'Competence-Based "Exit Profile" For Pre-Registration Mental Health Nursing'. It was evident at that stage that something innovative was needed to capture the complexities of mental health nursing and mental health nurse education in the twenty-first century.

It is not our intention to maintain a cliché nor to state an obvious truism when we echo the words of Martin Brown (Co-Director of the Northern Centre for Mental Health) when he said that 'tomorrows services will be run, managed and led by today's learners'. It is therefore essential that they receive the proper and timely preparation for their future roles and continual personal and professional development through lifelong learning. The competencies highlighted within this text are designed to show the starting point of the professional journey and will help educators plan curricula, which engage, encourage and enliven learners through a variety of educational activities.

The principle behind the development of the 'Exit Profile' was to ensure that there is consistency in the essential knowledge, skills and attitudes that mental health nursing students will acquire by the end of their educational programmes, while maintaining an acceptable level of flexibility to be responsive to local needs. The developers engaged a partnership approach to curriculum development, which meant that the Curriculum Development Team consisted of not only Mental Health Lecturers, but also clinicians from our local NHS Trusts, the views of previous student nurses and users and carers of local mental health services.

The development of the 'Exit Profile' acknowledges the drive for quality in the NHS, which includes the changing context of mental health care delivery described in the *National Service Framework for Mental Health* (DoH, 1999a). The domains and benchmarks within the 'Exit Profile' (See Appendix 1 of this text) are provided to assist curriculum and planning groups in the construction of contemporary pre-registration mental health nursing education programmes, which have an overall aim of preparing mental health nurses to be fit for practice, purpose and award upon registration.

With the publication of *Making a Difference* (DoH, 1999b), and *Fitness for Practice* (UKCC, 1999) the School of Health and Social Care within the University of Teesside was successful in being chosen as a pilot site to introduce the 'competency-based approach' to Pre-Registration Nurse Training. These reports along with the *Requirements for Pre-registration Nursing Programmes* (UKCC, 2000) provided a contemporary framework for the development of nursing and midwifery programmes based upon a new outcomes and competency approach. The recommendations published in these reports provide generic competencies for entry to the register that have been used as a foundation to construct specific benchmarks for the mental health branch of nursing.

In developing our curriculum we used the *Fitness for Practice* (UKCC, 1999, p 35) definition that described competence as the 'skills and ability to practice safely' and is 'fundamental to the autonomy and accountability of the individual practitioner and therefore to their code of conduct'. Therefore, this competency-based approach to education and the development of the 'Competence Based Exit Profile' (the nucleus and focal point for this text) will encourage the development of the knowledge, understanding, practical and technical skills, attitudes and values of the student nurses who, over a three year period, will work with, as well as support, all those professionals with a responsibility for developing and delivering pre-registration mental health nursing programmes.

Once successfully approved by our internal and external validation bodies it was clearly that the new 'Making a Difference' (MaD) (no pun intended!) Mental Health Student Nurse Training Programme was radically different to our previous programmes. The first two cohorts for this programme commenced (for the Degree Pathway) in September 2000 and (for the Diploma Pathway) in January 2001. These students, including one of this text's authors, are being monitored and evaluated by a national research programme, funded by the Department of Health and are due to qualify soon. But our intermediate evaluation is very positive with practitioners reporting a more competent and skilled student nurse working on the clinical areas. Therefore, this book, as well as being based upon the mental health competencies, is also a reflection of this innovative mental health student nurse pre-registration programme.

While the editors and contributors see the readership of this text as being (primarily though not exclusively) the mental health student nurse undertaking the Making a Difference Mental Health programmes, we also feel that this book is very useful to a wider range of other mental health clinicians – from the newly qualified nurse through to the experienced nurse who acts as a Practice Mentor for the aforementioned students when they undertake their practice. We also hope that this text will help coordinate the practice experience and assist clinical settings to develop their sites and to assist in enhancing further the students' learning experience.

The contributors (apart from those who provide education at the University of Teesside) are drawn from a range of specialities and services around the UK and range of clinical experiences.

Readers should be aware that while each chapter carries benchmarks (taken from the Exit Profile) which are indicative to the theoretical content, one domain was not included (Domain 1.1 *Professional Practice*), this is due to the fact that we feel that this domain and its inherent benchmarks are intrinsic to *all* the chapters in this text and therefore to include them in the tables at the head of each chapter would have been just added to the bulk of benchmarks already there, this is why the observant among you – those of you who intend to 'map' the chapter benchmarks to the framework (in the Appendices) you will not find these particular *benchmarks for achievement* highlighted as being specific to any particular chapter.

We hope that you, the reader, will find the contents of this book interesting, illuminating and provoking a variety of questions and a desire to find out more, which will motivate you to read further texts on the variety of subjects covered here. We are not intending to provide all the answers to questions, rather we would like you to use this book as a 'springboard' to further reading for your personal and professional development.

We hope you enjoy what you read from here forward.

Stephan D. Kirby, Gordon Mitchell, Dennis Cross & Denis A. Hart

References

Department Of Health (1999a) *National Service Framework for Mental Health*, London: HMSO.

Department of Health (1999b) *Making A Difference: Strengthening The Nursing, Midwifery and Health Visiting Contribution To Health and Health Care*, London: HMSO.

United Kingdom Central Council For Nursing, Midwifery and Health Visiting (1999) *Fitness For Practice*, London: UKCC.

United Kingdom Central Council For Nursing, Midwifery and Health Visiting (2000) *Requirements for Pre-registration Nursing Programmes*, London: UKCC.

Notes on the Contributors

Sheila Arnold: BSc (Hons), MSc, RMN, RGN, RNT, Cert Ed, Cert Coun, Dip Nursing, (PhD Student) is Senior Lecturer at the School of Health and Social Care, University of Teesside. She has over three decades of experience as a psychiatric–mental health nurse and educator. Sheila is a Registered Mental Health Nurse and Registered General Nurse and completed a Diploma in Nursing in 1980. In recent years her personal, professional research interests have been in relation to the experiences of nurses in the field of psychiatric care with a particular focus on 'therapeutic working' and 'therapeutic conversation'. Her Doctoral studies involve a discourse analysis of the experiences of nurses utilizing a psychosocial approach (PSI) to care of the individual and their families and carers.

Val Chapman taught modern foreign languages until she became a full-time carer in 1998. She now works as a volunteer with 'Rethink', the UK's largest mental illness charity, and is involved in carer support, campaigning for better services, and reducing stigma. She coordinates a support/campaigning group throughout County Durham, and is working in partnership with the local NHS Psychiatrist Trust to improve services to families. She has a particular interest in early intervention and has been involved in the Newcastle Early Psychosis Declaration, which is supported by the World Health Organization and is set to become an international benchmark for service providers. She has recently trained as an advocate and set up an advocacy service for members of the group.

Jan Connolly: BA (Hons), MA, RMN, PgCE, DPSN, RNT is Senior Lecturer in the School of Health and Social Care at the University of Teesside. Jan undertook her pre-registration training at the Maudsley Hospital, London and completed in 1982. She qualified as a Nurse Teacher in 1991. Her current role is Pathway Leader for the Advanced Diploma in Mental Health Nursing. She was formerly Clinical Nurse Specialist (Mood Disorders) and Honorary Lecture-Practitioner, Liaison Psychiatry. Specific professional interests include Cognitive Behaviour Therapy; Interpersonal Psychotherapy; Feminist approaches to Women's Mental Health Problems and Discourse Analysis.

Dennis Cross: TD, BA (Hons), BEd (Hons), MA, RMN, RGN, RNT, (PhD Student) (co-editor) is Principal Lecturer (Mental Health) School of Health and Social Care at the University of Teesside. He is currently completing his PhD in nursing education and mental health. He was the Project

Leader for the development of the 'Exit Profile' working closely with Elaine Readhead, on behalf of the Northern and Yorkshire NHS Workforce Development Group and the Northern Centre for Mental Health. During part of academic year 2002/3 he has been seconded to the Institute of Technology in Tralee, Ireland to help to introduce a new pre-registration degree in Mental Health Nursing.

Liz Desira: BSc (Hons), MSc, RMN, RGN, RCNT, Cert Ed is a Senior Lecturer in the School of Health and Social Care at the University of Teesside. She undertook her pre-registration Adult Nursing at Mount Vernon Hospital Middlesex, her Midwifery training at the Simpson Memorial Maternity Pavilion, Edinburgh and Mental Health training at The Middlesex Hospital, London and Hill End Hospital, St Albans. After a short period working as an operating theatre sister she returned to mental health nursing. Her current employment includes (as well as being Senior Lecturer (Mental Health)) her role as Examinations and Assessments Officer for pre- and post-registration nursing studies at the University of Teesside. Specific professional interests include care of the elderly and health promotion.

Mike Firn: BA (Hons). RMN is a Mental Health Nurse with nine years experience using the Assertive Community Treatment model in the UK. He is the Service Manager for 3 ACT Teams in South West London, as well as Home Treatment and Early Intervention Services. Mike is coordinator of the London Region for the National Forum for Assertive Outreach. He has co-authored with Prof. Tom Burns, the book *Assertive Outreach in Mental Health*, a manual for practitioners, published by Oxford University Press (2002).

Mike Fleet: BSc, MSc, RMN, RGN, PgCE, Dip Thorn is a Senior Lecturer, at the School of Health and Social Care, University of Teesside. Mike is module leader for several programmes including 'Integrated Approaches and Interventions with People with Serious Mental Illness and Their Families', 'Multidisciplinary Assertive Outreach for the Severely Mentally Ill' and 'Awareness of Psychosocial Interventions'. Previously Mike was Clinical Nurse Specialist with the South West London and St George's Hospital Mental Health NHS Trust's Assertive Community Treatment Team. He is currently developing a degree in 'Evidence-based Interventions in Mental Health and Social Care' to promote evidence-based practice at a clinical level. Mike is a member of the British Association for Behavioural and Cognitive Psychotherapies.

Gillian Green: BSc (Hons), RMN, Dip Nursing, (PhD Student) is the Specialist Clinical Practitioner at the Duchess of Kent's Psychiatric Hospital, Catterick Garrison, North Yorkshire. Her role has focused on psychological injury for the past six years. She has been instrumental in the establishment an ongoing development of a Defence Medical Services Unit dedicated to the assessment and treatment of psychological injury resulting from traumatic experiences. Her keen interest in the professional development of both herself and others has enabled her to design and implement an evidence-based six month rotational training programme for Registered Mental Health nurses in the assessment and treatment of psychological injury. In addition to this she has also developed and presented a number of workshops and educational packages focusing on various aspects of stress and trauma across a range of both health care and non-health care professionals. Gillian is also a member of the International Society of Traumatic Stress Studies (ISTSS), which has afforded her a number of opportunities not only to share her research interests, but also to present the model of care used by her and her colleagues on a national and international level. In addition she is also a member of the British Association of Behavioural and Cognitive Psychotherapy (BABCP).

Maggie Hadland: BA (Hons), MA (Ed), RMN, RGN, RNT, Cert Ed is a Senior Lecturer in the School of Health and Social Care at the University of Teesside. After obtaining a first degree in Sociology, Maggie trained in both Adult and Mental Health Nursing, and has worked in a variety of Acute Mental Health settings, including managing a 29-bed acute in-patient facility. Maggie is also a qualified counsellor, having received her Masters in Counselling from Durham University, and was responsible for implementing and operating a counselling service in five schools for children and young people aged 9 to 18. Maggie continues to practice counselling with children in a local primary school. Her current teaching includes providing the input on Humanistic Counselling approaches to the MSc in Counselling and Counselling Psychology, as well as teaching counselling skills to nurses and other health professionals. At the moment she is studying for a Post-Graduate Diploma in Psychology, and is researching changes in visual–spatial ability over the menstrual cycle. Other research interests are adult attachment and women and mental health.

Angela Hall: BSc (Hons), MA, RMN, RGN, RNT, PgCE, Cert Coun, App Dip (PhD Student) is a Senior Lecturer (Mental Health) in the School of Health and Social Care, University of Teesside. Angela is Programme Leader for the Joint Social Work/Mental Health Nursing framework at pre-registration, the first in the UK. Having qualified in both Mental Health and General Nursing she practised as a Community Mental Health Nurse, first within Primary Care and more recently as part of a Community Mental Health Team. She became a nurse educator in 1992 and her current interests are in Inter-professional Working and Education, Primary Mental Health Care and Psychosocial Interventions for People with a Serious Mental Illness. Her PhD studies are focused on the students development of a 'Shared Professional Identity'.

Celia Harbottle: BA (Hons), MA, CSS, Cert is a Senior Lecturer in Social Work/Learning Disability Nursing at the School of Health and Social Care, University of Teesside. She is also Programme Leader for awards offering both nursing and social work qualifications. Her research interests are integrated working, competency frameworks in vocational education and social care practice. She is also a fellow of the Royal Society of Arts.

Stephen Harrison: BSc Hons, RMN, Dip CAMH (ENB 603), Dip CMHN is a Nurse Consultant working at the Newberry Centre for Young People in Middlesbrough (Tees and North East Yorkshire NHS Trust). He took up the post in September 2002. Born and raised in Teesside, his career began as a Nursing Assistant working with teenagers in 1979. He trained at St Luke's Hospital and went on to study Nursing to Degree Level at the University of Teesside. Steve has nursed and managed in residential and community settings with young people as well as contributing to the Health Advisory Service Thematic Review – 'Together We Stand' – and contributing to the Department of Health's Children's National Service Framework. Steve is also a part time lecturer at the University of York teaching on the Child and Adolescent Mental Health Degree Pathway.

Denis A. Hart: MPhil, MA/CQSW, MA, BSc. (Soc), MBSA, (co-editor) is a Visiting Lecturer at the School of Health and Social Care, University of Teesside. Prior to this Denis was Houseparent at Kingswood School in the late 1960s and early 1970s before becoming House-warden at Tennal Assessment Centre from 1970 to 1971. He then entered academia and was Lecturer in Social Work (University of Bristol, 1971–73), he then became Deputy Head at Aycliffe Assessment Centre in County Durham (1973–81) becoming Head of the Centre between 1981 and 1985. In 1985 he returned once again to academia when he became Principal Lecturer at Trent Polytechnic. He moved to the University of Teesside in 1991 when he became the Principal Lecturer (Social Work) until 1997. From then to the present date, Denis has been a Research Associate working with the University of Teesside. As well as producing a wealth of Open Learning materials for a variety of programmes within the School of Health and Social Care, Denis is also a Trustee for the Resource Network for Disordered Adolescents, he monitors Bail support for NACRO and the Youth Justice Board and is working on developing protocols with the local Youth Offending Team.

Sue Jackson: RGN, BSc. (Hons), MPhil trained as an RGN in London and worked predominantly in head injury and neuro-oncology in London then moved to Addenbrookes in Cambridge where she completed the ENB 148 (Neuro-medical, Neuro-surgical Nursing). Sue has travelled and worked in Australia for 3 years. On her return, she studied for her BSc. (Hons) (Health Studies) at East Anglia Polytechnic University. Sue then moved to Newcastle and joined the Department of Psychiatry in 1995, where she has undertaken a number of research studies in mental health issues in nursing. Working with Prof. Phil Barker and Dr Chris Stevenson, she was involved in the 'Need for Nursing Studies'. Sue's MPhil Thesis 'What Do People Need Psychiatric and Mental Health Nurses For' was one of a collection of studies which formed the underpinning framework for the Tidal Model of Nursing (Barker, 2000).

Stephan D. Kirby: MSc, PgC (L&T), Dip MDO, RMN (PhD Student) (co-editor) is a Senior Lecturer (Forensic Health and Social Care) in the School of Health and Social Care at the University of Teesside. He has nearly three decades of experience working with the mentally ill, the largest part being within Forensic Mental Health Services. He is Programme Leader for a number of post-registration educational pathways as well as numerous other pathways and modules ranging from Level 1 through to Masters level. The research for his MSc Thesis looked at Cognitive Distortions in Child Sexual Offenders. Currently he is studying for his PhD, which is exploring the experiences of 'Life in a Category A Segregation Unit'. Steve is also the current Chair of the National Forensic Nurses' Research and Development Group (www.forensicnurse.org.uk) and is also (Non-Executive) Director of Nursing for Veritas Management Ltd. Veritas provides highly experienced staff to all types of healthcare services. It specializes in secure environments, especially Police Nurses, and HMP Service with the provision of Custody Nurses and Forensic Medical Examiners.

Anne Maidment: MA, BA, Cert Ed is a user of mental health services in the North East of England. She describes her mental illness (bipolar disorder) first becoming apparent after the birth of her son. She describes her interests and activities as: *Political* – has been a constituency Chair for 18 months and on the Executive for 8 years; *Trade Union* – regional Vice Chair and National Council Member for NATFHE and helped to establish the Retired Members Section; *Misc.* she has been a Community Health Council member for 6 years and a member of the Committee of Sunderland Art Studio. Anne is also a member of Headlight – Sunderland's Mental Health Resource Centre. She retired, on health grounds, in 1992.

Geoff Martin: RGN, RMN, BSc (Hons), MA has worked in Mental Health Nursing and with the care of older people in Leicester and Middlesex Hospitals before moving into education as Staff Development Officer at Bishop Auckland General Hospital. He joined the University of Teesside in the mid 1990s, and is presently Team Leader for the Adult Nursing Team. His research has been around empowerment of dying patients and more recently working with an audit programme in North Durham using Dementia Care Mapping. The project attempted to measure the level of person-centred care provided by the Mental Health Trust in the area and the work has been published in a series of papers in national nursing journals.

Peter Melia: BA (Hons), MA, RMN, PgCE, PgCPD is the Nurse Consultant (Forensic Service), at the The Hutton Centre, St Luke's Hospital, Middlesbrough (Tees and North East Yorkshire NHS Trust). He has worked in forensic mental health services for more than two decades and has considerable experience in both health service management and clinical practice. He has contributed significantly to the development of PSI type (poly-factorial) approaches in working with individuals who suffer serious mental illness and personality disorder.

Gordon Mitchell: BSc (Hons), MA, RMN, Dip Nursing, ILTM, (co-editor) is a Senior Lecturer and Pathway Leader for Pre-Registration Mental Health Nursing in the School of Health and Social Care at the University of Teesside. He has responsibility for the implementation of the Making a Difference programme for Pre-Registration Mental Health Nurse Training. Specialist areas for teaching, are Mental Health Law, Care of the Client in a Acute Mental Health Setting. He has been working with the local Mental Health Trust on a project to implement 'Essence of Care' and with the Older Person Unit, which successful achieved Practice Development Unit Status. Gordon's clinical background, since qualifying includes working with clients in an acute mental health setting until 1992, when he entered education, however he still maintains clinical links with an acute admission unit where he spends time working with staff and student nurses on the complexities of this client group.

Angela Morgan RGN, RM, Cert Ed, BSc. (Hons) MSc is a Principal Lecturer, currently working in the role of Learning and Teaching Co-ordinator in the School of Health and Social Care at the University of Teesside. She is a Nurse and Midwife and retains a commitment to facilitating learning for a wide range of health professionals in the field of research methods and evidence-based practice.

David Mudd: MSc, RMN, RNMH, Cert Ed, Dip CPN is the Principal Lecturer, for Learning Disability in the School of Health and Social Care, University of Teesside. His research interests include evaluating the influence of service-user involvement in the development, delivery and evaluation of health and social care educational curricula. He is currently involved in curriculum developments related to integrated approaches to health and social care and working across organizational and professional boundaries.

Elaine Readhead: BA (Hons), MA, RMN, Dip CPN is a Project Manager for the Northern Centre for Mental Health – A Regional Development Centre for the National Institute for Mental Health (England) (NIMHE). Elaine started work in the National Health Service in 1981 as a Registered Mental Nurse. She has a wide range of experience in a variety of community settings. She has also worked as a Mental Health Training Co-ordinator for a local Workforce Development Confederation. She currently manages projects relating to mental health education, training and workforce development. Elaine is also a Visiting Fellow at Teesside University.

Colin Rowley is a student nurse on the BSc (Hons) Nursing Studies (Mental Health) course at the University of Teesside and is due to graduate in 2003. He is a member of the first cohort to undertake the Making a Difference programme – which is underpinned by the Exit Profile explored within this text. At the time of writing he is in his third year, having lived through the experience of writing two portfolio's and is currently engaged in his third. His experience throughout the course has ranged from acute settings through to high and medium secure forensic settings. He sees his immediate future in acute nursing with a long-term view of working in community settings. He is currently undertaking his dissertation examining the interface between primary and secondary care.

Chris Stanbury: RMN, BSc (Psychotherapy), MEd is a registered mental health nurse and came into nursing as a psychology graduate and now has over 20 years of experience of nursing practice. She holds a second registration in psychodynamic psychotherapy and a Masters Degree in Education. She has special interests in clinical supervision and nursing practice development and has worked in nurse education and acute mental health as a Nurse Specialist. Her current post in the Mental Health and Learning Disabilities Trust in County Durham and Darlington is Deputy Director of Nursing.

Dr Chris Stevenson: RMN, BA (Hons), MSc (Dist), PhD is Reader in Nursing at the University of Teesside. The focus of her scholarship was on describing the nature of nursing, the nature of nursing research and scholarship and the nature of nurse education/training, from within the postmodern turn. Chris has a keen interest in social constructionism in relation to the practice of family therapy, especially with people in eating distress, a further research interest. She has worked closely with Prof. Phil Barker in developing and evaluating the Tidal Model of Psychiatric Nursing, which has a developing profile nationally and internationally. Chris has an extensive publication profile, which includes many papers that challenge received nursing wisdom.

Dominic Wake: BSc (Hons), MSc, RMN, RGN is a Senior Lecturer in the School of Health and Social Care, University of Teesside. Dominic worked for 3 years in Acute Psychiatry at Guy's Hospital where he developed an interest in substance use by instigating sessional work with heroin users in and around Deptford. He then joined the Community Drug Team which covered Lewisham & Southwark for 3 years. He then developed and managed a new Methadone Dispensing Programme before moving back to the North East, where he developed a three year alcohol home detoxification service. Dominic then managed the in-patient detoxification beds at Hartlepool General Hospital before moving to Guisborough to manage the Community Drug Team in Redcar & East Cleveland. For the past couple of years, his main interest has been with parents and families of drug-users and how services provide support for them.

James T. Watson: RGN, ONC, RCNT, RNT Dip Nursing, MBA, MA, BEd (Hons), Dip (Pg) is Senior Lecturer and Pathway Leader for the Management Pathway within the BSc (Hons) Promoting Practice Effectiveness at the School of Health and Social Care, University of Teesside. James' career in Nursing has covered a wide range of areas from General Nursing, Paediatric Nursing, Learning Difficulties to Mental Health care. In the latter part of his career he has focused on the subject of management applied to the NHS and Nursing. James' work within the Colleges of Nursing and over the past 10 years the School of Health and Social Care at the University of Teesside, has enabled him to teach a wide area of management subjects from Certificate to Masters level within the context of the NHS and in particular the Nursing Profession.

Lyn Williams: MSc, Dip HE, RMN, HNC is Consultant Nurse, Liaison Psychiatry for Tees and North East Yorkshire NHS Trust. She qualified as an RMN in 1992 and worked within acute inpatient admission areas for elderly mentally ill and acute general psychiatry. Lyn began working in Liaison Psychiatry in 1996 when Liaison Psychiatry was first established in Middlesbrough. Liaison Psychiatry is a relatively new concept of mental health nursing and today is increasingly being acknowledged as a specialism within mental health nursing. Within her current role she has developed partnership working within Cancer Care at the local Acute Trust. This work was undertaken in the form of project work initiating a 'nurse to nurse' fast track referral route for mental health assessment for patients diagnosed with breast cancer and presenting mental health problems. Other areas of interest include, the development of an Integrated Care Pathway (ICP) in conjunction with the local Acute Trust for those presenting following an act of deliberate self harm. The main aims of the ICP is to improve the quality of the patient journey through the Acute Trust, prevent repetition, identify those at high risk of suicide, identify new mental illness. Also, in light of the National Suicide Prevention Strategy, establishing a multi agency task force to address suicide on Teesside and finally developing national core competencies for nurses wanting to pursue a career in Liaison Psychiatry.

Neil Woodward: RMN; Cert Ed; RCNI has a long history of working in forensic mental health care and is currently responsible for the management of the 'Aggression Management Training Centre' for the Tees & North East Yorkshire NHS Trust. He is an experienced Trainer, practitioner and lecturer in aggression management techniques and theory and has provided personal safety and aggression management training to a variety of health care personnel, both nationally and internationally.

Introduction

STEPHAN D. KIRBY, DENIS A. HART, DENNIS CROSS AND
GORDON MITCHELL

The principal aim of this text is to provide student mental health nurses with the necessary foundation knowledge required to enable them to integrate theory and practice when evidencing competence. The text is further designed to provide current practice mentors with a contemporary knowledge base to enable them to both evaluate performable, and to assist those on the practice placements to develop the required theoretical, connections.

In recent years, mental health nurse training has developed significantly from hospital-based training to academically based Schools within the Higher Education Sector. With this transition mental health nursing was transformed from a day-to-day operational context to fully fledged graduate level training programmes.

This transition occurred quite rapidly and saw the development of bench-mark criteria as performance indicators of the competences to be developed and acquired. This has created a real void in terms of the adaptation of existing practical nursing knowledge and theoretical underpinning to focus specifically on enabling students to integrate theory, values and praxis into evidenced competence in practice.

The text begins by recognizing the need for the contemporary mental health nurse to work effectively in partnership with service users and their carers in keeping with the National Service Framework for Mental Health (Department of Health, 1999). The 'Background to Good Practice and Effective Learning' section therefore introduces the reader to these themes as they are developed, first, by the Chapter on 'The Recognition of Inequality and the Need for Empowerment', which seeks to encourage students to explore their own value bases and then apply new knowledge to appraise individual, cultural and structural discrimination. The theme is continued when we explore the importance of service-user involvement in research within mental health is demonstrated in 'How Can Nurses Meet the Needs of Mental Health Clients?'. This chapter is based on a funded research study and we feel that its inclusion offers the reader a balance within the text between the theory and competency driven chapters. This reports a study that explored how mental health professionals, service users, ex-service users and carers perceived the needs of people in the psychiatric system. The section closes with valuable insights into contemporary mental health services and its practice from both a service user and a carer of a mental health service user.

Although assessment is a key theme throughout the text, the authors recognize that this is a pre-requisite to any form of intervention or treatment. In Part II 'Prevention and Health Promotion, the chapter on 'Common Mental Health Problems' provides learners with a typology of conditions to enable them to make assessment evaluations that encapsulate need, risk and self-determination as well as the aetiology of the presenting problems. The themes of collaborative working, explorations of values and patient-centred care are continued through the chapters on 'Mental Health Promotion' and 'A Positive Approach to Mental Health Nursing: Role, Values and Attitudes'. The chapter 'Risk Prevention' addresses the need to balance, the rights of the patient, the needs of the patient and the potential costs to others, when determining an appropriate care plan. As mental health nurses work in the community as well as in residential settings the final chapter of the section addresses the crucial aspect of 'Creating and Maintaining a Safe Environment' without differentiating between patient or staff showing that the issues raised within the chapter are important to all of us within mental health services.

The third Part 'Continuum of Treatment' helps to provide a robust framework for effective practice and is further developed by revealing the key modalities of service delivery based upon appropriate diagnoses notably, 'Treating Post-traumatic Stress Disorder', 'Psycho-social Interventions for People with Serious Mental Health Problems', 'Brief Psychological Therapies' and 'Using Counselling in Mental Health Practice'. As risk is an additional theme that transcends contemporary practice there is a strong emphasis on the management of individuals in a variety of settings, hence this section also looks at 'Mental Health Nursing Within Secure Conditions', 'Assessing and Engaging People with Personality Disorder', 'Assertive Community Treatment . . .' and 'Interdisciplinary Approaches to Community Mental Health Practice'.

Given the need for both students and qualified mental health practitioners to engage in evidence based practice, this final Part deals with 'Using Effective Learning to Develop Reflective Practice' and how the student and their practice mentors can use the Competency Based Exit Profile to monitor the acquisition of new skills and to assess student practice. This section looks at issues as wide as 'Management for Practice' and 'Learning: from Self-development to Competency'. It also includes a 'hands on' perspective from a student of the first cohort of Making A Difference students, who offers his views on completing the competency based programme in 'A Framework for Success: A Students Perspective'. This Part, and the text, finishes with a collection of lived experiences from three senior practitioners from varied services, who are offering the reader 'A Day in the Life of . . .'.

Throughout the text the emergence of the Multi-Agency Public Protection Panels (MAPPP's) are identified and the revised Mental Health legislation is anticipated and there is an emphasis on early intervention and public safety building upon the powers already contained in the Mental Health (Patients in the Community) Act (Department of Health, 1995).

We hope this text will not only provide students with the necessary under-pinning knowledge in one central point to enable them to become effective practitioners but that furthermore the text will assist mentors in their task of ensuring quality of the workforce and maintaining high standards of practice for the benefits of the public, carers, and most importantly the patients themselves.

References

Department of Health (1995) *Mental Health (Patients in the Community) Act*, London: HMSO.

Department Of Health (1999) *National Service Framework for Mental Health*, London: HMSO.

PART I

BACKGROUND TO GOOD PRACTICE AND EFFECTIVE LEARNING

This first Part begins by focusing on the student as a learner as the first chapter explores the development of the competency approach and its relationship to the exit profile. Other chapters build upon this perspective beginning with the chapter on the 'Recognition of Inequality and the Need For Empowerment' and developing this further in Chapter 3 'How Can Nurses Meet the Needs of Mental Health Clients' by examining research undertaken into the contemporary mental health nurse role. The researchers concluded that it is essential to involve service users and carers throughout the mental health system and consequently Chapter 4 is an appraisal from the service user's point of view while Chapter 5 is an appraisal of mental health services from a carer's point of view.

CHAPTER 1

Developing a Competence-based 'Exit Profile' for Pre-registration Mental Health Nursing

DENNIS CROSS AND ELAINE READHEAD

The project at the centre of this chapter and the topic it covers, which lies at the fundamental heart of the complete text, relates to the development of a competence-based exit profile for mental health student nurses (Northern Centre for Mental Health et al, 2000). This project was a collaborative venture between Service Providers, the University of Teesside and the Northern Centre for Mental Health (NCMH). The Northern Centre for Mental Health was established in 1999 by the Northern and Yorkshire Regional NHS mental health service providers to support a Regional modernization programme through project work and is affiliated to the Sainsbury Centre for Mental Health.

This chapter will introduce the reader to how and why the 'exit profile' for pre-registration mental health nursing was developed. This background will be important to all educators, practitioners and users of services who are charged with constructing and delivering 'Making a Difference' (DoH, 1999a) programmes for mental health nurses. The development of this 'exit profile' acknowledged the drive for quality in the National Health Service (NHS), which included the changing context of mental health care delivery described in the National Service Framework for Mental Health (NSF) (DoH, 1999b).

The benchmarks within the 'exit profile' were intended to provide assistance for curriculum-planning groups in the construction of contemporary pre-registration mental health nursing education programmes. They were also expected to aid the commissioners of pre-registration mental health education determine what a contemporary mental health nurse education programme would include. The overall aim being to prepare mental health nurses to become fit for practice, purpose and award upon registration.

Competencies for Entry to the Register

The United Kingdom Central Council for Nursing, Midwifery and Health Visiting (UKCC) *Competencies for Entry to the Register* (UKCC, 1999b) were used in the development of the 'exit profile' as a foundation to construct specific benchmarks for the mental health branch of nursing. The aim of developing an 'exit profile' was to produce a point of reference to ensure national consistency in the essential knowledge, skills and attitudes which mental health nursing students are expected to acquire by the end of their educational pathway.

For many years, a number of concerns had been expressed regarding the quality of mental health nurse training (see particularly Dodd, 1973; UKCC, 1986), notably poor educational standards, skills development, service delivery, recruitment and retention. These highlighted the deficiencies in the delivery of programmes and identified factors that were suggested as barriers to educational improvement. Camiah (1998, p 369) suggested that until the introduction and implementation of Project 2000 (P2K) in 1986 nurse education was: 'organised along an apprenticeship model of education and training which was characterised by embodying conventional teaching methods and learning styles'.

The original Project 2000 proposal document *A New Preparation for Practice* (UKCC, 1986) identified required changes to the funding and delivery of nurse education. This encouraged a more adult learning orientated educational philosophy. The process of learning was facilitated by the recognition of each student's individual potential and worth, which included the development of a portfolio to encourage self-evaluation and critically reflective practice. This entails the student 'logging' their own development and needs and this process thereby becomes an important part, not only of learning, but also of assessment, for as Jowett et al (1994, p 4), rightly observed: 'the emphasis in the relevant documentation should be consistently student-centred'.

The aim of P2K was to influence the status of nurse education by reforming the nursing curricula and the reorganization of nursing knowledge. This would be delivered by a Common Foundation Programme (CFP) for the first 18 months, followed by specialization in one of four branches for a further 18 months (adult nursing, mental health nursing, learning disabilities nursing or children's nursing). It also: dictated a move from hospital-based education into higher education establishments; provided supernumerary status for students; and gave them a Diploma level qualification. Academic work and practice placements were to be evenly divided across the programme, while the teacher–student relationship moved from one of lecturer–tutor to that of mentor and facilitator of learning.

The new format, however, did not receive universal acclaim. Cuthbertson (1996, p 38), for example, claimed that: 'Project 2000 nurses were not well prepared, particularly in relation to having enough practical skills.' In response, the UKCC established a commission for education, chaired by Sir Leonard Peach, that was given 12 months to: 'Prepare a way forward for pre-registration nursing and midwifery education that enables fitness for practice based on health care need' (UKCC, 1999a, p 2).

This study culminated in the *Fitness for Practice Report* (UKCC, 1999a), which made 33 recommendations building on the P2K framework. The report recognized the Government's prioritization of economic and social factors, notably an ageing population and the changes in the expectations of the workforce.

The Department of Health responded by producing *Making a Difference* (DoH, 1999a), stressing that: 'nursing and midwifery are no longer routine, task orientated roles; they are patient and client centred based on holistic partnership approaches to care' (ibid, p 17). The recommendations were implemented by the creation of 16 'Partnership' sites, each to include a Higher Education Institution (HEI), a pre-registration nurse education provider and a Commissioner of Nurse Education or Education Consortium (now the Workforce Development Confederation).

The UKCC operationalized *Making A Difference* in its *Requirements for Pre-registration Nursing Programmes* (UKCC, 2000). This established a contemporary framework for the development of nursing and midwifery programmes using a competency-based approach, which could be used to evidence eligibility for entry to the register for all four branches of nursing. However, some practitioners and educators felt this not to be sufficiently specialized to appraise ability in a specific area of practice. A group of mental health practitioners argued that the proposed UKCC generic nursing 'skills' needs to be further defined to make it specifically relevant to the acquisition of mental health nursing skills. Barnett (1994, p 76) supported this when he stated that: 'We cannot teach skills as such, we have to specify the skills in mind.'

The competency approach in its entirety hasn't gone unchallenged. Barnett (1994), Edwards & Usher (1994) and Hyland (1992) have all raised issues. Barnett (1994, p 76) in particular, was concerned that as competence focuses upon: 'action and behaviour as such, the ways in which in professional life, at least action is saturated with thought, understanding and reflection is entirely neglected'.

While practice-based competence is essential to safe clinical practice, the changing day-to-day environments in which these competencies are applied will require thought and understanding in order to adapt them to new situations, for as Schön (1983) explained we should recognize that professional practice is a matter of reflection-in-action and knowledge in use. Similarly, Birch (1998) argued that the graduate employee will need to show an interest in making links between the world of pure understanding and the world of action. This action focus is considered to be central to the perception of the nurse in the modernised mental health service since: 'action without insight, we might say is blind' (Barnett, 1994, p 84).

Furthermore, it was suggested by Edwards and Usher (1994, p 2) that competence could be used as: 'a means of producing consent without the need for oppression and force in the reproduction of social order', which would clearly conflict with the nursing education philosophy that it should be 'based on humanistic and holistic principles with the student as the central focus' (Jowett et al, 1994, p 4).

There are, however, advocates for the competency-based approach (Jessup, 1991). Even Barnett (1994) stated that there can be no objection in principle to the application of the terms of competence and outcomes to the educational processes, however, he goes on to state (1994, p 71) that: 'Characterising educational processes primarily in these terms and deploying these terms as criteria by which educational processes are to be designed and evaluated are matters of concern'.

The journey to construct a competence-based 'exit profile' for mental health pre-registration nurses began. The Development Group believed that it was not the educators alone who should identify the competence statements but rather a collaborative partnership of all stakeholders, educators, and commissioners and practitioners from the mental health service providers. The stakeholders were identified, according to Weiss (1986), as persons affected by the implementation of policy. While Jessup (1991, p 150) set the curriculum for the context by stating that: 'Outcome statements can be created for all learning that is considered important or what people want. You cannot say what you require, how can you develop it and how do you know when you have achieved it?'.

The Development Group addressed this by ensuring the stakeholder partnership was reflected in the construction process and by identifying the processes used in the construction of an 'exit profile' plan (see Figure 1.1).

The process began by asking all stakeholders to identify the proposed skills that mental health nurses require to enter the nursing register as fit for practice, followed by an identification as to how feedback would be defined, analysed and presented as a cogently argued response to the exercise. This approach has been endorsed by Robson (1993, p 23) who argued: 'There is much to be said for regarding this initial stage of research as a group process and enlisting the help of others.'

The consultation process relied heavily on qualitative data, which did not appear to fit precisely into any one style of educational research, but which promoted the need for practical reflection (Elliott, 1987; Stenhouse, 1983) and the critical theorist concepts of Carr and Kemmis (1986). Although it was felt that the study appeared to be similar to Elliott's (1987) perspective, central to which is the idea that the practitioner: 'Develops a personal interpretative understanding from working on practical problems and that theoretical understanding is constitutive of practical action and discourse' (Elliott, 1987, p 157).

Undoubtedly the main limitation of the study was the very short timescale imposed (three months) in which to construct the 'exit profile'. This was as

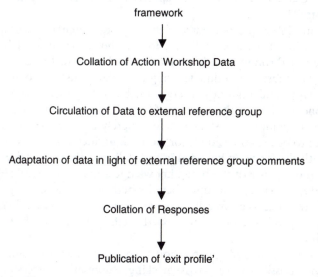

Identification of work already undertaken by others with regard to competencies of mental

health workers

↓

Collation of work to date

↓

Production of working paper, which includes collated information for circulation prior to

Action Workshop

↓

One day Action Workshop, to include all stakeholders, to develop an initial competency

framework

↓

Collation of Action Workshop Data

↓

Circulation of Data to external reference group

↓

Adaptation of data in light of external reference group comments

↓

Collation of Responses

↓

Publication of 'exit profile'

Figure 1.1　The processes used in the construction of an 'exit profile' plan

a result of pressure placed by the 'Fitness for Practice' partnership sites who required validation of the revised nursing curricula by September 2000. One key question used in the initial consultation was, 'what should the development of the "exit profile" contribute to the formation and development of independent, informed mental health nurse practitioners?' The groups' vision was that it would be a modernized framework of mental health nurse education that would deliver nurses who were fit for practice. This thinking was similar to that of Lester (1995, p 45, cited in O'Reilly et al, 1999) who described his proposed model of professional development as: 'self-managed, intelligent practitioners capable of advancing their practice and operating effectively in environments of uncertainty and change'.

The group concluded that the needs of the modern mental health practitioner could not be realized with a list of competencies or actions and behaviours of what they ought to be able to do but should further consider the fact that: 'competent professionals should be able not simply to cope with change but actively to shape change' (Barnett, 1994, p 73). This addition necessitates the encouragement of an enquiring, critical and creative approach to learning at the same time as meeting the statutory bodies' requirements of pre-registration nursing curricula. Lester (1995, p 46, cited in O'Reilly et al, 1999) rightly points out that: 'practice characterised by technical knowledge, standards and professional boundaries is by itself inadequate for professional work at the close of the 20th century'. He goes on further to suggest that what is required is: 'a moving up a level from the frameworks offered by professional bodies and curriculum designers and seeing them as perspectives or frames of reference from which to approach the territory rather than as the territory itself'.

Chapman (1999, p 134) stated that: 'the competency-based approach to nurse education is an indisputable reality but the curriculum needs to be constantly viewed through a critical lens if excellence is to be realised. Nursing competencies must only influence or guide, they must not control the curriculum.' Thus, utilizing both 'interpersonal' and 'intrapersonal' strategies the group concluded that the 'exit profile' must not be a purely technical-rational list of competence standards that merely measure performance as this would lead to professional education becoming: 'increasingly narrow and specialised with the focus on knowledge and skills specific to practice of the profession at the expense of the broad knowledge and perspectives' (Haggerty & Early, 1992, p 29). The group debated whether this was exactly what it was doing. Narrowing the overall nursing curricula to mental health-specific benchmarks, and it therefore questioned itself, had the concept been grasped incorrectly?

The group considered this method to be more inclusive and particularly valued the possibility of cross-checking summative assessment against the development of clinical competence. Cross-checking was first raised by Partlett and Hamilton (1972) within their approach to evaluation, which they described (p 14) as: 'different techniques are combined to throw light on a common problem. Besides viewing the problem from a number of angles, this triangulation approach also facilitates the crosschecking of findings'.

In relation to clinical assessment, Clifford (1994) and Duke (1996) recommended that clinical assessors need to be properly educated and thoughtfully mentored themselves to perform this expert role.

The outcome of clinical evaluation decisions has serious implications for students in terms of self-esteem and protection of their rights to pursue a livelihood; for the patients and clients with regards to protection from unsafe practice; and for teachers concerned with potential charges of unfair evaluation practices and the legal repercussions of decisions where students are wrongly failed (or passed) on a clinical practice course. (Cohen et al, 1993, p 14)

The Development Group responded by recognizing that assessment is a powerful concept and has a key role in ascertaining fitness for purpose. Involving significant others in the assessment process could thus be seen as a two-edged sword. On the one hand it could lead to key stakeholders such as service users claiming that a potential practitioner was acting badly or inappropriately simply by denying them services or by using authority appropriately but with an outcome perceived by them to be detrimental. While, on the other hand, as Birchenal (1999, p 431) has rightly pointed out: 'the success of nurse education depends on open and transparent relationships with service providers.'

The group recognized throughout the development process that collaboration presented both a challenge and an opportunity to embrace individual learning as part of creating an effective learning environment. This collaborative analysis, which leads to a deeper critical understanding, is termed higher order thinking (Vygotsky, 1978).

Aherne (1999) suggests that clinical learning is at the heart of the educational experience for nursing students and that their mentors and clinical assessments form the quintessence of clinical learning. Therefore, the group construed that the assessment of clinical learning had particular importance in relation to the new nursing curricula, as well as the construction of the 'exit profile' which was primarily due to the practical placement assessment being equal to the weight given to the academic components of the course. The group concluded that this change needed to be openly shared with both pre-registration mental health nursing students and clinical assessors alike to clarify the purpose of the introduction of the 'exit profile' benchmarks and to minimize the disenchantment that accompanies so many new initiatives.

Hargreaves (1982) explores in depth how formative assessment innovations can lead to frustration and a reduction in motivation rather than the original intention of the development of autonomous, competent, confident practitioners. The learning experience for the group at this time was in understanding the ripple-like effect that change can cause and highlighted the need to work collaboratively with all stakeholders to ensure the changes were successfully put into practice. Mahara (1998) suggested that it is insufficient to rely on students acquiring competence by unstructured exposure during clinical placement and acknowledges the need to review the current system for skill acquisition.

The precision with which the 'exit profile' identifies the skills and various assessment methods to measure the requirement of pre-registration mental health nurses, the group envisaged, would add structure to the clinical assessment. This was supportive of Harris et al (1995, p 165, cited in Mortimer, 2000) when they discussed that: 'they should be specified as rigorously as possible if students are successfully to use their experience as the basis of learning'.

The idea of defining learning outcomes and their assessment methods has increasingly become associated with work-related curricula (Harris et al, 1995, cited in Mortimer, 2000). Learning outcomes have been described as possessing several strengths, which include: providing a way to support the development of learner autonomy and self-discipline; and improving the quality of teaching and learning (see Mortimer, 2000, p 165).

The group recognized the need to marry up these principles to the context of service delivery as defined in National Service Framework for Mental Health (DoH, 1999b) and that the benchmarks produced needed to relate directly to these standards. This threw up the challenge as to how the competency-based approach could be best linked to reflexive theories of learning. Guile and Young (1999) have described a connective model of pedagogy and learning in work-based contexts, which seems to perfectly suit mental health nurse education. The aim is to allow learners to conceptualize their experiences in different ways and for this conceptualization to serve curriculum purposes. Furthermore, it helps learners to experience different combinations of theoretical and practical learning, enabling them to relate their formal programmes to work organizations. The goal of the model is to encourage students to develop critiques and alternatives to existing practice and to apply them in the process of developing their capabilities. This descriptive model mirrors the development of the variety of both knowledge and practice-based assessments identified within the 'exit profile', which moves away from a technical-rational list of purely competence-based statements.

Conclusions

The development group began by adopting a pure reductionist approach to competence, seeing it as a technological exercise where pieces of appropriate performance are evidenced, rather than as an integrated exercise whereby underpinning knowledge is provided, learning opportunities are offered for reflection and the development of skill and the 'entire behaviour' is underpinned by appropriate values. The development group evolved by recognizing the need for a better coordinated and integrated approach, and we hope that this current text will facilitate your development in a similar way.

References

Ahern, K. J. (1999) The nurse lecturer role in clinical practice conceptualised: helping clinical teachers provide optimal student learning, *Nurse Education Today*, 19, 77–82.

Barnett, R. C. (1994) *The Limits of Competence, Knowledge, Higher Education and Society*, Buckingham: Open University Press.

Birch, W. (1998) *The Challenge To Higher Education*, Buckingham: Open University Press.

Birchenal, P. (1999) Learning and teaching beyond 2000, *Nurse Education Today*, 12, 431–2.

Camiah, S. (1998) Current educational reforms in nursing in the United Kingdom and their impact on the role of nursing lecturers in practice, *Nurse Education Today*, 18, 368–79.

Carr, W. & Kemmis, S. (1986) *Becoming Critical: Education, Knowledge and Action Research*, Lewes: Falmer Press.

Chapman, H. (1999) Some impact limitations of competency-based education with respect to nurse education, *Nurse Education Today*, 2, 129–36.

Clifford, C. (1994) Assessment of clinical practice and the role of the nurse teacher, *Nurse Education Today*, 14, 272–9.

Cohen, G. S., Blumberg, P., Ryan, N. C. & Sullivan, P. L. (1993) Do final grades reflect written qualitative evaluations of student performance? *Teaching and Learning in Medicine*, 5(1), 10–15.

Cuthbertson, P. (1996) Attitudes to Project 2000: a survey of a qualified nurse, *Nursing Standard*, 11(11), 38–41.

Department of Health (1999a) *Making A Difference: Strengthening The Nursing, Midwifery and Health Visiting Contribution To Health and Health Care*, London: HMSO.

Department of Health (1999b) *Modern Standards and Service Models: Mental Health National Service Framework, NHS Our Healthier Nation*, London: HMSO.

Dodd. A. N. (1973) Towards an understanding of nursing, Unpublished PhD thesis, University of London, in S. Jowett, I. Walton & S., Payne, (eds), (1994). *Challenges and Change in Nurse Education: A Study of the Implementation of Project 2000*, Berkshire: National Foundation for Educational Research in England and Wales.

Duke, M. (1996) Clinical evaluation-difficulties experienced by sessional teachers of nursing: a qualitative study, *Journal of Advanced Nursing*, 23, 408–14.

Edwards, R. & Usher, R. (1994) Disciplining the subject: the power of competence, *Studies in the Education of Adults*, 26(1), 1–14.

Elliott, J. (1987) Educational theory, practical philosophy and action research, *British Journal of Educational Studies*, 35(2), 149–69.

Guile, D. & Young, M. (1999) The question of learning and learning organisations, occasional paper from Post 16 Education Centre, London: Institution of Education, University of London.

Haggerty, B. & Early, S. (1992) The influence of liberal education on professional practice: a proposed model, *Advances in Nursing Science*, 14(3), 29–38.

Hargreaves, D. (1982) *The Challenge For The Comprehensive School: Culture, Curriculum, Community*, London: Routledge and Kagen Paul.

Hyland, T. (1992) Expertise and competence in further and adult education, *British Journal of In Service Education*, 18, 23–8.

Jessup, G. (1991) *Outcomes: NVQ's and the Emerging Model of Education and Training*, London: Falmer Press.

Jowett, S., Walton, I. & Payne, S. (1994) *Challenges and Change in Nurse Education: A Study of the Implementation Of Project 2000*. Berkshire: National Foundation for Educational Research in England and Wales.

Mahara, M. S. (1998) A perspective on clinical evaluation in nursing education, *Journal of Advanced Nursing*, 28(6), 1339–46.

Mortimer, P. (2000) *Understanding Pedagogy*, Buckingham: Open University Press.

Northern Centre for Mental Health, Cross, D. & Readhead, K. (2000) *A Competence-Based Exit Profile For Pre-Registration Mental Health Nursing*, Durham: Northern Centre for Mental Health.

O'Reilly, D., Cunningham, L. & Lester, S. (1999) *Developing The Capable Practitioner: Professional Capacity Through Higher Education*, London: Kogan Page.

Partlett, M. & Hamilton, D. (1972) Evaluation as illumination: a new approach to the study of innovatory programs, occasional paper 9, Edinburgh: Centre for Research in the Educational Sciences, University of Edinburgh.

Roberts, P. M. (1998) Nurse education in competitive markets: the case for relationship marketing, *Nurse Education Today*, 18, 542–52.

Robson, C. (1993) *Real World Research, A Resource for Social Scientists and Practitioner Researchers*, Oxford: Blackwell Publishers Ltd.

Rogers, C. (1983) *Freedom To Learn For The 80s*, New York: Macmillan, now Palgrave Macmillan.

Schön, D. A. (1983) *The Reflective Practitioner*, London: Temple Smith.

Spouse, J. (1998) Scaffolding student learning in clinical practice, *Nurse Education Today*, 18, 259–66.

Stenhouse, L. (1983) *Authority, Education, and Emancipation*, London: Heinemann.

United Kingdom Central Council For Nursing, Midwifery and Health Visiting (1986) *Project 2000: A Preparation For Practice*, London: UKCC.

United Kingdom Central Council For Nursing, Midwifery and Health Visiting (1999a) *Fitness For Practice*, London: UKCC.

United Kingdom Central Council For Nursing, Midwifery and Health Visiting (1999b) *Competencies for Entry to the Register*, London: UKCC.

United Kingdom Central Council For Nursing, Midwifery and Health Visiting (2000) *Requirements for Pre-registration Nursing Programmes*, London: UKCC.

Vygotsky, L. (1978) *Mind in Society*, Cambridge: Cambridge University Press.

Weiss, C. H. (1986) The stakeholder approach to evaluation: origins and promise, in E. R. House (ed.), *New Directions of Educational Evaluation*, London: Falconer Press.

Young, M. F. D. (1998) *The Curriculum of the Future*, London: Falmer Press.

CHAPTER 2

The Recognition of Inequality and the Need for Empowerment

DENIS A. HART

This chapter has been written to provide the reader, particularly mental health nurses with the necessary underpinning knowledge in accordance with the following Benchmarks for Mental Health Nursing.

Indicative Benchmark Statements

- The impact of own attitudes to mental health and social care

- The impact of stigma on mental health service users, their families and carers, and the motivational basis of prejudice

- The need to work in mental health and social care settings in a non-discriminatory way

- The need to develop non-judgemental, non-blaming and non-punitive attitudes to users of mental health services and their carers

- How to assist mental health service users and their carers in making informed choices about their care through the provision of culturally appropriate forms of communication

---

Introduction

In this chapter we will take you on a journey to empowerment whereby we will look at:

- prejudice and the oppression of mentally ill people;
- how discrimination and oppression take place at both the level of individual practice and at the structural level of service delivery;

- how some groups of patients are more vulnerable than others; and
- the need for mental health nurses and social carers to understand the processes involved so that they might effectively counter them.

Prejudice and discrimination

Mentally ill people, whether in the community, or in hospital attract negative images whereby they are seen as 'less worthy', and this perception gets in the way of providing appropriate treatment. Thompson (1997, p 33) described prejudice as: 'an opinion or judgement formed without considering the relevant facts or arguments: a biased and intolerant attitude towards particular people or social groups, an opinion or attitude which rigidly and irrationally maintained even in the face of strong contradictory evidence or in the persistent absence of supportive evidence.'

As professionals we are not exempt from holding prejudicial attitudes and indeed we are in a position whereby we could potentially turn our prejudices into discrimination by virtue of the power we hold over the patients for whom we provide care. Thompson (1997, p 32) describes the process whereby prejudice (a state of mind) develops into discrimination (an actual act) in his definition of discrimination, being the: 'unfair or unequal treatment of individuals or groups; prejudicial behaviour acting against the interests of those people who characteristically tend to belong to relatively powerless groups within the social structure.' Clearly mentally ill people meet this criteria and are thereby likely to be victimized.

This has now been recognised by the Department of Health who in *A National Service Framework for Mental Health* (DoH, 1999, p 21) include, as part of an action plan, the need to clarify and endorse: 'Key skills and competences required throughout mental health services to ensure services which are non-discriminatory, and sensitive to the needs of all service users and carers regardless of age, gender, race, culture, religion, disability or sexual orientation'.

Three levels of discrimination

Thompson (1997) has argued that discrimination occurs at three separate, but interrelated levels:

- the personal or psychological level;
- the cultural level; and
- the structural level.

P (personal or psychological) level

This is the individual level of thoughts, feelings, attitudes and actions which relates primarily to: *practice* – individual workers interacting with individual patients; and *prejudice* – the inflexibility of mind that stands in the way of fair and non-judgemental practice.

Burton (1993) presents an example whereby a nurse was told that a person of a particular religious faith could only wash using running water. The nurse chose to fill a jug and run up and down the corridor so the patient would indeed get 'running' water. Not only does this behaviour reflect prejudice (an intolerance of other people's religious beliefs and practices) but it is also unacceptable practice because the behaviour is offensive to that patient. Furthermore, the nurse's conduct is in breach of Competence 1.3 requiring registered nurses to:

> Practice in a fair and anti-discriminatory way, acknowledging the difference in beliefs and cultural practices of individuals or groups.

Allport (1954) identified a scale of prejudice, each stage increasing the intensity of the one before:

- *Verbal rejection* – openly verbalizing dislike of certain groups of people.
- *Discrimination* – denying equality of treatment to people with certain 'characteristics'.
- *Physical attack* – targeting certain groups for physical violence.

As part of professional training nurses and social carers should keep a 'Learning journal' which includes recording ways in which the student has developed personally as well as professionally. Personal attitudes are to some extent 'controlled' by the Requirements of professional bodies. CCETSW, (Central Council for the Education and Training of Social Workers) now TOPS (The Training Organization for the Personal Social Services (England) http://www.topps.org.uk/welc_fs.htm), has a specific Values Requirement, whereby all students qualifying must demonstrate:

- the value and dignity of individuals;
- the right to respect, privacy and confidentiality;
- the right of individuals and families to choose; and
- the need to recognize the strengths and skills embedded in local communities.

(*Source*: Adapted from CCETSW, 1995)

Anti-discriminatory practice begins by becoming aware of our own prejudices so that we can take action within ourselves to prevent these permeating through into actual behaviours. Ogle (1990, p 12) provides a helpful personal statement on the subject of caring for mentally disordered offenders:

> The population to which I provide health care are persons that have committed crimes, some of those crimes being horrendous. Personally I do not want to know the crimes committed, I want to be able to provide quality health care to the inmates of the institution. It is not my job to judge them. Society and the Judicial System make those decisions.

Non-judgementalism is thereby an important component of our own commitment to anti-discriminatory practice as it makes us aware as to how labelling and stereotyping take place. Whitehouse (1986) studied court reports written by probation officers on black offenders and discovered they contained many racist assumptions which led to negative consequences for their clients. Whitehouse (1986, p 117) concluded that: 'if the social worker has stereotypical expectations and attitudes, he or she will tend to select the information to confirm them.' Whitehouse went on to observe that whenever black offenders picked up the stereotypical expectations of the interviewer they: 'withdrew from the interaction, gave as little information and collaboration as possible' and consequently, this became, 'interpreted by the more powerful in the interaction as uncooperative behaviour or having "something to hide"'. The basis for professional bodies having values requirements is that personal prejudice is no longer solely about attitude once that person holds a position of power.

Ahmed (1990, p 31) explains further: 'It is well acknowledged that Mental Health professionals have power to enforce controlling functions, including the law. The correlation between over-representation of Black People in Mental Health services and exposure to social control is not hard to identify.'

Having seen how prejudice is a state of mind, and discrimination the implementation of prejudice in practice we now move on to look at Thompson's second stage of discrimination.

C (the cultural level)

Thompson uses this term to describe the shared ways of seeing, thinking and doing, and relates primarily to:

- *commodities* – values and patterns of thought and behaviour;
- *an assumed consensus* – as to what is right and what is 'normal';
- *conformity* – lays down the expectation to abide by the norms; and
- *continuity* – ways are created to ensure that the 'cultural' messages are transmitted and reinforced.

As part of its 'policy', a secure treatment ward decided to ban certain substances on the grounds of safety. One long-term patient had always bleached her hair but was informed that she could no longer do so as products contained in the bleach were included in the ban. Staff on the wards handle far more toxic substances than those contained in hair bleach. The solution is actually quite simple: issue the bleach to the patient as and when she needs it and allow her to bleach her hair under supervision.

The problem here is that the ward is developing a culture that fails to recognise individual need. Burton (1993, p 116) points out:

> in a place which people are detained and locked up, a place where residents do not *choose* to live, there are going to be rules . . . But within these limitations it is especially important that residents learn how to manage their own lives and relationships better, and here the imposition of extra rules doesn't help.

It was precisely this process which led Goffman (1961, 1963) to write his definitive texts *Stigma* and *Asylums* whereby he argued that rules are used to reinforce power differentials between patients and staff and how this leads to degrading and dehumanizing experiences.

Cultural oppression however is not confined to the hospital setting. In community care it can take a number of different forms. Bean (2001, pp 3–4) cites a Department of Health circular which is particularly telling:

> Care in the community has failed. Discharging people from institutions has brought benefits to some. But it has left many vulnerable patients trying to cope on their own. Others have been left to become a danger to themselves and a nuisance to others. Too many confused and sick people have been left wandering the streets and sleeping rough. A small but significant minority has become a danger to the public as well as to themselves.

Here prejudice abounds:

- There is no mention of the under-funding of Community Care, how hospitals were closed so rapidly that no Community Mental Health Team could have reasonably been expected to keep up and no one thought about 'suitable' accommodation. It is perhaps really no surprise then that people have been left, wandering the streets and sleeping rough but it begs the question 'who's to blame' the people or Government Policy?
- The sick, the confused and the dangerous are all lumped together to justify the need for more assertive action to protect the public. The traditional fayre of the prejudiced, generating irrational fears is well evidenced.

But this is no simple prejudice for it is no less than the Department of Health which Bean quotes. The body responsible for shaping policy and which seems keen to emphasize *assertion* and *compulsion* as its value base rather than *care* or *compassion*.

The C element is therefore evidenced when we want to use medication as control, when we try to define all acts of non-conformity as dangerous, and when we, not as individuals, but as entire teams begin to afford mentally ill and recovering mentally ill people as less worthy and as having less rights than others. Rogers and Pilgrim (2003, p 9) confirm the relevance of this to mental health practice:

> Psychiatric knowledge has developed in a social context that has been far from politically neutral. It has been legitimised by some interest groups and attacked by others, who have challenged the notion of a free standing 'disinterested' or 'objective' body of medical knowledge which simply informs social research.

S (the structural level)

> Oppression and discrimination cannot be explained simply by reference to personal prejudice. Katz's (1978) notion of 'prejudice plus power' takes us in the direction but ultimately confuses more than it clarifies. (Sibeon, 1991)

Discrimination is a reflection (and a reinforcer) of structural inequalities. The fact that we live in such a highly stratified society means that inequalities are part and parcel of the social order – inevitably there are winners and losers. 'Oppression does not derive simply from individual actions or "praxis". It can be, and often is built into structural and institutional patterns and organisational policies' (Thompson, 1997, p 24).

Dominelli (1997, p 26) confirms that here we are no longer talking about personal views or cultural ideologies but rather about institutional oppression whereby: 'the entire organisation has been set up in such a way as to disadvantage or discriminate against certain categories of people.'

Care of mentally ill people

In the same way non-judgmentalism, self-awareness and a commitment to professional values is the antidote to individual discrimination and oppression, care offers a practical first step when exploring institutional oppression. Here care should not be confined to just physical aspects but rather should address *all* matters which relates to:

- respect for persons as individuals; and
- respect for persons Human and Civil Rights.

Care is an over-arching concept that should include:

- emotional care;
- respect for culture;

- respect for religion; and thereby
- respect for people's self-identity.

Care in this sense is inextricably linked to Anti-Discriminatory Practice rather than to equality. It is about providing what is *relevant* to the needs of the individual and not a blanket approach to all in the name of some misguided principle of equality. As nurses we need to be conscious of our legal General Duty of Care and interpret this widely and holistically. In so doing we are setting our practice in a more appropriate context, which should address the concerns about institutional racism (Fernando, 1991) and institutional sexism (Women in Secure Hospitals, 1999).

Nevertheless, as Perkins and Repper (1998) point out, psychiatry continues to seek to address the needs of the 'whole' population and hence the *specific* needs of individuals and minority groups can easily be overlooked. The result is that: 'services become organised around the most dominant and demanding group in the population. In the case of people with severe on-going mental health problems this group comprises of young men with diagnoses of schizophrenia' (Perkins and Repper, 1998, p 6).

To avoid such a pitfall we will now look at particular aspects of mental health as they affect black people, women and gay and lesbian people.

Racism and mental health

Chakraborty (1990, p 15) believes that racism in constructed upon: 'a set of beliefs, or a way of thinking, within which groups identified on the basis of real or imagined biological characteristics (skin colour, for example) are thought to possess other characteristics that are viewed in a negative light'. Dominelli (1997, p 7) defines institutional racism as consisting of: 'customary routines which ration resources and power by excluding groups . . . and . . . pathologises excluded groups for their lack of success within the system and blames them for their predicament'. Racism, like all other aspects of oppression is located in the assessment, treatment and care of patients.

Acharyya (1996) expressed concerns that the assessment tools used by psychologists, mental health nurses and psychiatrists were not always fair. Intelligence tests, for example, rely heavily on language and can easily lead to a person for whom English is their second language, performing less well. Models of psychiatric interpretation such as Freudian psychoanalysis are riddled with Western cultural assumptions.

Rogers and Pilgrim (2003, pp 9–10) develop this effectively:

Cultural and cross national diversity pose a particular problem for psychiatric knowledge. On the one hand modern psychiatry aspires to be universal in its authority about moral abnormality. At the same time lay and professional judgements about the latter are situated in time and space. A compromise has been made by 'comparative' or 'transcultural' psychiatry to claim the existence of two concurrent versions of psychopathology – the 'emic' and the 'etic'.

The *emic* refers to culturally specific disorders, while the *etic* refers to universal ones. 'Any substantial professional concession to the importance of "emic" disorders threatens to undermine psychiatry as a universally applicable form of medical science, but to deny their existence immediately invites accusations of Western intellectual imperialism or racism' (ibid, p 10).

As Cheng (2001) explains, psychiatrists have tended to substantiate the emic to the etic rather than abandon efforts at making standard and universal diagnoses. To move mental health on, and to ensure a fairer and more appropriate treatment of black people, Acharyya (1996, p 343) suggested:

> perhaps it is important for us, when attempting to understand 'the patient', to concentrate harder on actually listening to what the patient is saying in their own terms – whether verbally or non-verbally and to take special note of the particular cultural dimensions that make up personhood.

Barker (1997, p 17) reminds us that: 'Assessment tries to gain an *overall picture*: one that describes positive characteristics as well as problems. A full assessment describes the skills, assets and other positive features of a person.' This approach has an attractive superficiality about it but fails to recognize that black people have had a life-long accumulation of negative experiences from the ways many white people have treated them. This is because until recently we, as white people, have failed to recognize this:

> This unarticulated nature of racism . . . enables white people to define racism as the crude, irrational beliefs and actions manifest by a few National Front supporters instead of a normal feature of interaction between black and white people. This enables them to acquire a self concept which is not racist. Hence, white people generally take exceptional umbrage at being called racist and become extremely defensive if it is suggested that they live in an inherently racist society. (Dominelli, 1997, pp 10–11)

Racism in assessment in mental health has been specifically confirmed by a number of researchers. Ranger (1989) has established that *Cannabis psychosis* is a label attached to Afro-Caribbean people when British psychiatrists are perplexed by their behaviour. Bhugra et al (1997), Harrison et al (1988; 1997) and King et al (1994) have confirmed that young black people are frequently misdiagnosed as schizophrenic when the real tension has been that they have been raised by black families to live in a society that only recognizes 'white values'. Black workers have rightly complained that where a black child has been placed with white foster carers without appropriate identity work being undertaken then the confusions the child faces on reaching adulthood will be conducive to the development of schizophrenic like symptoms.

Fenton and Sadiq (1996, p 252) have shown how Asian women are frequently misdiagnosed as having clinical depression: 'In the language of western psychiatric medicine, the term "depression" is used to describe a specific mental and emotional state with particular symptoms, and is treated, in part by anti-depressant drugs.' However, the Asian women interviewed revealed that: 'While their suffering always began as a completely natural and normal response to some terrible personal shock . . . this turned into a virtually unmanageable state of mental and emotional distress' (ibid, p 252).

They also found that the women studied had little support nearby and saw themselves as socially isolated. They did not see the professionals as knowledgeable or understanding as to their culture and as a result they became more confused. As one woman stated 'What should I do? Go on taking anti-depressants or go to Pakistan'. As they established, racism is not only inherent in mental health's assessment processes but also in the way it dispensates treatment.

Fernando et al (1998), among others, have established that black people are treated in a more coercive and punitive way within the psychiatric system than white people, and that Afro-Caribbeans are over-represented in locked wards, secure units and the Special Hospitals.

Littlewood and Cross (1980) found that black patients were more likely to:

- be given major tranquillizers and intra-muscular medication; and
- be seen by junior medical staff.

McGovern and Cope (1987) pointed out that some psychiatrists defend racist practices on the grounds that the stronger interventions black people are subjected to, is in response to them being more ill and as being perceived as more likely to become violent. What they found especially concerning was that, there is little real empirical evidence to support such stereotypical views.

Pilgrim and Rogers (1999, p 51) set out clearly the need for the development of Anti-Racist practice in mental health as currently: 'the mode of referral, diagnosis, compulsory admission and psychiatric management of patients indicates that black people (particularly young black men) are subjected more to the harsh end of mental health services than white people'.

Sexism in mental health

The definition of sexism contains similar elements to that used to identify racism. For example Bullock and Stallybrass (1977) have defined sexism as: 'a deep-rooted, often unconscious system of beliefs, attitudes, and institutions in which distinctions between people's intrinsic worth are made on the grounds of their sex and sexual roles.'

Carlen and Worrall (1987, p 3) looked at the consequences of sexism for women and at the expectations society places on the 'normal' woman,

> Being a normal woman means coping, caring, nurturing, and sacrificing self-interest to the needs of others. It also means being intuitively sensitive to those needs without them being actively spelt out . . . Femininity is characterised by lack of control and dependence. Being a normal woman means needing protection . . . It means being child-like, incapable, fragile and capricious.

It is easy to see from this definition how mentally ill women are expected to acknowledge their failure and how dependency is thereby encouraged.

We have already seen how Asian women are more likely to be misdiagnosed as clinically depressed but furthermore research has established that:

- women are over-represented generally in terms of mental health referrals;
- women are far more likely to be prescribed minor tranquillizers; and
- women are more likely to be regarded as 'dangerous to themselves' while men are more likely to be regarded as 'dangerous to others'.

Sheppard (1991) discovered that GPs were much more likely to refer women for compulsory admission to hospital than men, while mentally disordered women who offend are far more likely than men to end up in hospital rather than in prison.

Again sexism permeates throughout mental health practice whereby: 'sexism in psychiatry has its roots in, and can be transmitted by, the type of knowledge, diagnostic categories and practices followed by the profession which can still be called "patriarchal" even when used by women doctors' (Pilgrim and Rodgers, 1999, p 51). Perkins and Repper (1998, p 7) point out that the problem for female patients is similar to that of black people whereby psychiatry continually seeks to address the needs of the 'whole' population and that it is wholly inappropriate to fail to recognize problems specifically experienced by women:

> Women with serious mental health problems may have experienced numerous social disadvantages and pressures prior to the onset of their difficulties. Some such as poverty and unemployment, may be shared by their male counterparts, others are more specifically – but not exclusively – associated with women's lives. These include sexual abuse in childhood (Williams and Watson, 1994), rape and violence as an adult, domestic violence, raising children single handed and looking after other relatives.

Sexuality and mental health

We need to be clear at the outset that every person whether mentally ill or not has the right to choose their own sexuality. Therefore we can easily establish that homosexuality is *not* part of any mental illness we need to address (Golding, 1997) nor should it constitute the grounds for a diagnosis of mental illness (McFarlane, 1998). Males who rape women do not have their hetero-sexuality addressed as 'a problem' but rather it is the person abuse of women and misuse of power which gives us genuine grounds for involvement. A man who abuses children may not be gay and so when working with a paedophile it is important we confine our concerns to the patient seeking out vulnerable young males for sexual gratification who are powerless and by virtue of age, unable to give informed consent to the patient's advances.

What we are doing here effectively is to sort out:

- the person;
- their rights to be who they want to be; and
- in this case their criminality (the serious abuse of young boys).

Wilton (2000) explains:

> In terms of professional responsibility to lesbian or gay service users, there are two key implications . . . First, both an understanding of the degree to which sexuality is a factor in socio-political exclusion, and an acceptance that discrimination is still widely present in public service provision, become increasingly important in the context of interprofessional care management and delivery. Indeed there are some circumstances in which the responsibility to provide effective care may well require the informed professional to take an active role in challenging such discrimination (Royal College of Nursing, 1994).

Anti-discriminatory practice

Society has tended to see 'equal opportunities' as the panacea for all prejudice, discrimination and oppression. However, this view is built upon a false premise. We know for example that middle class people have a greater life expectancy than working class people and hence there would have to be considerable action taken in order to increase the life expectancy of working class people as this is linked to:

- differential abilities to purchase health services;
- differential knowledge as to the impact of certain key factors, e.g., drugs, alcohol, tobacco on health, and a preparedness to incorporate this knowledge into life styles; and
- differential environments whereby working class homes tend to be nearer to industrial conurbations with a greater level of pollutants and toxins in the air.

Real change is only brought about by a commitment to recognizing existing equalities and then taking appropriate positive action to counter these. This process is called anti-discriminatory practice whereby the practitioner seeks to: 'reduce, undermine or eliminate discrimination and oppression, specifically in terms of challenging sexism, racism, ageism and disablism' (Thompson, 1997, p 33). Anti-discriminatory practice is: 'an attempt to eradicate discrimination and oppression from our own practice and challenge them in the practice of others and in the institutional structures in which we operate. In this respect, it is a form of emancipatory practice' (ibid).

However, before anyone decides to go out and positively discriminate to counter years of negative action, be careful – positive discrimination is *unlawful*. Supposing you are working in a Community Mental Health Team where the majority of your patients are female but the staff are nearly all male. You may feel that there is a need to redress the balance and seek to appoint a woman should any of the team leave. By law, unless the post is specifically exempt, you cannot do this but rather you *must* appoint the most suitable person for the job regardless of their gender.

Upon reflection this is quite common-sensical as, in long term we are likely to simply exchange one victimized group for another. If we believe, for example that pornography is degrading to women, we shouldn't counter it by making pornographic images of men socially acceptable as this will eventually become degrading to men. What we can do, however, is to embark upon a policy of positive action.

Positive action and anti-racism

Once we recognize that the processes whereby black people are treated and assessed are prone to bias or are not appropriate the logical next step is to address the problem. Fernando (1989) pointed out that the beginning of anti-racist practice is to recognize that there are different cultures and that people from other cultures have alternative views of the world and different needs. This in turn means we will recognize racism in our practice and in our agencies' practices and procedures.

Bhugra and Bhui (1997) develop this and highlight the need to develop cross-cultural assessment tools, which would recognize different cultural backgrounds as part of a process of *contextualizing* assessments. Such an approach would certainly help to reduce the misdiagnosis of young Afro-Caribbeans as schizophrenic and Asian women as clinically depressed as pathological behaviour would be explained in terms of socio-cultural expectation, i.e. situational factors and the point of labelling for such individuals would be far further down the road of personal pathology than it is at present.

There is an obvious need to recruit more social carers, mental health nurses and doctors from black and ethnic minority backgrounds. This means going out to the communities where potential candidates may live and encouraging them to think about mental health work and for professional bodies and academe to think much more pro-actively about how such people can be helped to access training opportunities.

Treatment modalities also need to recognize and embrace difference and diversity and find ways to communicate effectively with black and ethnic minority service users rather than resort to Sectioning and sedating them (Browne, 1996). As Acharyya (1996, pp 340–1) writes:

> One of the problems for a patient from a minority cultural group may be that what the patient presents as a problem, and the way it is presented, does not fit easily into the standard European text-book classification that the doctor has so meticulously absorbed, categories which are themselves taken to be culturally-free.

However, the positive suggestion is proposed (p 343) that:

> The preconceptions about each other that both doctor and patient bring to the consultation will have to be examined and a dialogue can then take place which may go towards alleviating the patients' distress. In mutually divesting the other . . . the doctor has a special role in allowing the patient to feel that they have the power and the right to present their own view of what is wrong.

Positive action and anti-sexism

Similar principles apply when constructing anti-sexist practice as to the ones we have just used to look at anti-racism. Doyal et al (1994) and Berer (1998) have drawn attention to the fact that clinical disclosure presumes the male body to be the norm, with the result that we have less information about women's health than we do about men's. Moreover, the medical concern has been primarily with women in terms of their reproductive function so women's mental health has been given low priority to men's. This has been further compounded by the notion we explored earlier that men are perceived as a danger to others while women are only a danger to themselves.

Part of the remedy is appointing more women as mental health nurses and psychiatrists but it is important that they are *not* subject to professional acculturalization whereby they are expected to suppress their gender in the name of professional neutrality. Organizations such as 'Women in Secure Hospitals' are important for supporting female patients but there may be a need for a similar group to support female mental health nurses and psychiatrists.

As Monahan (1988) wrote: 'The nurse may be able to determine the coping ability of the service user by asking what they see as the biggest stressors in their lives and how they cope with them.' But given, for example, that 90 per cent of domestic violence is committed by men on women it seems imperative that the assessment is either: conducted by a woman; or by a man who has been specifically trained to understand the impact of abuse on women and the fear and suspicion they may harbour when being assessed by a man who they may believe may himself be abusive, or at best, not really be able to understand.

This was precisely the process revealed by Fenton and Sadiq (1996) as it affected Asian women. Having been made to leave the family home by an abusing husband, they were then ostracized by the local Asian community and left isolated and vulnerable. When they went to the GP for help his/her concern was about physical symptomotology being unable to comprehend exactly how oppressive this feeling of isolation would be for that woman.

Even therapeutic work with rape victims can be undertaken by men given the right training and the right disposition. Gardner (1996, p 315) for example describes a case where an analyst in training couldn't get the patient to engage at an emotional level and so he:

> worked on imagining through reading and then empathising with what the patient had undergone, and talked with her about the trauma not about 'libidinous feel-ings'. He was taking the rape so seriously that the patient felt able to get in touch with a whole range of emotions about the abuse, which eventually relieved her depression.

Advocacy, empowerment and user involvement

Anti-discriminatory practice begins by recognizing power imbalances. Rogers and Pilgrim (2003) have identified four specific areas:

1 the power imbalance created by professional knowledge;
2 psychiatric knowledge, medical dominance and individualization;
3 normative knowledge and social control; and
4 knowledge and status differentials in the mental health professions.

Once recognized, anti-discriminatory practice goes on to recognize the need to redress this by a series of processes aimed at empowering service users and increasing their involvement in their own care and treatment. However, ini-tially some patients are too unwell or incapacitated to be fully involved and for them the first step is for somebody to advocate on their behalf.

Advocacy tends to be used whenever someone is unable to represent them-selves and essentially is a vehicle for someone else to get the patient's point of view across (Thompson, 1998). The mandate for this can be found in the objectives of the NHS and Community Care Act, 1990 (DoH, 1990) which is, 'to give people a greater say in how they live their lives and the services they need to help them do so'.

Trevithick (2002) sees advocacy as having four components:

1 supporting clients to represent themselves;
2 arguing client's views and needs;
3 interpreting or representing the views, needs, concerns and interests of clients to others; and

4 developing appropriate skills for undertaking these different tasks such as listening and negotiating skills, empathy, assertiveness skills, being clear and focused and so on.

Advocacy is the initial point of putting awareness of the patient on the agenda, next comes empowerment.

> A central feature of anti-discriminatory practice . . . is that of *empowerment*. This involves seeking to maximise the power of clients and to give then as much control as possible over their circumstances. It is the opposite of creating dependency and subject clients to agency power. (Thompson, 1997, p 8)

Byrt and Dooher (2003) identify four domains to empowerment:

1 individual or psychological empowerment in which the individual experiences increased power and control;
2 service-initiated empowerment where the professionals or managers enable service users or carers to increase their power;
3 achieving actual change in health services; and
4 social inclusion.

Breeze (2002, p 109) points out that this will not be easy as nurses seem to feel obliged to 'take control',

> The constraints of structural power can render feelings of powerlessness in nurses as well as service users . . . the ethical dilemmas produced by the conflict of individual right to autonomy versus the duty of care and the proposed changes in mental health law and policy, such as Community Treatment Orders, may serve to exacerbate this feeling, especially in relation to people with multiple and complex needs.

Gutierrez (1990) maintains that empowerment is not only essential as it reflects appropriate values, but it is, in itself, part of therapy whereby patients move away from apathy and despair to a sense of personal responsibility thereby:

- increasing self-efficacy;
- developing group consciousness;
- reducing self-blame; and
- assuming personal responsibility.

This also means we too have to adapt so as to:

- accept the client's definition of the problem;
- identify and build upon the existing strengths of individuals;

- engage in a power analysis of the user's situation; and
- mobilize resources and, where needed, advocate on behalf of users.

This cannot be achieved overnight, as Trevithick (2002, p 143) explains: 'it takes time to help people empower themselves, and to find ways to move their lives forward, not least because the very nature of oppression means for some, the confidence and courage to explore new areas and to take risks feels beyond their reach.'

By contrast:

> many recipients of health services, particularly those concerned with mental health, describe themselves as 'survivors' . . . there are many survivors' accounts which challenge the (often serious) oppression, stigmatisation and denial of rights which they have experienced (Byrt and Dooher, 2003, p 91).

Social inclusion, the fourth dimension of Dooher and Byrt's empowerment typology, often involves regarding people as stakeholders, yet even though patients have at long last been recognized as stakeholders in the National Service Framework for Mental Health (DoH, 1999), 'Clinical research in the area of mental health has tended either to exclude the views of patients or to portray them as passive objects of study' (Pilgrim and Rodgers, 1999, p 193), while the Medical Research Council's priorities for the funding of schizophrenia research emphasizes genetic and biological study and: 'evaluation of services to patients is number eight out of ten priorities and user evaluation of services and treatment is not mentioned at all' (Pilgrim and Rodgers, 1999, p 193).

Dooher and Byrt (2003, pp 278–9) conclude their text with a planned strategy:

1 *Clear concepts, aims, goals, policies and strategies:* essentially we cannot empower others unless we ourselves are clear about what we are doing, what we hope to achieve and how we expect to achieve it.
2 *Service users, carers and organizational participants with power:* we need to pinpoint the sources of power and be realistic as to when, how and where we will share it.
3 *Professionals, managers and Government Departments:* we need to identify individuals involved in the process and develop attitudes and communication skills that reflect active listening.
4 *Specific areas:* Dooher and Byrt list nine specific areas:
   - awareness of the specific components of empowerment/participation to be increased;
   - efforts to ensure social inclusion and life opportunities;
   - identification of anticipated and actual benefits and problems;
   - awareness and choice of the most appropriate methods;

- identification of specific resources needed e.g.: funding, appropriate venues;
- evaluating and monitoring of initiatives;
- making information available on successes and failures;
- awareness of organizational culture, which constrains, and the provision of cultures that facilitate empowerment/participation; and
- awareness of the stages at which carers/service users can be involved.

As we stated at the beginning of this chapter, empowerment is the end of the journey for the anti-discriminatory practitioner, the point where we relinquish control while retaining responsibility. It is a place where we know 'letting go' is essential but we remain anxious and fearful because the transfer of power to another always will entail a removal of some power from ourselves. Having seen the benefits to users of 'letting go', we hope you will now be confident to *share* power and responsibility in your own practice:

> A central feature of anti discriminatory practice is that of *empowerment* . . . it is the opposite of creating dependency. (Thompson, 1997, p 8)

References

Acharyya, S. (1996) Practising cultural psychiatry: the doctors dilemma, in T. Heller, J. Reynolds, R. Gomm, R. Muston & S. Pattison (eds), *Mental Health Matters*, Basingstoke: Macmillan – now Palgrave Macmillan Ch 42, 339–45.

Ahmed, B. (1990) *Black Perspectives in Social Work*, Birmingham: Ventura Press.

Allport, G. W. (1954) *The Nature of Prejudice*, Reading, MA: Addison Wesley.

Barker, P. J. (1997) *Assessment in Psychiatric and Mental Health Nursing*, Cheltenham: Stanley Thomas.

Bean, P. (2001) *Mental Disorder and Community Safety*, Basingstoke: Palgrave – now Palgrave Macmillan.

Berer, M. (ed.) (1998) *Reproductive Health Matters (special issue: sexuality)*, 6(12).

Bhugra, D. & Bhui, K. (1997) Community care planning approach, *Advances in Psychiatric Treatment*, 3, 236–43.

Bhugra, D., Leff, J., Mallett, R., Der, G., Corridan, B. & Rudge, S. (1997) Incidence and outcome of schizophrenia in Whites, African Caribbeans and Asians in London, *Psychological Medicine*, 27, 791–8.

Breeze, J. (2002) User participation and empowerment in community mental health nursing practice, in J. Dooher & R. Byrt (eds), *Empowerment and Participation*, Wiltshire: Quay Books.

Browne, M. (1996) Needs assessment and community care, in J. Perg-Smith (ed.), *Needs Assessment in Public Policy*, Buckingham: Open University Press.

Byrt, R. & Dooher, J. (2003) Service users and carers and their desire for empowerment and participation, in R. Byrt & J. Dooher (eds), *Empowerment and the Health Service User*, Wiltshire: Quay Books.

Bullock, A. & Stallybrass, O. (1977) *Dictionary of Modern Thought*, London: Fontana.

30	*Mental Health Nursing*

Burton, J. (1993) *The Handbook of Residential Care*, London: Routledge.

Carlen, P. & Worrall, A. (1987) *Gender, Crime and Justices*, Buckingham: Open University Press.

Central Council for the Education and Training of Social Workers (1995) *DipSW Rules and Regulations for the Diploma in Social Work* (Revised), London: CCETSW.

Chakraborty, A. (1990) *Racial Prejudice*, Buckingham: Open University Press.

Cheng, A. T. A. (2001) Case definition and culture: are people all the same? *British Journal of Psychiatry*, 179, 1–3.

Department of Health (1990) *NHS and Community Care Act 1990*, London: HMSO.

Department of Health (1999) *A National Service Framework for Mental Health*, London: HMSO.

Dominelli, L. (1997) *Anti-Racist Social Work*, London: BASW.

Dooher, J. & Byrt, R. (2002) *Empowerment and Participation*, Wiltshire: Quay Books.

Doyal, L. et al (1994) *AIDS: Setting a Feminist Agenda*, London: Taylor and Francis.

Fenton, S. & Sadiq, A. (1996) Asian women speak out, in T. Heller, J Reynolds, R. Gomm, R. Muston & S. Pattison (eds), *Mental Health Matters*, Basingstoke: Macmillan – now Palgrave Macmillan Ch 30, 252–9.

Fernando, S. (1989) *Race and Culture in Psychiatry*, London: Croom Helm.

Fernando, S. (1991) *Mental Health Race and Culture*, London. MIND.

Fernando, S., Ndeqwa, D. & Wilson, M. (1998) *Forensic Psychiatry, Race and Culture*, London: Routledge.

Gardner, F. (1996) Working psychotherapeutically with adult survivors of child sexual abuse, in T. Heller, J. Reynolds, R. Gomm, R. Muston & S. Pattison (eds), *Mental Health Matters*, Basingstoke: Macmillan – now Palgrave Macmillan Ch 38, 309–18.

Goffman, E. (1961) *Asylums*, New York: Anchor Books.

Goffman, E. (1963) *Stigma*, London: Pelican Books.

Golding, J. (1997) *Without Prejudice: Lesbian, Gay and Bisexual Mental Health Awareness Research*, London: MIND.

Gutierrez, L. M. (1990) Working with women of colour: an empowerment perspective, *Social Work*, 35(2), 149–53.

Harrison, G., Glazebrook, C., Brewin, J., Cantwell, R., Dalkin, T., Fox, R., Jones, P. & Medley, I. (1997) Increased incidence of psychotic disorders in migrants for the Caribbean to the United Kingdom, *Psychological Medicine*, 27, 799–806.

Harrison, G., Owens, D., Holton, A., Neilson, D. & Boot, D. (1988) A prospective study of severe mental disorder in Afro-Caribbean patients, *Psychological Medicine*, 19, 683–96.

Katz, J. (1978) *White Awareness*, Norman, OK: University of Oklahoma Press.

King, M., Coker, E., Leavey, G., Hoar, A. & Johnson-Sabine, E. (1994) Incidence of psychotic illness in London: comparison of ethnic groups, *British Medical Journal*, 309, 1115–19.

Littlewood, R. & Cross, C. (1980) Ethnic minorities and psychiatric services, *Sociology Health and Illness*, 2, 194–201.

McFarlane, I. (1998) *Diagnosis: Homophobic – The Experience of Lesbians, Gay Men and Bisexuals in Mental Health Services*, London: Pace.

McGovern, D. & Cope, P. (1987) The compulsory detention of males of different ethnic groups, *British Journal of Psychiatry*, 150, 505–12.

Monahan, J. (1988) Risk assessment of violence among the mentally disordered: generating useful knowledge, *International Journal of Law and Psychiatry*, II, 249–57.

Ogle, B. (1990) What is forensic/correctional nursing? *The Florida Nurse*, June/July, 12.

Perkins, R. & Repper, J. (1998) Taking women's mental health seriously, *Mental Health Practice*, 2(3), 6–10.

Pilgrim, D. & Rodgers, A. (1999) *A Sociology of Mental Health and Illness*, Buckingham: Open University Press.

Ranger, C. (1989) Race, culture and cannabis psychosis: the role of social factors in the construction of a disease category, *New Communities*, 15(3), 35–69.

Rogers, A. & Pilgrim, D. (2003) *Mental Health and Inequality*, Basingstoke: Palgrave Macmillan.

Sheppard, M. (1991) Good practice, social work and mental health sections: the social control of women, *British Journal of Social Work*, 21, 663–83.

Sibeon, R. (1991) *Towards a New Sociology of Social Work*, Aldershot: Avebury.

Thompson, N. (1998) *Anti-Discriminatory Practice*, London: BASW/Macmillan – now Palgrave Macmillan.

Trevithick, P. (2002) *Social Work Skills: A Practical Handbook*, Oxford: Oxford University Press.

Whitehouse, H. (1986) Race and the criminal justice system, in V. Coombe & A. Little (eds), *Race and Social Work*, London: Tavistock.

Wilton, T. (2000) *Sexualities in Health and Social Care*, Buckingham: Open University Press.

Women in Secure Hospitals (1999) *Defining Gender Issues: Redefining Women's Services*, London: WISH.

CHAPTER 3

How Can Nurses Meet the Needs of Mental Health Clients?

SUE JACKSON AND CHRIS STEVENSON

Introduction

Defining health problems and their treatment has always been the responsibility of the health professional although, of late, changes within health care services have encouraged individuals to see themselves as much more active consumers than passive recipients (Audit Commission, 1991; DoH, 1991; DoH, 1993). Putting a name to peoples' health problems has always been the role of the health care professional (Peplau, 1987). As a result of this shift towards a more consumerized health care system, nurses need to relate to the client in a significantly different way to that previously expected (May, 1995), by giving them a voice in the definition of their own needs.

The user movement grew in strength during the last decade. Up until this point service users' expectations of mental health services were rarely sought. In fact people with mental health problems were often precluded from research studies because they were thought to be irrational due to their mental health status (Clifford et al, 1991). Rogers et al (1993) and others broke with this tradition, undertaking comprehensive studies of user perceptions of mental health services. Increasingly, service users have opportunities to discuss their satisfactions and dissatisfactions without the fear of compromising the care they receive, for example, Rose (2001).

Nursing practice has also undergone a period of rapid change. It has moved away from practical task-orientated labour to a more reflexive involvement with individuals, as recommended by Schön (1987). This human approach, 'New Nursing' as it has been coined (Smith, 1992), has made it more diffi-cult for mental health nurses to define their role accurately, since many of their skills are employed while working alongside clients within ordinary settings. These 'invisible' skills make the true nature and value of psychiatric nursing difficult to recognize (Michael, 1994). While there has been much debate as to what psychiatric and mental health nurses do and what they ought to do, little has been written regarding the extent to which these roles meet the needs of service users. A study was therefore undertaken to explore how mental health professionals, service users, ex-service users and carers perceive the needs of people in the psychiatric system, and the psychiatric nursing activity meeting those needs.

How the study was organized

The principles of grounded theory as proposed by Glaser and Strauss (1967) underpin the study. Grounded theory is an inductive approach that relies on a systematic process to arrive at a theory about basic social processes. Theory was inducted from the actual words of the study participants. These words were captured through focus groups conducted with service users, their friends and family, and professionals working within mental health services. The strength of the focus group lies in the collection of data from group interaction (Morgan, 1988). Through engaging with one another new ideas are generated. In addition, Kitzinger (1994) notes that people are more comfortable discussing sensitive topics as focus group participants support one another. Each focus group contained between 6 and 12 participants, in accordance with the recommendations of Basch (1987), Kreuger (1988) and Kitzinger (1994). Interviews were held in two sites in England (North and South), two sites in Northern Ireland (East and Midland) and two sites in the Republic of Ireland (East and Midwest). A total of 92 people participated.

Flannagan's (1954) Critical Incident Technique (CIT) was used as the framework for the focus group sessions. CIT allowed group discussion, which was more focused on the purpose of the study but was not likely to limit the generation of data. Flanagan (1954, p 327) describes CIT as 'A set of procedures for collecting direct observation of human behaviour to solve practical problems'. Focus group members were asked just two questions. First, to think of a situation where they felt that a nursing intervention had been effective. Second, to think of a situation where nursing had not been as effective as they might have wished. For both situations, the group generated ideas of what the needs of the person in distress were and what nursing activity might have been instrumental in meeting those needs.

Data analysis

Focus group meetings were tape recorded and transcribed verbatim (with full permission). The researcher used a process of constant comparison in coding initial interviews. With constant comparison, the text subsumed under each code was compared for internal consistency. In addition, the text was compared across codes to ensure that each code represented a distinct phenomenon. These codes then provided the framework for analysis of all transcripts with the help of QSR NUD*IST, a computer package that assists with the organization of qualitative data. Alongside open coding, more detailed exploration of some categories began to take place (axial coding, Strauss and Corbin, 1990). The axial coding phase encouraged the development of a descriptive story that identified the essence of the research and helped the researchers to choose a core category that seemed to best describe the central phenomenon. The core category was related to other categories and developed as a theoretical narrative, that is a 'story' that wove together the different threads into a coherent account.

Findings and discussion

The theory of what people need psychiatric and mental health nurses for articulates around the core category 'Knowing you, Knowing me' (see Figure 3.1). Nurses had to be able to read what the client expected from them at any given

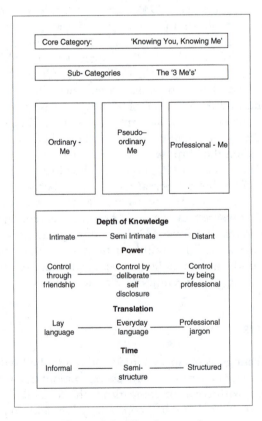

Figure 3.1   The three me's

moment in time. There is some resonance with the concept of accurate empathy (Rogers, 1961) here. However, accurate empathy involves an understanding of the person's understanding of the state in which they currently exist. 'Knowing me, knowing you' involves a predictive dimension, in which the nurse can second-guess how the patient wants the nurse to respond *given* the patient's particular understanding of their life world. For example, the nurse, on detecting a very subtle change in the patient's mental state, may choose to step back from that person for a while in order to provide them with a little more space to think through their problem. In a sense, it is not only to do with the communication of the nurse's understanding of the person's situation but it is also linked to the behaviour that the nurse chooses to take. The researchers chose to call this 'Accurate Actioning'.

The three sub-categories relating to the core category (the 3 Me's) are ordinary-me, pseudo-ordinary or engineered-me and professional-me. These describe the kinds of professional performance a nurse needs to employ to meet client needs. The ordinary-me performance domain implies a natural ordinariness that Brandon (1982) described as akin to that of being a friend in everyday life. The pseudo-ordinary or engineered-me domain involves consciously presenting a picture of oneself to the client who is a friendly face but not allowing the intimacy that ordinary friendship involves. Professional-me indicates that the nurse draws on theoretically based practice in order to do what the nurse perceives are best for the client.

Each sub-category has four dimensions (or properties); depth of knowing, power, time and translation. Depending on which 'Me' the nurse is operating within, the relationship with the patient will be different. For example, with ordinary–me, depth of knowing is intimate while within the professional-me domain it is distant.

Categories, sub-categories and dimensions of categories are discussed in depth below. Where appropriate people's own words have been used to illustrate the theory.

Knowing you, knowing me

The study suggests that the users of mental health services wanted nurses to anticipate and recognize their needs at any given time. Nurses were expected to know what the client wants even if the client is unable to express this verbally. The clues enabling the nurse to do this are not always clear and clients' needs are forever changing. According to Peplau (1987), people transmit messages to each other through verbal and non-verbal cues, patterns and variations of behaviour. Bryman (1988) states that the interpretation of interactions is a mutual and continuous process. Goffman (1959) suggests that information about the individual tells others how best to act in order to produce the desired response from them. For example, in this study, the consensus among clients *was* that nurses should relate to them as a friend, sharing personal experiences in a two-way relationship based on reciprocity and respect. But clients also expect the nurse to provide them with expert knowledge about their condition. This involves the nurse moving across the domains that range from being 'ordinary' with the client, to being more distant and professional.

Many of the activities undertaken by nurses are dependent on there being time in which to execute them. Time only becomes important when there are activities that need to be performed within it. These activities make time explicit. The description of time will depend upon which of the 3 me's the nurse is operating as. For example, within professional-me, time is seen as something to be structured by appointments with clients to deal with specific problems via professional intervention. Within ordinary-me, time will need to be more available in order to meet clients' need for friendship.

Depth of knowing

All members of the professional groups interviewed agreed that nurses know most about the client. This they attributed to the fact that nurses spend more time with clients than any other members of the mental health care team. According to Kirby and Slevin (1992) the time nurses spend with clients is what makes nursing unique. Nurses agree with this statement, yet they also recognize that their knowledge is not necessarily of the in-depth level that others believe they have. They do not claim to understand what the patient is experiencing. People's own experiences provide the basic material for their imagination therefore it is very subjective and limited. A nurse who has not experienced mental illness personally cannot know what it feels like. Even if they themselves have experienced mental health problems they still cannot know what it feels like for that particular client.

It seems from the data that clients like to talk to others who have experienced similar forms of distress. Professional help would seem to be even more effective if the nurse admits to having experienced a mental health problem. The Pathfinder project in London has actively sought nurses with mental health problems (Davidson, 1997) to work with clients in this way with successful outcomes. However, in the light of the Clothier Report (DoH, 1994) into the case of a paediatric nurse who caused death to four children in her care, Davidson (1997) notes that nurses are unlikely to admit to mental health problems to colleagues or clients for fear of dismissal.

Ramos (1992) has shown that too much emotional involvement from the nurse is non-productive for both parties. Yet, the clients in this study hoped that nurses would share intimate information with them within the 'ordinary-me' domain. The client initially, may be the sole provider of information within the nurse–patient relationship. But as time passes the client will not feel inclined to give any more to a one-sided relationship. Titmus (1973) described gift relationships within which there is a significant obligation to give and to repay. As time passes after a gift has been given the notion of credit becomes more imposing in that the nurse then owes the client a return gift (an exchange of personal information). Nurses operating within the ordinary-me domain are happy to tell the client about themselves just as friends would be comfortable to share knowledge and confide in each other. However, some nurses indicated that too much knowledge about the client as a person became a burden on their emotional budget, leading them to relate to the client on a more professional level at times.

Within 'pseudo-ordinary' or 'engineered-me' nurses do divulge information about themselves but they reported tailoring it to a level at which they feel comfortable. Here the nurse uses pseudo-ordinary or engineered-me to allow the client reciprocal surface knowledge about them so that the client feels valued: 'I tell them about myself, you know. Not things that are dangerous but more about things that have happened to me. You could be a cardboard cut out if you don't share this with people' Nurse (Group A).

Relationships within the professional-me domain are likely to be unequal, since it is the professional who has the specialized knowledge that will allow clients access to services that they require. As Peplau (1987) has pointed out, the professional keeps or owns the purpose of the relationship.

The respondents in the study saw nurses as having a special kind of knowledge about clients. Doctors actively seek the nurse's opinions because they are aware that they have a greater knowledge of the patient, according to Mackay (1993). Other professional groups use nurses' knowledge as a point of reference by which to monitor the client's mental status. For this reason, the nurse's experience of clients is highly regarded within multi-disciplinary meetings. 'They [the nurse] also know the client in a different way to me and this can be an effective role for any discipline in the team context. It's great to be able to share like this. You also get the observation and insight which nurses can bring to cases' Psychologist (Group M).

Psychiatric nurses try to maintain ordinary relationships with people who have been described as acting or reacting in extra-ordinary ways (Hill & Michael, 1996). Nurses, it would seem, are more willing to do ordinary things for the client than other groups within the health care team. For example: 'If I saw an old person that didn't have coal I see myself taking them down to the shop and putting coal in the boot, putting it out the back and filling up their bucket. I wouldn't leave a house without coal or bread. Those are small things but they are a big part of patient care' CPN (Group F).

Some see their role firmly within the professional-me domain. These relationships are much more focused and allow the client little or no insight into the professional's life. As one psychiatrist said: 'I think you have to be clear in your mind how you are doing that relationship, because obviously you are starting to get into dodgy ground in a professional relationship when you start and have this warm, human type relationship, as opposed to this so called cold professional type relationship. You must still have clear boundaries in your head' Psychiatrist (Group C).

The different depths of knowing the client can be seen in the situation where a client is being observed closely by nursing staff. Some nurses follow the client saying nothing while others are more comfortable talking with them while observing them: 'There are two types of close [observation] as I saw it. Some do closes [close observations] nicely. They talk to the patients like a friend and still carry out their duties. But others are like robots. When the patient moves they follow like zombies' Client (Group B).

Power

Caring for someone was seen as an activity within the ordinary-me domain. While caring about someone relates more to the pseudo-ordinary-me domain. However, De Swaan (1990) suggested that caring encourages a dominance of the carer and disempowerment of the cared for. This was not thought to be of benefit to the client or to the nurse.

On two occasions a doctor and a social worker described the role of a nurse as having been that of a 'motherly' figure to the client and the benefits of this discussed:

> This particular nurse was positively encouraged by the consultant to act as a mother figure and to actually mother vulnerable, distressed patients. I have to say that I was struck by how incredibly effective it was. She needed to have time and she was constantly forming very good relationships with patients and there was a lot of normalising or whatever going on. She was ideal, you know, if you had someone rather upset then she was really good to go along and make them a cup of tea and chat with them or take them for a walk round the ward. She was one of the most positive assets in that unit. Psychiatrist (Group C)

A 'mother figure' conjures up the image of the traditional view of a nurse as that of nurturing the client and protecting them from harm. This role suggests that the nurse has personal knowledge about the client within the ordinary-me domain implying that the nurse is accepting of the responsibility for the client and is, likewise, accepting of the effect on the nurse's emotional budget. Through its protective function and ownership of intimate knowledge, the role of mother in western society is implicitly powerful. The analysis presented is congruent with the need expressed by the clients interviewed that while in distress they wanted to hand over their concerns to the nurse until they felt able to cope again.

One client said that he felt relieved to be admitted to hospital when feeling unwell: 'They make sure you get disciplined medication and they make sure that you eat. Hospital is not always a healing place but a place of safety' Service user (Group B).

When the client eventually feels more able to cope the nurse will need to adapt their position accordingly on the power continuum. But not all service users want to be mothered and they do not want to have responsibility removed from them. Previous studies have suggested that some clients actively resist nurses who want more involvement with them (for example, Latimer, 1994). Coleman (1996), a service user, when a speaker at a conference said: 'You care for us don't you? We don't want you to; we want you to care about us. If you care about us you can take risks. We don't want you to work on us anymore; we want you to work with us and that means on our terms.'

Leinginger (1984) located caring at the heart of interpersonal professional work and says that caring is the essence of nursing. Yet, there are situations where the nurse is subject to professional constraints such as the need to protect the client from themselves and others from injury. In these instances the nurses is beholden to the legal responsibilities of the Mental Health Act (1983) or the United Kingdom Central Council for Nursing, Midwifery and Health Visiting (UKCC, 1996) *Guidelines for Practice.*

Working inductively from the data, both intimate knowledge and professional control can be disempowering for the client. Intimate knowledge because it encourages the client to hand self-responsibility to the nurse, and professional control because clients are prevented from having any self-responsibility. Conversely, caring for the client enough to allow them to take risks was thought to be empowering for the client by giving them much more control of their situation. The nurse needs to strike a balance between trusting the client and professional judgement without stifling the client.

How much control the client is given within the ordinary-me domain was also affected by the nurse's knowledge of the client:

> A person came into the office and asked if he could have permission to go out and buy cigarettes. To that person I was able to say, 'You don't have to ask me at all, you are a sensible guy.' You just do it because it was in the parameter of reasonable timing like it wasn't the middle of the night. Nurse (Group K)

It is possible to argue that nurses have a great deal of control within the pseudo-ordinary-me power domain. By actively making the client feel comfortable by behaving in a friendly manner, the nurse is able to win the client's confidence, which in turn enables the nurse to work with the client on therapeutic issues (Strang, 1982). The nurse is most likely to set the agenda. Unlike some of Bowers' (1992) subjects, the nurses interviewed for this study did not form friendships with clients they worked with. But, they did acknowledge that they were 'friendly' with clients:

> I think that you can be friendly without building up a friendship and the relationship is basically a therapeutic one rather than a social reason. Although the patient may use it as social and may enjoy the company of the nurse calling and talking to them. But we are not using it. Our main role isn't to socialise. There is a goal and

we must look for it. I don't see a problem with being friendly to achieve some other goal. Nurse (Group F)

Time

Time is very important to those trying to maintain an ordinary-me relationship with the client just as spending time with a friend is important. However, time is not an absolute concept. If you think of time as a glass of cordial, then time available for the client can be diluted by the other tasks for which the nurse is responsible. As other duties and distractions are added to the drink it becomes weaker until there is little of the original flavour remaining. The client could prevent this drowning of their time if only they would demand time with the nurse. But it would seem that clients are reluctant to disturb nurses who appear to be busy:

> I think that people who are in emotional distress don't have a good opinion of themselves and they are just not going to demand things. They are not going to be well enough to go up to a nurse and say 'excuse me, but this is your job to listen to me.' Very very often people try to talk to the nurse and the nurse will say 'later'. Service user (Group A)

The more senior the nurse the greater the dilution seems to be, suggesting they have less ordinary-me, intimate knowledge. Other professionals imagine the most senior nurse to hold the key to the client's personal knowledge when in reality this may not be the case. Knowledge of the client may be limited to more junior or untrained nurses who may know more about the client but have less experience. Indeed, Mackay (1993) found that patients and their relatives were most comfortable confiding in support staff, probably because they saw them the most frequently.

The less time the nurse has with the client the more removed they become from intimate knowing and so become more similar to other professional groups who maintain a distance from the client. Although not all nurses operate an appointment system, nurses can physically remove themselves from the client's presence. For example there were many references to nurses not being available to clients because they spent a lot of their time within the office: 'Sometimes I don't get to see a patient all day what with arranging things, paperwork, staff problems, meetings and so on' Nurse (Group I). Once nurses were in the office clients needed to knock to get attention: 'They sit in the office and the patients are outside and whether going through distress or whatever, you knock on the door and say can I see somebody' Client (Group A).

Time, although important, does not necessarily correlate with the depth of knowledge a nurse has about a client. It may take a client a long time to feel comfortable with the nurse. 'I think it is important that an easing in process happens before the actual clinical or intervention begins' Nurse (Group K). This comment suggests that the nurse was aware of the client's needs at that time and was monitoring the client's progress from the pseudo-ordinary-me domain. At this point the nurse would know very little about the client as a person so by waiting for the client within the relative safety of this domain the nurse could adjust their position as required by the client. The nurse's position within the pseudo-ordinary or engineered-me domain is of the nurse standing on a seesaw. It offers the nurse the best vantage point for moving towards a more professional-me or ordinary-me should it be required. Which way the nurse decides to move depends greatly on the moves of the client and the nurse's interpretation of their need at any given time.

Although the CPN has a large caseload and probably spends less time with the client over the day, their time with the client is less diluted with fewer distractions. They will understand more about the client's family circumstances, accommodation and social functioning. This may result in them feeling more responsible for the client. Going into someone's home forces a more informal and friendly approach to the relationship (Bowers, 1992). This suggests that clients are more receptive to the nurse's therapeutic advances. But the downside may be the loss of professional control over the relationship.

Having time available for clients allows spontaneity within the relationship. Being able to sit down with a client for a chat and a cup of tea was highly valued. There were frequent referrals to a cup of tea, both positive and negative, within the entire users', carers' and nurses' groups. This was also apparent within the pseudo-ordinary or engineered-me domain but rarely within the professional-me domain.

Within the ordinary-me domain the cup of tea represents a symbol of ordinary humanness and civility. It is something familiar in an unfamiliar situation and represents a welcome that seemed to make clients more comfortable: 'It's a very human thing; you can put your arm round them and make a cup of tea' Nurse (Group B). This spontaneity does not always occur within pseudo-ordinary or engineered-me domains. Nurses are acutely aware of the familiarity of making and sharing tea with somebody and this situation can be utilized within a setting in order to make a client comfortable. When offered a cup of tea by the client the nurse is in a position to take it or to refuse it. If they feel it better to concentrate on the therapeutic side of the relationship then tea will be politely refused. If, however, the nurse feels it would help the client relate to the nurse then tea is accepted. Tea within the professional-me domain is rarely accepted since it is thought inappropriate in a focused and goal driven relationship.

Translation

In the ordinary-me domain, service users wanted nurses to be honest with them just as telling the truth within a friendship is important.

Operating in the professional domain, nurses sometimes put a positive spin on medication or simply tell the patient what the doctor wanted them to hear:

> The doctor prescribes it and we give it so we are in there with the doctor. The patient often sees us in this way. Sometimes I say that I don't prescribe it, I only give it. It's embarrassing though, saying it is the doctor who prescribes this and that and it is the doctor who said it is going to do you good and that I have to agree with that. Nurse (Group B)

The nurse is expected to listen and to help the client obtain their own goals and to interpret professional knowledge and language. Sometimes this would involve making decisions for the client based on what they know about the client and the client's family and giving advice more like that of a friend ('if I were you'). Conversely, some users of services interviewed also wanted the nurse to provide information about drugs, about welfare and their future health. This suggests a more professional approach is required from the nurse.

The nurse needs to be multilingual to converse with the client and with the other professional staff. The nurse translates information from the client to the medical staff. In this way the nurse moves across the domains and dimensions. The notion that nurses are able to communicate across professional and lay dimensions is not new. Tracy (1938) described the nurse as a 'bridge' between the physician and the patient.

This translating role has meant that: 'Nurses are not only the blocks; they are the cement as well' Psychologist (Group K), because they piece together all the information from other professional groups in order to form a complete picture they think the client will understand.

Conclusion (and implications of the study)

People with mental health problems expect nurses to relate to them as both friend and professional. They need nurses to anticipate their ever-changing needs and to react accordingly. Nurses are expected to share their lives with clients while still being able to provide professional advice. The nurses we spoke to placed themselves within the pseudo-ordinary-me domain that offered them the best freedom of movement to meet the client's needs. Other professionals within mental health services appreciate and value the closeness that nurses have with clients and they rely upon nurses to provide them with information that will inform their professional judgement. Nurses are the most flexible and accessible work force available to clients to bridge the gap between intimate and professional knowledge and, in so doing, cement mental health services together.

From this summary the research implications for practice follow:

- The psychiatric nurse must be visible and accessible to patients/clients.
- The psychiatric nurse must be able to move across domains of language in order to act as an interpreter to fellow professionals and patients/clients.
- The psychiatric nurse must be able to establish and sustain friendships with patients that are intimate beyond the level of closeness that psychiatric nurses customarily offer.
- Given the above, there will be the need and opportunity to develop the form and function of clinical supervision in support of the nurse's role.

In terms of policy, a clear implication is in nurse education. The study challenges current wisdom that friendships and close relationships with patients erode the boundaries of professional behaviour (*Nursing Standard*, 1997). An emphasis on nursing as an interpersonal process at different levels, and the theory and skills associated with the process, would be the core of education and training. There is a sense of going back to the future here, in that Altschul (1972), Peplau (1952, 1988, 1994) and Travelbee (1969) have consistently advocated the interpersonal relationship to be the proper focus of psychiatric nursing. This does not mean that mental health nursing needs to be de-professionalized in favour of the more ordinary task being performed by less-well-trained generic mental health workers but rather it serves to stress the value of nurses who are able to move across domains and dimensions in response to needs.

Note

The grant holder for the study reported in this chapter was Professor Phil Barker.

References

Altschul, A. T. (1972) *Patient–Nurse Interaction: A Study of Interaction in Acute Psychiatric Wards*, Edinburgh: Churchill Livingstone.

Audit Commission (1991) *The Virtue of Patients Making Best Use of Ward Nursing Resources*, London: HMSO.

Barker, P. J. (2000) The tidal model, a holistic approach to psychiatric and mental health nursing, online at: http://www.tidalmodel.co.uk

Barker, P., Jackson, S. P. & Stevenson, C. (1999) The need for psychiatric nursing: towards a multidimensional theory of caring, *Nursing Inquiry*, 6, 103–11.

Basch, C. (1987) Focus group interview: an under-utilised research technique for improving theory and practice in health education, *Health Education*, 14, 411–48.

Brandon, D. (1982) *The Trick of Being Ordinary*, London: Macmillan/Mind Publications.

Bryman, A. (1988) *Quantity and Quality in Social Research*, London: Routledge.

Bowers, L. (1992) Ethnomethodology II: a study of the community psychiatric nurse in the patient's home, *International Journal of Nursing Studies*, 29, 69–79.

Clifford, P., Leper, R., Lavender, A. & Pilling, S. (1991) *Assuring Quality in Mental Health Services: the QUARTZ System*, London: Research and Development for Psychiatry in Association with Free Association Books.

Coleman, R. (1996) *The Politics of the Illness Model of Voices*, Department of Psychiatry, University of Newcastle, 'The Construction of Psychiatric Authority', June 20–21, Longhirst Hall, Northumbria.

Davidson, B. (1997) Mad to work here, *Nursing Times*, 93, 26–30.

Department of Health (1991) *The Patient's Charter*, London: HMSO.

Department of Health (1993) *A Vision for the Future. The Nursing, Midwifery and Health Visiting Contribution to Health and Health Care*, London: HMSO.

Department of Health (1994) *The Allitt Inquiry: Report of the Independent Inquiry Relating to Deaths and Injuries on the Children's Ward at Grantham and Kesteven General Hospital During the Period February to April 1991* (The Clothier Report). London: HMSO.

Department of Health/Home Office (1983) *Mental Health Act (1983)*, London: HMSO.

De Swaan, A. (1990) *The Management of Normality*, London: Routledge.

Flannagan, J. C. (1954) The critical incident technique. *Psychological Bulletin*, 51, 327–58.

Glaser, B. G. & Strauss, A. L. (1967) *The Discovery of Grounded Theory*, New York: Aldine Publishing Company.

Goffman, E. (1959) *The Presentation of Self in Everyday Life*, Harmondsworth: Penguin.

Hill, B. & Michael, S. (1996) The human factor, *Journal of Psychiatric and Mental Health Nursing*, 3(4), 245–8.

Kirby, C. & Slevin, O. (1992) A new curriculum for care, in O. Slevin & M. Buckingham (eds), *Project 2000: The Teachers Speak: Innovation in the Nursing Curriculum*, Edinburgh: Companion Press.

Kitzinger, J. (1994) The methodology of focus groups; the importance of interaction between research participants, *Sociology of Health and Illness*, 16, 1.

Kreuger, R. (1988) *Focus Groups: A Practical Guide*, London: Sage.

Latimer, J. (1994) Writing patients, writing nursing: the social construction of nursing assessment of the elderly patients on an acute medical unit, unpublished PhD thesis, Edinburgh: University of Edinburgh.

Leininger, M. (1984) Care, in M. Leininger (ed.), *The Essence of Nursing and Health*, New Jersey: Slack Inc.

Mackay, L. (1993) *Conflicts in Care: Medicine and Nursing*, London: Chapman Hall.

May, C. (1995) Patient autonomy and politics of professional relationships, *Journal of Advanced Nursing*, 21, 83–7.

Michael, S. (1994) Invisible skills, *Journal of Psychiatry and Mental Health Nursing*, 1, 56.

Morgan, D. L. (1988) *Focus Groups as Qualitative Research*, Newbury Park, CA: Sage.

Nursing Standard (1997) Relationships with patients, *Nursing Standard*, 11, 23–4.

Peplau, H. E. (1952, 1988, 1994) *Interpersonal Theory in Nursing*, Basingstoke: Macmillan – now Palgrave Macmillan.

Peplau, H. E. (1987) Interpersonal constructs for nursing practice, *Nurse Education Today*, 7, 201–8.

Ramos, M. C. (1992) The nurse–patient relationship: theme and variation, *Journal of Advanced Nursing*, 17, 496–566.

Rogers, A., Pilgrim, D. & Lacy, R. (1993) *Experiencing Psychiatry: Users Views of Services*, London: Macmillan/Mind Publications.

Rogers, C. R. (1961) *On Becoming a Person*, Boston: Houghton, Mifflin.

Rose, D. (2001) *User's Voices*, London: Sainsbury Centre for Mental Health.

Schön, D. A. (1987) *Educating the Reflexive Practitioner*, San Francisco, CA: Jossey-Bass.

Smith, P. (1992) *The Emotional Labour of Nursing*, London: Macmillan Press – now Palgrave Macmillan.

Strang, J. (1982) Psychotherapy by nurses – some special characteristics, *Journal of Advanced Nursing*, 7, 167–71.

Strauss, A. & Corbin, J. (1990) *Basics of Qualitative Research*, London: International Professional Publishers.

Titmus, R. (1973) *The Gift Relationship*, Harmondsworth: Penguin.

Tracy, M. A. (1938) *Nursing: An Art and a Science*, St Louis: Mosby.

Travelbee, J. (1969) *Intervention in Psychiatric Nursing: Process in the One-to-one Relationship*, Philadelphia: FA Davis Co.

United Kingdom Central Council for Nursing Midwifery and Health Visiting (1996) *Guidelines for Practice*, London: UKCC.

CHAPTER 4

User Perspective – The Good Psychiatric Nurse

ANNE MAIDMENT

Just before breakfast time on an acute Psychiatric ward a Nurse shouted at me, threatened me and really frightened me. I was then in the early depressive phase following a manic episode. If I didn't immediately get up and dressed, she yelled, I'd be in serious trouble. As I almost fell over trying to get my underwear on, she called me lazy and worthless. In my heavily drugged state she showed no compassion or understanding at all. She was hateful.

But was she real? Did I dream her? She was certainly the opposite of a good psychiatric nurse. Even now 13 years after that morning drama, I really don't know and that's rather alarming.

I have read enough to know that historically the 'carers' of the mentally ill could be brutal, sadistic, taunting, ignorant and frightening. The whole concept of the treatment of the 'mad' was to incarcerate and contain. Recently mentally ill people, as in *Speaking Our Minds* (Read & Reynolds, 1996) proudly adopt the term 'survivors' as their rallying cry, who tend to despise 'psychiatry', drug therapy, ECT and all in-patient care. I can't wholly believe in their resentment, anger and pain. How much is real, how much is exaggerated, how much is posturing for effect, how much hallucination?

That considerable pain is involved in the healing process of a mentally ill person there is no doubt, I have to state my own position at this point as a woman whose 30 year experience of bipolar disorder has lead to a viewpoint very different from 'the survivors'. I believe in the efficiency of most drug therapies, which have improved greatly in my time as a diagnosed manic depressive. I have benefited from courses of ECT. I have been fortunate in the five psychiatrists I have seen as an in-patient and out patient I have met many caring and conscientious psychiatric nurses and very few impatient or lazy ones. My misery was one of the trigger causes of my illness not, except for the 'dream' the treatment I received. In 1973 the charge nurse of the ward I was on at that time, who told me of the death of my father, was courteous, caring and gentle; it was the sudden death itself, so soon after my husband's desertion, which was the understandable pain.

So, my research for this chapter on the good psychiatric nurse has revealed a catalogue of bad behaviour on the part of mental health professionals; but the qualities of the effective nurse of the mentally ill are much more than the absence of the cruel traits. As an initial example of the Nurse who is remembered for good, I quote a patient's memories of one such: 'When I was a day patient, there was a very caring nurse, she never talked down to me, she always treated me as an equal and I also trusted her to tell me whenever I was making progress or deteriorating, Basically, I trusted her' (Rogers et al, 1993, p 43).

I have used this testimony in full as only then can trust be seen as the vital element in this staff–patient relationship. The nurse's conduct is the reverse of the non-therapeutic 'them and us' professional, she will not blandly reassure the patient if her condition is worse. She is 'very caring' but she is wholly truthful. This seems a good place to start, in concentrating on a description of the good nurse.

I read part of a survey published by MIND in the early 1990s (MIND, 1991) before concentrating on the charity's Nov. 2000 report (Barker, 2000). I was amazed at the difference between the two. The earlier work was much longer, but it was harder to extract patients' views and feelings. The 2000 report – *Patient's Views of Conditions on Psychiatric Wards* – was well produced and statistics were clearly presented. The overall effect was of a woman who had carefully and logically researched her material and her findings could be trusted to be accurate. Sadly though, in the report's introduction the researcher states, 'results of this survey . . . point to the fact that examples of good practice, are not the common experience.'

The majority of people receiving treatment in a Psychiatric Hospital are there voluntarily; for a patient admitted for the first time the environment can be very frightening. A patient (from the South East) comments, 'Staff did not explain where you were or why.' Fifty-seven per cent of patients said they didn't have enough contact with staff, 82 per cent said they had 15 minutes or less each day. Yet a patient (from Wales) declares that he could not have recovered without the ward. Blame for the lack of contact on the wards is apportioned as follows:

Staff shortages	51%
Overcrowding	29%
Lack of funding	29%
Negative staff attitudes towards patients	67%
Management of the ward	44%

It is clear, then, that several reasons given for staff distancing themselves from the patients on their wards are still matters of finance and political will, for the individual nurse though, the percentage of people questioned who cite the negativity of attitudes towards them, should be worrying. Linked closely to this finding are the comments that the ward environment has 'a sense of hopelessness, is custodial and uncaring' (from the South East), has 'a general atmosphere of boredom' (from the North West). Some staff made patients feel like 'nuisances'.

Respondents who spoke of good practice gave their experiences of very supportive and understanding staff who actively aided recovery. The patient wishes to build a relationship with staff and time spent is of the essence; friendliness and patience is needed if this contact is to be therapeutic. The most frightening example of bad practice, in relation to staff apportioning time is given by a South East patient: 'I was left to care for an extremely anxious woman for two hours, as staff would not come to help her. In the end the woman was clinging to me.' To talk to the patient and to help her with her distress is central to good nursing. It appears from the 2000 MIND (Barker, 2000) survey, that the best feature of the good psychiatric nurse is being there, when help is needed. It is consoling, therefore, to read this comment from a South East patient: 'The staff were always there when I needed someone to talk to.' Another South East contributor, though, writes: 'Those who did care just had so little available time.'

Time, or rather, lack of it, is commented on most frequently by the ex-patients who replied to MIND's questionnaire. It is as if the psychiatric nurse has not enough time for caring, helping, being there. Lack of interest when present on the ward, is also given as a grave failing. But this is obviously not a general answer. It is clear from the reports that different staff had quite different perceptions of their role: 'One of the staff members was brilliant . . . others were appallingly rude with serious attitude problems' (No Address).

Good nurses, it seems, can adapt their time to prioritize patients' needs. Not one patient reply seemed to show unreal expectations of the nurse's availability. Allowances were made for the lack of adequate funding, the short staffing, the overcrowding or the ineffective management styles. Yet the one to one care is seen as essential. Patients can understand that staff are sometimes stressed and tense. Yet without 'proper communication and support a patient can feel s/he is in Hospital to be punished, not helped' (from the North East). A respondent (from the South East), blamed 'changing shift patterns, casual staffing (especially at night) and a "them and us" culture' for the lack of caring. The same former patient said that they felt like 'an animal in a zoo' and had overheard one nurse talking about 'mixing with the low life'. She blames a lack of proper training for this unacceptable attitude.

The reasons, or excuses, given for bad conduct by some nurses rarely means that the patient's treatment was universally bad. I find the most moving example of this 'mixed' culture on the ward is given by a patient from the West Midlands: 'Some staff members were excellent – open, knowledgeable and supportive. Others were indifferent in a frightening way – cold, distant and even threatening in a quiet watching way. A few were sarcastic and bullying.'

To attempt to adjust to such opposites in behaviour causes a great deal of upset to an ill person. We can only be relieved that they did experience good practice from some nurses as the description of the others leads us to question their employment in any psychiatric care. Although such damning indictments of psychiatric nursing practice appear, other former in-patients show that poor and indeed, cruel behaviour is not the norm, 'My key worker (and to a lesser extent a few others) was a good deal of help to me *and trying to help facilitate change*' [my emphasis] (from Trent and Yorkshire).

In order to help and support a patient, the initial and continuing training a psychiatric nurse undertakes, must enable them to be more than a warder. As well as administering any prescribed drug therapy, the nurse will want the patient to benefit from the ever developing behaviourist therapies. This will be further considered when recent individual interviews are recorded later in the chapter.

One of the most moving tributes to a good psychiatric nurse is from a Welsh patient, 'When I was deep down, they gave me hope to keep going.' And similarly, 'One Nurse was kind – he spent some time talking to me about why I had felt suicidal.'

It's clear that though the occasional complaint is made about staff spending too much of their shift in the office, the nurse who achieves the satisfaction of seeing the patient's health improve, is the one who gets to know the patient on the ward. As well as talking and giving advice when they can, the good nurse *must* be a good listener. This takes time, patience and consideration. It's no use at all for the nurse to *appear* to be listening; this will only cause resentment, even anger, if the nurse cannot later differentiate between the life events the patients describe. A nurse who only *seems* to empathize with the patient, can be more despised than one who makes no pretence to understand.

In the Reports section on the 'Environment' of the psychiatric hospital or unit, it is evident that most questionnaire respondents link the good quality ward conditions with the high morale and good practice of staff. When describing a dismal ward, a patient outlines a 'sense of hopelessness, custodial and uncaring' (from the South East). Good conditions on a ward can help both staff and patients. Describing a new women's ward, a patient described it as 'safer, calmer and the staff were more understanding and more concerned – they took me seriously, were helpful, more relaxed and cheerful'. Mixed wards are being phased out as part of Government policy and this woman has evidently had some bad experiences of them. In her linking of surroundings and staff good conduct she names several important qualities of the good nurse. The 'calm' of the pleasant ward transfers to staff attitude. The staffing ratio appears satisfactory as nurses have time to care and to understand. They are not dismissive of the patient's views. Their manner is unhurried, their demeanour pleasant. Certainly in this woman's experience, the ward conditions and the staff's attitude seem automatically connected.

It is evident that poor staffing levels mean that staff on wards have little chance of achieving the relationships with their patients that the latter appreciate. Stricter styles of ward management can also impede a friendly approach. When the ward is seen by patients to be managed for *them* and not for the convenience of the staff, staff morale is also seen to be higher, 'the Nurses spent much of their time with patients on the ward, chatting or assembling groups to play board games, or sometimes sitting apart completing paperwork' (from the South East). The respondent considers that in this way nurses could be vigilant without being overbearing and this negated the need for locked doors.

The skills mix in wards as well is seen as vital, if appropriate care is to be delivered. Throughout the MIND (Barker, 2000) survey the following essential attributes of the good psychiatric nurse are often repeated, 'they must be attentive, a good listener, caring and ready to help.' The respondents do not have unrealistic work patterns in mind for their carers. They are quite aware that the most helpful and supportive of nurses will have routine tasks to carry out. But several responses made it clear that there is much more to be done on the ward than the obvious routines, for example, 'I think there needs to be much more emphasis on the healing powers of being able to talk, not just dishing out medication and sitting in the office all day – with extra support then for staff who see people's distress' (No Address).

Even allowing that a disturbed patient will see their needs as central and compelling it's clear that a good psychiatric nurse will be very well trained in personal interactions; so much can be gained by a few minutes of talking *and* listening. Several former patients have suggested that good staff training should definitely include *user* involvement in the training of would-be professional nurses, as well as listening carefully to their views. This is being implemented in some training courses, but despite Government good intentions, as yet, plays little part in Hospital Trust decision making.

In her recommendations, Barker links the ward's environment and conditions to people's recovery. Even more important, however, is the value of a higher staff:patient ratio. She too reiterates the need for an input by service users in care staff training. She feels this would encourage flexible recruitment and retention with the aim of building a diverse workforce and ensuring an appropriate skills mix. She comments that, 'there needs to be a culture change that respects patients and therefore begins to recognise the daily indignities that too many patients of acute wards endure' (Barker, 2000). Barker stresses the need for a public policy framework that aims to put patients at the centre of service delivery. Better quality services need to involve patients.

The anthology of patient's accounts of their illnesses – *Speaking Our Minds* (Read & Reynolds, 1996) at first seemed as though it would be a useful source of material to outline service users views of the good psychiatric nurse. It did not prove to be so. The stories were very personal and revealed many aspects of mental distress but for the most part the traditional patterns of psychiatric healing are shunned, even loathed. One example of a person 'acting mad' in a department store actively seeking admission to a psychiatric unit, finally reveals her motive – she is in need of free accommodation!

There were bound to be *some* useful sections of this anthology, but in keeping with the 'survivors' description at the beginning of this chapter, we have to work with mainly negative viewpoints. One description ('A Survival Story' by Patricia Brunner) (Brunner, 1996) of the way in which a patient often has to conform to the staff's notions of recovery in order to get out of hospital is a clear pointer to nurses to take an individual's personality into account before reporting the worst to their doctor. Why is it that the psychiatric inpatient, who feels and expresses the full range of human emotions, is in danger of having them interpreted as a symptom of their mental illness?

I can vouch for a clear example of this! On the wards, a few of us put some pop records on and began to dance. The others tired of it before I did and I was left, quite happily dancing on my own. This 'evidence' of still being 'high', when reported by nurses to my psychiatrist cost me weekend leave substituted with day release only. But they would *never* have seen me quietly knitting at the side of the ward!

The writer I found most illuminating was Peter Campbell in the chapter 'Challenging Loss of Power' (Campbell, 1996). His examination of his own illness and its treatment led him to believe that the psychiatric system is founded on inequality and that the user is at the bottom of the pile. He feels that when admitted to hospital he is treated not as Peter Campbell, but as a manic depressive. While the resources of the medication trolley are over used, the human resources of those living and working in the psychiatric unit are consistently under used. The environment, declares Campbell, prevents nurses from exercising their most important human skills, their creativity, their caring, which were the very reasons for most of them entering their chosen profession. Psychiatry, Campbell continues, must be more than custody and care – 'talk should be of creativity and change not control and illness' (Campbell, 1996, p 62).

The comfort and cosiness of the nurse's office is described by Clive in 'I've got Memories Here' (Clive, 1996). Having been a 'serial patient' for years, he now has his own flat in the community. This he finds very lonely and isolated. His nostalgia and longing for the safety of the hospital ward is marked, 'If you had a nightmare you'd get up and go into the Nurse's Office and they would reassure you!'. There is no automatic 'Hospital – bad', 'Community – good'. Clive regards the world outside the Hospital grounds as threatening and dangerous.

So far, the hospital-based psychiatric nurse has been the object of study. There are many service users and carers, though, who reject the 'psychiatrist dominated hospital scene' (Lindow, 1996) in favour of the CPN's visits and several of the people I talked to while preparing this chapter, regarded the CPN best known to them as a wonderful benefit, a great improvement on in-patient care. It is also obvious that a CPN can only be of use to the person who will allow them to be so. When CPN's started their peripatetic work, my late husband would elude his with great ease! Only a few weeks in hospital, usually on a Section, served to stabilize him.

In order to find out some current opinions about nursing care in mental health, I talked to several people closely affected by standards of performance. I made it known at Sunderland's recently opened Mental Health Resource Centre – Headlight – now a registered charity – that contributions on the subject would be welcomed (I'm a member myself, but I do very little compared to others). One carer member wrote a full assessment for me which I shall shortly examine. Also two other service user members proffered valuable material as well as a paid worker at Sunderland MIND. It was of interest to compare the views of the people I talked to (no discussion was formal enough to be termed an 'interview') with the books and reports already considered. Overall the people I spoke to had more positive, forward looking views than those expressed in the report material.

David Brooke (pseudonym)

Diagnosed schizophrenic, a number of years ago, the memory of being an inpatient is like a nightmare to David. However, over the years I have known him, through Community Health Council and political work, he has always spoken very favourably of his community psychiatric nurse. David has been fortunate enough to have had the same CPN visit his home for a number of years now. He praises the nurse's communication skills, his patience, his ability to work out medication guidelines *with* his patient, not dictate to him. Although David has a range of interests, he always makes his CPN's visits a priority. At the present time, David speaks highly of psychosocial intervention and believes it will do good as it is further developed.

Walter Ragg (pseudonym)

Walter spent a period of time in the same acute psychiatric ward as I did 13 years ago. He is a very able creative man, an accountant, teacher, writer and poet. However, though the symptoms he displayed in hospital were very close to mine, he refuses to accept the 'bipolar disorder' label and finds that for him, prescribed medication has severe side effects. Through continuous community pressure he has now been offered a place in a hospital specializing in homeopathy and alternative treatments. For him, nurses experimenting with alternative techniques have been of most help to him. Sunderland Social Services, in their Mental Health Forums have introduced a number of people to alternative medicine.

Jan and Simon Hardy (pseudonyms)

The most comprehensive response I reviewed in preparing this survey was a written commentary from a woman I first met about 10 years ago at a

Sunderland Mental Health Forum. She has been active in the local Carers Centre Branch and is now Secretary of Headlight, the Resource Centre previously referred to. Jan's son, Simon, was diagnosed as having schizophrenia in his late teens. He is now a man of about 30. So Jan's piece about experiences of psychiatric nursing staff is an overall view, though she admits that it was difficult for her to write. I quote Jan and Simon's present position, in her own words, as it is so hearteningly positive, 'My son now has treatment Monday to Thursday from the Assertive Outreach Team and everyone involved is marvellous. The main reason and the big factor is that they have TIME! (her emphasis)'.

Jan states that the CPNs Simon has had in the past have been very good (with the exception of one). His present CPN, she describes as, excellent. Through the 'talking treatment' he now receives, Simon has been enabled to change from a recluse, when only his family seemed to have time for him. He is now engaging with people at football, talking, going to social clubs. This confidence in Simon gives respite to his family, delighted at the progress he has made. Jan believes that now her son receives treatment and time in the community; before the current team began to visit, it was often a 10 minute visit 'while I give you an injection'.

Before she lists the good qualities so apparent in Simon's present CPN, Jan makes an alarming statement, 'Hospital staff and community staff are a world apart, more so now. The gap is widening by the day.' I shall return to this at the end of the chapter. Throughout her praise for Simon's CPN, the good Psychiatric Nurse, Jan stresses his 'common sense approach'. The positive qualities stated include: 'positive attitude'; 'enthusiasm and commitment'; 'time to talk and communicate meaningfully'; 'flexibility (to patients' needs)'; 'empathy'; 'listening skills'; 'accessibility'. There is consistency in the team's approach but this does not encourage dependency as the care workers have a sensible system of rotation. From a carer's point of view, Jan comments that this is the first time she and her husband have had confidence in the staff 'because we have access if necessary'.

The good nurse, Jan declares, does not just listen to problems, but will come up with a plan of action and help carry it through. With Simon's and his carers' full cooperation, the teams' planning abilities have enabled a full care programme to be drawn up and information is available for out of hours help. Because the psychiatric nurse now has time, he gives encouragement to use the service. Jan states that they now have few concerns about Simon's treatment in the community and because of this confidence, they no longer feel the need to intervene in the decision making, on Simon's behalf. The realistic goals set by the community team and the ability of the CPN to use his own initiative are reassuring. Jan ends her account thus, 'PS: my son has just said he has a new set of friends (at the football social clubs). He was not talking about nurses, but people he is meeting and being able to meet.'

But, throughout Jan's writing there is a bogeyman lurking. Her son's social contacts, which the family feel are so important, have expanded; he is clearly much more content and more fulfilled. But there is a 'what if?' which greatly troubles them. It is really necessary to use Jan's own words for this, 'Our confidence is growing with Simon's but we fear for him if he has to go back to Hospital!!!!! (Brigadoon as we call it).' Since Jan's testimony was only written in July 2002, it can't be dismissed as poor hospital care of long ago. It is an indictment of hospital inpatient provision, which is the very opposite of her praise for community services.

Brenda McAvoy (pseudonym)

Brenda is a paid officer at the Sunderland Branch of MIND (Sunderland MIND were especially helpful to me when my former husband was killed by a youth in December 2000). My association with MIND ensured that this was a friendly mutual exploration of ideas, rather than 'an interview'. In many ways Brenda's opinions on what constitutes a good psychiatric nurse, although she was speaking primarily about inpatient care, linked closely with those of Jan Hardy. The nurse's aim, wherever possible, was 'being there'. Their work should concentrate on confidence building. Listening and chatting should be calm and unhurried. There should always seem to be the 'spare' nurse available – one who is not always seen to be bustling about on specific duties on the ward. Only so, will the patient be relaxed enough to talk freely.

The bleak saying, 'time is money' really seems to be at the core of psychiatric care. In the vision of so many witnesses, their main criticisms stem from the nurses being too busy and too short with them to establish any useful relationship. It must be the main role of the Trust Boards, researchers, lecturers and former patients, to press for more staff, both in the hospitals and in the community. Nurses themselves must insist on more staff among the many other demands on Government funding. It should not be hard for those wishing to be psychiatric nurses to extract from the testimonies recorded, the essential qualities of the good nurse. These desirable features are repeated throughout this chapter. If nurses are granted the requisite time, they will be able to be friendly, patient, caring, skilled in talking and listening, able to negotiate, enthusiastic, realistic and positive.

I began this chapter by describing a nurse who might well have been a dream. I close by mentioning one who definitely wasn't. Jill had the nursing qualities already listed and she helped me a great deal when I was last an inpatient on an acute ward. She boosted my confidence and never talked down to me. A couple of years after my discharge, I met her in town. I was pleased that she remembered me. When I began to thank her, she interrupted – 'I had to leave' she said, 'I've got a new job. I found I just couldn't work as I wanted to work.' This was 10 years ago. It was (and is) a sad reflection on NHS priorities.

References

Barker, S. (2000) *Patients' Views of Conditions on Psychiatric Wards*, London: MIND.

Brunner, P. (1996) A survival story, in J. Read & J. Reynolds (eds), *Speaking Our Minds: An Anthology*, Basingstoke: Palgrave – now Palgrave Macmillan, pp 16–22.

Campbell, P. (1996) Challenging loss of power, in J. Read & J. Reynolds (eds), *Speaking Our Minds: An Anthology*, Basingstoke: Palgrave – now Palgrave Macmillan, pp 56–62.

Clive (1996) I've got memories here, in J. Read & J. Reynolds (eds), *Speaking Our Minds: An Anthology*, Basingstoke: Palgrave – now Palgrave Macmillan, pp 126–8.

Lindow, V. (1996) What we want from community psychiatric nurses, in J. Read & J. Reynolds (eds), *Speaking Our Minds: An Anthology*, Basingstoke: Palgrave – now Palgrave Macmillan, pp 186–90.

MIND (1991) *Survey of Patients Care*, London: MIND.

Read, J. & Reynolds, J. (eds) (1996) *Speaking Our Minds: An Anthology*, Basingstoke: Palgrave – now Palgrave Macmillan.

Rogers, A., Pilgrim, D. & Lacey, R. (eds) (1993) *Experiencing Psychiatry*, Basingstoke: Palgrave – now Palgrave Macmillan.

CHAPTER 5

Carer Issues in Mental Health

VAL CHAPMAN

What I notice the most about the care of people who are mentally ill is the fragmentation of it. I see this as a carer; the mother of a 22-year-old son with a diagnosis of severe and enduring paranoid schizophrenia; and also as a coordinator for the county branch of 'Rethink' (formerly the National Schizophrenia Fellowship).

Despite the emphasis now being on joined-up, multi-disciplinary care, social workers don't seem to know what nurses do or think; hospital staff seem to disregard the social workers; psychiatrists see families as a nuisance; families think psychiatrists don't listen to them; people who are ill think their relatives are in league with the doctors; consultants who don't do research make jokes about those who do . . . you could go on like this forever.

Attitudes between different groups of stakeholders are confrontational and suspicious, with carers feeling like 'piggy in the middle', passed over by every-one. Yet they have been described as the 'glue that holds the system together' (Chapman, 1997). The extent of the responsibility given to carers is well documented, and no one can ignore the ever-increasing family role implicit in the current emphasis on community care and home treatment. Studies showed that 40–60 per cent of people with schizophrenia return to live with their families (Brady, 1996; Norton et al, 1993) and 1.5 million people in Britain spend 20 hours a week or more looking after someone with a mental illness and save the Government something in the region of 3 billion pounds (Berry, 1997). And no one questions the fact that in taking on this huge responsibility, carers also take on a very heavy burden, which is different from that of a carer of someone with a physical illness:

> although their sickness might dramatically disrupt the logistical routines of every-day family life, physically ill people are ordinarily deeply involved in getting well and returning to their pre-sickness roles. In contrast, mentally ill people often cannot abide by the usual rules of social settings, may engage in behaviours considered socially repugnant, sometimes deny that they are ill, and frequently treat their care-givers with hostility instead of gratitude. (Karp & Tanarugsachock, 2000)

On top of this, the person who is ill may well hold the carer directly responsible for the illness. The influence of R. D. Laing persists in the populist view of madness, ie: that it is a culturally conditioned, internal conflict, a reaction to poor relations among family members. When, in desperation, eight months after my son had been diagnosed as having schizophrenia, I asked his social worker 'So what exactly is it, this illness?' he gave me a printout of something which explained that it was *probably* caused by over-dominant mothers. This was at the end of 1998, when knowledge about schizophrenia had moved on, but the social worker didn't know that, and that printout did me no good at all. No wonder families are scared to meet with practitioners when they feel they're being judged like this, condemned without a hearing. By then (my son was just 18) I was used to being the guilty party.

Not every professional made the kind of unwarranted assumption I once found in his school file ('Mother very unstable'), but there were certainly enough to make me unable to trust anyone. Another spin-off from the Laing era, equally damaging for carers, is the anti-psychiatry movement, which from the late 1960s was the basis for the formation of campaigning groups such as the British Network for Alternatives to Psychiatry. Again, this attitude persists in some organizations, and I think many practitioners, particularly psychiatrists, assume that anyone who asks questions is under the same umbrella, and consequently feel threatened. This anti-psychiatry view also provides ammunition for mentally ill people who are refusing medication, and this is a huge problem for carers who are convinced that the medication is the starting point for recovery. My son has had to be sectioned under the Mental Health Act three times, the last twice being only a few days after he decided to stop taking his Clozapine. When he takes this medication he is unafraid, sociable, living a more-or-less normal life; as soon as he stops it he is delusional, terrified and angry. Nothing will ever persuade me that he has no need of chemicals.

Getting medication into someone who sees no need for it is only one of the problems, of course. One of our carers is so desperate that she puts her son's tablet into his tea every day; she knows she shouldn't do it, and is well aware of the risks if he realized, but can't bear to see him so tormented. There are plenty of other difficulties. These can be categorized under the headings of objective and subjective burdens (Chapman, 1997), with objective burdens including physical or logistical problems associated with financial hardship or disruptions to household and social functioning, and subjective burdens covering feelings of anguish, guilt and loss.

Rebecca Reay-Young (2000) points out that there is general consensus in the literature as to the nature of both the objective and subjective burdens placed on carers of people with schizophrenia. Neither I, nor any of the carers I know, need the literature to tell us this. We all have the same problems, with the imposition of a chaotic lifestyle that you never asked for and certainly don't want and the unpredictable nature of mental illness taking away your ability to plan for the future. First, it is unbelievably difficult to live long-term with someone who sleeps most of the day and is up all night, even if you don't have to go to work the next day.

Sleep deprivation is apparently one of the commonest forms of torture for political prisoners, which is what I sometimes feel I am. When my son is well, he's the kindest, most considerate person there is, but when he's ill you have no chance of appealing to his better nature as he just doesn't have one. I know all about keeping down the levels of expressed emotion; but at 3 o'clock in the morning, when he's telling me that the problem is that I'm just a light sleeper and should do something about myself, being a saint is quite beyond me. And of course you can't go out during the day because you can't leave alone someone who is in a deep medicated sleep and who wouldn't smell a fire, or who, if he woke up to find the house empty, would be terrified. How do you ask someone to baby-sit for a man of 22, and who could do it anyway? Also, these sleep patterns make it difficult to fit in with the needs of the rest of the family, difficult to have visitors, and difficult to do ordinary household chores.

People with severe mental illness have problems with planning and organization, so when my son is finally out of bed he expects me to drop everything to meet some need he sees as urgent. Cooking a meal with someone pacing round and round the kitchen table needs a fairly skilful kind of choreography, and if you're not a smoker yourself the full ashtrays and permanent fug in the atmosphere are really unpleasant. Normally smoking is something we don't allow in the house, but it is such a need for my son that it seems cruel to refuse him. All these add up to a huge amount of irritation. No wonder that 70 per cent of carers feel that their physical health has suffered because of their caring role. (Hogman and Pearson, 1995)

Another consequence is the reduction in social networks, which again has been well-documented (Brady, 1996; Chapman, 1997). It's difficult to organize a night out, (even if you can afford it); I wish to discuss further on the economic impact of mental illness on families. We are very lucky in that most of our friends are totally sympathetic to our situation, although there are one or two who have just stopped communicating completely. However, I still feel reluctant to mix socially because my son's illness is always uppermost in my mind; I can't be bothered to talk about other things and at the same time I know that I'm being a real bore. What other carers tell me about (frequently) is how desperately irritating are the friends who make 'helpful' suggestions without understanding anything about the illness. Then they feel guilty for being so annoyed – as if there isn't enough guilt already.

The worst of these is the 'Tell her it's time she pulled herself together' message, closely followed by 'You shouldn't give in to him, he just needs a bit of discipline', 'I'll have a good talk to her, we've always got on well, I'll sort her out', or 'Have you thought of hypnosis or aromatherapy?' One of the main reasons carers join support groups is to replace the social network they used to have with one where people understand enough not to make such comments. Stigma, too, is an issue here. Society tends to blame families or partners, and although mental illness is slowly becoming more accepted, it's impossible to predict what people's reaction will be. When my son was sectioned for the third time, amidst great noise and drama, I was massively encouraged by the genuinely caring response of his neighbours. 'Why didn't you tell us, we'd have kept an eye on him?' 'Let us know what we can do to help when he comes out of hospital?' 'Come in for a cup of tea whenever you're up this way.' They were all young people, so perhaps this is a generational change.

Family relationships can be affected in a similar, but more distressing, way. One of our carers, whose son is now well and living a happy and fulfilled life in his own home, has lost a daughter, son-in-law and two grandchildren; the daughter blames her for allowing the illness to take hold and then for forgiving the behaviour it produced, and has completely severed relations. In many other families I know, there are regular arguments about how best to manage not only the illness itself but also the practitioners involved in the care. It has to be remembered that families often begin to deal with the *illness* only after very long periods of incomprehensible, unmanageable behaviour, which will have already set up deep-rooted patterns of conflict and stress between many of its members. It is sometimes a relief to have a diagnosis. I have been told that 40 per cent of parents of a child with mental illness separate. I don't know where the statistics for this come from, but it seems very likely. I know that it is particularly difficult in families where there is a stepfather, who is more likely to leave, or who will stay but may distance himself from the situation. This effectively leaves the mother to cope as a single parent, while still expected to fulfil all her wifely duties as if nothing had happened. With mental illness being such a costly thing to manage, the problem is compounded for mothers who are financially dependent on a stepfather.

The situation with regard to siblings is even more complex, and has more serious long-term implications. Siblings are not generally considered by practitioners, despite literature which emphasizes the difficulties they face (Gerace et al, 1993). Parents worry about what is happening to the well sibling but their time and energy is taken up with the child who is ill. Children recognize the stress parents are under and feel anxious about it. When my younger son was 13, well before we had a diagnosis for his brother, he said to me 'I wouldn't bother you with my problems, Mum, because I think you've got enough to worry about with my brother.' His reaction is one that is often found with siblings. He has always tried too hard to be good, suppressed feelings he should have been able to talk about, and ended up with huge anxieties which seemed to be about something else, mostly school work, but which were really about his brother's illness. We were lucky enough to be able to pay for counselling for him, which saw him through A-levels although with a much-reduced achievement, and he has managed to put some of the worries behind him during his first year at university. I am sure he worries about whether he will develop schizophrenia himself, and who is going to care for his brother when we are too old (which is also a major concern to us, of course). It has been suggested that sibling caregivers provide less help, but suffer a greater burden, than parental caregivers (Tennakoon, 2000).

Other siblings I know have taken the route of resentment, withdrawing from the family and taking refuge with friends; in one case I know, because of the choice of friends, this led directly to some fairly delinquent behaviour, compounding the problems the family already had. Brothers and sisters may well feel embarrassment, guilt because they have a better life than the sibling who is ill, difficulty in accepting the fact that they themselves receive less attention. When children reject a sibling who is mentally ill (and they have good cause for doing this), it adds to the parents' distress. We have often tried to protect our youngest son from knowing exactly what was happening, but this has never worked. Not knowing was worse for him, as it left too much to his imagination, and he always found out in the end. The last time my son was sectioned, I knew it was going to happen. I left my younger son revising for exams, said nothing, and planned to explain after the exams were over. But while the police were breaking into his flat, big brother, in terrible distress, made a phone call to little brother with a blow-by-blow account of events as they were unfolding. My younger son failed his exam and reproached me for keeping things from him. It's much better to keep other children informed. We once asked if our younger son could attend a ward round. Staff were puzzled, but agreed, and I think it helped him to have a picture of what went on and to be able to put faces to the names we had mentioned. With the current recognition of the importance of psychosocial and family interventions for optimal recovery, there will hopefully be a much greater involvement of, and consideration for, the other children in the family.

It has to be said, though, that in all this issue of social and family networks the experiences can be very positive. If people can manage to stay together their relationships are strengthened and their abilities for caring and understanding increased. My youngest son seems to have become a sort of 'agony aunt' for friends at university, and this must surely have something to do with his raised capacity for sympathy. I myself feel privileged to know many of the carers and workers I've met through my involvement with support groups, almost to the point of guilt (yet again!) that I am gaining some benefit from my son's illness.

The final, and possibly most damaging, element of the objective burden is the economic one. For families, schizophrenia must be the most expensive illness there is. Most of the time now our son is cared for in an area 80 miles away from home – a situation which I shall talk about later; consequently much of our spending has been on travelling this distance. But since the first episode of psychosis, at least a *quarter* of our income has been spent on coping with his mental illness, and I suspect that the financial commitment most families have to make is in this kind of proportion, no matter what the level of earnings. The money has gone on travelling to visit; buying meals out when we couldn't get home; sometimes hotels; paying for presents, 'toys' and activities to keep our son occupied in an attempt to drive away the delusions; replacing all the clothes (at times socks and underwear every week for weeks on end) and possessions lost in the chaotic lifestyle; postage on the five hundred or so letters I've had to write to ensure adequate care; a fax machine for when we had to send documents urgently; hours and hours of telephone calls; therapy for his brother; setting up an inheritance trust; expensive (and often vain) attempts to cheer ourselves up; paying workmen to do jobs we would normally have done ourselves. And of course there's my lost salary; it's impossible to make a commitment to a job when you are coping with an illness which needs such immediate responses. At the same time, while you're struggling to make your own money do ten times what it's capable of, you're likely to be trying to manage a relative who is being wildly profligate with his own, and probably harming himself in the process. It's extremely difficult to obtain Disability Living Allowance – it takes at least two hours to complete the form even if you know what you're doing – but if you are successful then the person you care for can end up with quite large amounts of cash, especially if they're in residential care.

My son once received over £2000 in backdated benefits, which massively increased his popularity with the drug users and alcoholics he'd become friendly with. His bank book shows a withdrawal of £100 every day for an 11-day period, at the end of which – when he had no food, no sleep, no medication, but plenty of vodka and cannabis – he had to be sectioned for the second time. I managed to become an appointee for receipt of the benefits, which is not much of a solution when you see the resentment and conflict it sets up. Every carer I know has to spend vast amounts of time, and often of their own money, sorting out the financial problems of the person they're caring for.

The subjective burden is far more difficult to discuss. It is well documented in the literature (Berry, 1997; Brady, 1996; Chapman, 1997) and everyone accepts the theory of the stages carers go through – shock, denial, anger, bargaining, acceptance – and the resulting feelings of anxiety, stress, fear, depression and confusion. Few of the theorists mention that you often experience all these stages and all these feelings simultaneously. Knowing all this sometimes helps practitioners to avoid dealing with the carer issue; they know that anger is an expected reaction, but don't distinguish this from justifiable anger about, say, mishandling of care, and therefore they take no steps to improve things. They know carers have emotional distress, so they express glib sympathy without realizing that this is just not enough. But it seems impossible to put across the global awfulness of what is happening, the incomprehensible surrealism of it, the way it takes over everything else.

Where there has been a death of someone else in the family, carers may find it impossible to grieve because there are no spare feelings for that. Sometimes I am appalled at my own lack of response, such as once when my son attacked another patient and I felt no shock or horror at all. The embarrassment, too, is very hard to tolerate, particularly when it occurs in a sexual context. The survey by the National Schizophrenia Fellowship for their 'Only the Best' campaign (2001) showed that for people on anti-psychotic medication the two most feared side effects were weight gain and sexual dysfunction. Children don't usually share their sexual fears or fantasies with their parents, especially in public, so mothers are very uncomfortable when, to give some real-life examples, a son removes all his clothes in full view of the neighbours, or asks for help with an impotence problem. Of course the guilt and the grief are impossible to describe. However much you tell yourself, on a rational level, the theory behind the causes of schizophrenia, the gut feeling remains that you should have done *something* to prevent it. Mothers are supposed to protect their children from harm, kiss it better, whatever it is, drive the bogeyman away – and you've failed miserably. A friend who has two sons with schizophrenia, and who is unbelievably well informed, an active campaigner and educator, laughs at herself for once thinking that the boys developed the illness because she ate brandy mince pies when she was pregnant. I suspect that underneath she still holds to the mince pie explanation. As for the grief: you can put it out of your mind most of the time, especially if you fill the time with support groups and campaigning, as I do, but when you do happen to touch the tripwire in the minefield, then it 'Whispers the o'er fraught heart and bids it break' (Shakespeare, *Macbeth*, Act 4 sc. 3)

Staff on hospital wards usually see families at a time of emergency. They focus on the patient, on the acute care of a crisis situation and tend to forget, or be unaware of, the day-to-day, ongoing treadmill which persists for the families after the crisis has subsided (Atkinson & Coia, 1995). What I am sure nurses don't realize is that their first response to the family is pivotal in determining the subsequent course of management by the carers after discharge from hospital. A ward culture which puts families in a separate room, leaves them to wonder what on earth is happening, and makes no attempt to explain anything, is setting up a situation which disempowers and disables the very people who can bring the most benefit to the person who is ill. Sixty-one per cent of young people believe that a caring family is the best protector of mental health (Ayerst, 2001). Carer presence is a key determinant in preventing escalation of substance abuse and suicide (Ayerst, 2001). If the wrong messages are given at the start, it will be almost impossible to put these right later. Carers will need, over a very long period of time, assistance with managing the objective burdens; in this context professionals could provide information about the illness and treatments, specific suggestions for dealing with behaviour, plus details of the Care Programme Approach, benefits, housing, respite care, etc.

In terms of coping with the subjective burdens, there needs to be, first, a huge emphasis at every stage that the family is not the cause of the illness; this will do a great deal to assuage the guilt. Beyond that, emotional factors can be enormously helped with peer support, sharing experiences, realizing that you're not alone, so I think it is the *duty* of hospital staff to help carers access people with similar problems. Currently very few carers (probably only 1 or 2 per cent) engage with formal support groups and there needs to be some very imaginative and proactive work done at the front line if this is to change. It would also assist in finding more carers for the vast amounts of carer consultation now being sought at every level. But it has to be borne in mind that the help offered to carers has to be appropriate to the stage they've reached in the adjusting process.

I mentioned before that my son now lives 80 miles away from us. We had nine months of care in a hospital in the North East of England, then, with help and advice from the National Schizophrenia Fellowship (now Rethink), managed to have him transferred to a hospital in the North West of the country. The culture of these two hospitals could not have been more different. In the first, we were completely excluded. Our son became a piece of NHS property, with the rules of confidentiality being misapplied as a means of keeping us away. He was suddenly none of our business, despite the fact that he was barely 18, had been our total responsibility for all his life until then, and was still turned over wholly to our care even though none of the care team was communicating with us. An obvious question here is whether or not hospitals would be allowed to discharge patients to a registered care home which had untrained staff they never talked to? It is obvious to any carer, and well recognized by *good* practitioners, that families or friends are the *real* experts when it comes to describing and monitoring the behaviour of someone who is mentally ill. Time and time again carers say to me 'They've only seen him for a few hours; how can they possibly know what he's like?' Or 'Why don't they believe me? I know she won't manage.' Or 'She manages to hide her funny thoughts while she's with the nurses; they seem to think I'm making it up when I tell them what she says to me.' After the attitudes we'd found in the first hospital, it came as a total shock to have a team who not only valued the information we could provide, but also treated us as equal partners in delivering the care. It is no coincidence that this hospital has a spectacularly high success rate and far fewer revolving doors. And I can't emphasize enough what this kind of respect does to increase the self-esteem of someone who spends most of her time wondering how she could have been such a useless parent.

This week I've had occasion to revisit the ward in the first hospital, nearly four years after my son left it. It hasn't changed. It is perhaps one of the worst examples, but not so very different from many other hospitals I've heard about. You wait on the ward, not knowing where to go, and people with badges go up and down, to and fro, avoiding eye contact, not smiling, with body language that tells you they haven't got time for you and don't want to know anyway. You approach the office; the person on the phone, safe behind the closed door and glass fortifications, sees you coming and turns his back. A carer I know recently took her son to be admitted as a voluntary patient. They waited three hours while, what seemed like, every employee in the hospital passed along the corridor. Finally she plucked up courage and asked someone 'Are you a nurse?' The person replied that she was a doctor and walked away. I've sometimes felt like the Invisible Man and wondered whether I'm hallucinating about my own existence.

In the second hospital, the ward layout reflects the philosophy, with a central administration desk accessible to everyone (no door, no glass!) surrounded by a large area where staff, patients, visitors all sit and, apart from the badges, are indistinguishable one from the other. I've formed several valuable friendships with families met here. When you arrive the nurses ask how you are (not as an imposed ritual but as if they really mean it) and listen to what you say. There is always a discussion about how your relative is doing, and questions about how you find him. If there are any upsetting incidents, families are comforted and reassured before they leave. Staff are proactive about passing on information about such things as support groups, and this is done verbally. Putting up posters is just not enough, and again conveys the wrong message; *real* partners communicate with speech, not with pieces of paper stuck on a wall. It is easy to contact staff on this ward and their tone of voice on the telephone is welcoming, friendly and concerned. The significant point about this comparison is that family sensitive practice *has* to be built into hospital protocols and underpinned by a real commitment from their leadership. It has to be a central and rewarded core component of service delivery.

Every piece of recent policy from the Department of Health (*NHS Plan* (DoH, 2000); *The Capable Practitioner* (Sainsbury Centre for Mental Health, 2001); *Modernising Mental Health Services* (DoH, 1998); *Mental Health Task Force Mission Statement* (DoH, 2001a); *Mental Health Information Strategy* (DoH, 2001b); *Workforce Development Confederation Remit* (DoH, 2002) acknowledges the importance of involving carers, not just as passive recipients of well meaning but useless sympathy (what I like to call the 'Indian head massage' syndrome) but as full partners in a truly collaborative care package. Practitioners are increasingly accepting that they must make use of carer expertise, but there is still a long way to go before the therapeutic role of carers is fully recognized, despite the current insistence on family interventions as an essential component of care. Professional training seems to focus on dealing with people who are dependent, and perhaps some practitioners are more comfortable with this relationship. But carers need tools far more than they need crutches and professionals need to grasp the extra dimension of carers as essential implements in the delivery of care. We live in a climate where doctors are no longer put on a pedestal and where people have far more information about treatment and rights. There is no need for professionals to feel threatened by this, nor for families and patients to scavenge for reasons to complain. More and more stakeholders are realizing that we all share the same task and must work for the same goal and if this trend continues I am optimistic that the glue will be strong enough to hold the fragments together.

References

Atkinson, J. M. & Coia, D. A. (1995) *Families Coping With Schizophrenia: A Practitioner's Guide to Family Groups*, New York: John Wiley & Sons Inc.

Ayerst, G. (2001) A dual diagnosis multiple needs toolkit, paper written for the National Schizophrenia Fellowship.

Berry, D. (1997) *Living with Schizophrenia*, London: Institute of Psychiatry.

Brady, A. (1996) A study on the effects of schizophrenia on carers, Dublin: (unpublished thesis), Department of Psychology, University of Dublin.

Chapman, H. (1997) Self-help groups, family carers and mental health, *Australian and New Zealand Journal of Mental Health Nursing*, 6(4), 148–55.

Department of Health (1998) *Modernising Mental Health Services*, London: HMSO.

Department of Health (2000) *NHS Plan*, London: HMSO.

Department of Health (2001a) *The Journey to Recovery: Mental Health Task Force*, London: HMSO.

Department of Health (2001b) *Mental Health Information Strategy*, London: HMSO.

Department of Health (2002) *Workforce Development Confederation Remit*, London: HMSO.

Gerace, L. M., Camilleri, D. & Ayers, L. (1993) Siblings' perspectives on schizophrenia, *Schizophrenia Bulletin*, 19, 637–47.

Hogman, G. & Pearson, G. (1995) *The Silent Partners: the Needs and Experiences of People who Care for People with a Severe Mental Illness: National Schizophrenia Fellowship Survey*, London: National Schizophrenia Fellowship.

Karp, D. A. & Tanarugsachock, V. (2000) Mental illness, caregiving and emotional management, *Qualitative Health Research*, 10(1), 6–25.

National Schizophrenia Fellowship (2000) *A Question of Choice: National Schizophrenia Fellowship Survey*, London: National Schizophrenia Fellowship.

Norton, S., Wandersman, A. & Goldman, C. R. (1993) Perceived costs and benefits of membership in a self-help group, *Community Mental Health Journal*, 29(2), 143–60.

Reay-Young, R. (2000) Support groups for people living with a serious mental illness: an overview, *International Journal of Psychosocial Rehabilitation*, 5, 56–80.

Sainsbury Centre for Mental Health (2001) *The Capable Practitioner*, London: Sainsbury Centre for Mental Health.

Shakespeare, W., *Macbeth*, Act 4 sc.3.

Tennakoon, L. (2000) King's College London Institute of Psychiatry Department of Psychopharmacology, Davos: 10th Winter Workshop on Schizophrenia.

CHAPTER 6

Working with People who have Special Needs and Disabilities and Mental Health Problems

CELIA HARBOTTLE AND DAVID MUDD

Indicative Benchmark Statements

▪ Identification of the impact of stigma on mental health service users, their families and carers, and the motivational basis of prejudice

▪ Ability to assist mental health service users and their carers in making informed choices about their care through the provision of culturally appropriate forms of communication

▪ Ability to work in mental health and social care settings in a non-discriminatory way

▪ Critical awareness of own competence and needs for future mental health nursing professional development

▪ Support peers and others with special needs when working in mental health and social care settings

Introduction

This chapter aims to acknowledge the difficulty in defining disability. It includes an analysis of the ways in which disability influences identity and how that, in turn can have significant impact on an individual's mental health (both positively and negatively). Consideration is given to the mental health issues that arise from a social construction of disability. We will also examine the psychological effects of being or becoming disabled in a society which values health, beauty and youth. This takes cognizance of the impact of prejudice, discrimination and perceived associated social disadvantage in relation to mental health. We believe that to work effectively with people who have special needs and disabilities and mental health problems, workers need to understand the social context in which care is provided and the prevailing attitudes in society. To develop such an awareness will enable workers to examine their own perspectives, which will enhance their contribution to the care of this service user group.

It is posited that the only true understanding of living with a disability can originate from disabled people themselves. It is acknowledged in the Government publication *The Expert Patient: A New Approach to Chronic Disease Management for the 21st Century* (DoH, 2001) that often the person living with a long-term disability understands their condition better than many health and social care workers. The task for professionals, therefore, is to engage with and learn from this expertise.

A critical review of definitions of special needs, disabilities and mental health and the limitations imposed by language

The language that we use to describe and define ourselves has different shades of meaning that reflect our attitudes, values and life experience. The language is culturally located and referenced to the situational context. Language is also located within a time frame. For example, words which were used to describe people 50 or so years ago were once acceptable but would now be deemed offensive. Some organizations have amended their name to reflect these changes in attitudes. For example in 1994 The Spastics Society took the decision to relaunch itself under the name of 'Scope'. Language, it could be argued, is at the forefront of discrimination. It is the vehicle for prejudice and positive communication is seen to lie at the heart of anti-discriminatory practice. To function and communicate effectively however, we need to use terms of reference and to share understandings. Terms such as 'special needs', 'disability' and 'mental health' are used as descriptors which could have both negative and positive connotations. 'Special needs' for example is used as a term to describe people who need additional support. However, 'special' in this context appears to be robbed of its more positive overtones. 'Special' in this situation infers 'different', 'problematic', "difficult". 'Disability' is a word that emphasizes deficit. It implies inability rather than different abilities. For example, Townsend (1979, p 691) gives the following definition: 'Disability itself might be best defined as inability to perform the activities, share in the relationships and play the roles which are customary for people of broadly the same age and sex in society.'

However, there is an alternative view: 'I'm not disabled. There are just some things that I cannot do.' This is the definition provided by a man who has lived with the effects of polio all his life but his focus is on recognizing and maximizing opportunity. This is his perception however he has faced a life long battle against prevalent negative attitudes in society to his physical differentness. The social constructionist approach argues that disability arises not from the disability itself but rather from the barriers of prejudice and discrimination.

Disability has been socially constructed through the meanings attached to physical and learning disabilities and defined in terms of personal disadvantage. Impairment is therefore equated with a deficit, which is at the root of negative images held by the able bodied and should not be a point of reference within a disabled identity. The difficulty a social model faces is the creation of what has been referred to as an untenable separation between the body and culture, impairment and disability (Hughes & Patterson, 1997).

Self-image is the perception that an individual has of him or herself which derives from interface with the environment and feedback from others. The person's attitude to their self-image makes a contribution to their level of self-esteem. Through their self-image, individuals develop an idea of how attractive they are to others. This is necessary for psychological well being and high self-esteem and is, therefore, closely related to the individual's own sense of their worth and potential.

Mental health could be defined as having a feeling of control over oneself and the environment in a way that balances individual need with the demands of the society in which one lives. As a definition, the terms mental health and mental illness are used often used interchangeably. Frequently, when people are asked to define 'mental health' they adopt a negative, reductionist and medical stance which highlights symptomology, for example depression, schizophrenia. Mental illness is the converse to mental health and could be best defined as an inability to adjust to and respond accordingly to the demands of social and emotional life and is associated with emotional and psychological dysfunction. The societal view of a psychologically healthy person is someone who has a positive body image, high self-esteem and a positive self-concept. By society's definition, this means that an individual who does not possess these characteristics is psychologically unhealthy.

The social model of disability and its relevance to mental health nursing practice

So what disables people? Is it their physical or psychological capacity or is it society's response to the needs of individuals. There are two main understandings of disability – a medical model and a social model. Initially there appears to be polarity between these two perspectives. We argue that that is too simplistic an explanation. The medical model appears to refer to disability as an individual attribute for which the person is solely responsible. The medical model has associations with the 'personal tragedy' perspective proposed by Oliver (1996) in which the perspective of the general public was to emphasize the disability and believe that there was a desire among people with a disability to be 'able bodied' and 'normal'. This reinforces the notion proposed by Blaxter (1990) who argues that there is a moral dimension to health and well being and can be seen in terms of willpower, self-discipline and self-control. The medical model places emphasis on the individual who experiences mental health problems being regarded as abnormal and dependent on the interventions of others to be able to cope with their psychological and emotional distress.

The social model of disability however claims that it is society, its structures and provision that disables people because it does not take into account different abilities. It is insensitive even to the implications of ageing where the once fit and agile can no longer independently access services and amenities. Oliver (1990 cited in Drake 1998) illustrated the differences between the two perspectives. The OPCS Survey (1986) of disabled adults asked (for example) 'does your health problem/disability make it difficult for you to travel by bus?' Oliver replaced this with his own question: 'Do poorly designed buses make it difficult for someone with your health problems to use them?'

The social model of disability emphasizes the concepts of choice, power, independence and opportunity and can be defined more accurately as the social and economic exclusions experienced by people who are living with a disability. (Becker, 1997).

Historically, educational programmes related to nursing were wedded to the medical model whereas social work students would be more exposed to the social model. This has contributed to the enduring philosophical differences (real or imagined) between the two professions. For example, some texts examining the social constructionist perspective argue that interventions driven by the medical model focus on rehabilitation and the provision of specialist services which segregate and isolate people. Kelly et al (1998) argue that operating within a medical model requires a relatively lower degree of practitioner autonomy because individuals are directed to comply with pre-prescribed instructions. The perspective of practitioner autonomy could be regarded as central to the ethos of social work practice. This would reinforce the belief that the medical model is restrictive, blaming and reductionist whereas the social model is liberating, creative and empowering. In consequence, the service user is seen to be liberated, enabled and imbued with choice-making powers and thus by definition, increasingly autonomous. The danger here is that the practitioner then abdicates responsibility for and to the newly autonomous client. The drawback with this approach is that the choice offered may be seen as an attempt to vindicate the practitioner should the individual be perceived to make the unhealthy or unwise choice. Naidoo (1984) describes this concept as 'victim blaming' and suggests that practitioners could argue 'I have advised you. If you choose to ignore my advice then it is you who have chosen the harmful behaviour.'

This raises the question does the total acceptance of the social model of disability have any negative implications. Can it always be regarded as a positive stance? To deny the credibility of the medical model of disability might, in turn result in denying the rights of the individual with a disability. For example, an individual living with schizophrenia whose psychotic symptoms are all-pervasive and untreated will be unable even to consider making choices about housing, employment, education and leisure needs. In effect, they would be unable to live independently, access opportunities and have a social life. Effective and positive mental health nursing practice therefore needs to operate as an amalgamation of both perspectives to consider the individual needs of service users and to enable working effectively across professional boundaries. This is especial important in view of the recent advances towards integrated and multi-agency working.

The evolution of contemporary attitudes to people with disabilities

Historically, people with disabilities have been described, perceived and treated in less than equal ways. The assumption was (and it would be fair to say, in some quarters, still is) that they needed special care and protection which resulted in segregation from their community. The expectation for development and gaining experience were limited and emphasis was placed on deficit rather than strengths and abilities. Wolfensberger (1972) identified that there were historical perceptions about people who were perceived to be different. These perceptions gave explanations for people's difference that set parameters beyond which people who have disabilities were excluded. For example, Wolfensberger stated that people with disabilities were regarded as sub-human. It was denied that these people had the same emotional and physical needs as the rest of the population. Provision of services reflected this and deprived disabled people of privacy, choice and dignity. People with disabilities were described in animal or vegetable-like terms and even when acknowledged as human, many behavioural interventions did not reflect this but were akin to the techniques used for training animals. Another perception was that people with disabilities were a menace and a serious threat to society. Reinforced links were made between physical and mental disabilities and crime and deviance.

Wolfensberger also linked historical perceptions with religion and superstition. Explanations for incidents of disability ranged from punishment for sins to gifts from God. Even in our scientific age, supernatural explanations still hold currency as people try to explain the inexplicable finding reasons for fate or life chances. Other historical perceptions cite people with disabilities as being objects of shame, ridicule, pity and charity. Society can therefore mock their differentness and scapegoat those who it regards as being outside the norm or it can bestow kindness on these individuals thus validating its capacity to define those it accepts and those it rejects. Wolfensberger's explanations are perceptive because none of us find them unacceptable or unintelligible. We may not embrace each individual explanation yet somehow, they touch an understanding in us all. We may have evolved away from such explanations but only because they initially informed our understandings. Historical perceptions can be seen in any analysis of the evolution of care service delivery and still inform every aspect of negative and oppressive practice. Historical perceptions have cast people with disabilities into social roles with limited opportunity and this has been mirrored in services designed to meet their needs: It is a well established fact that a person's behaviour tends to be profoundly affected by the role expectations that are placed upon him [sic] . . . This permits those who define social roles to make self fulfilling prophecies (Wolfensberger, 1972, p 15). Although the historical perceptions identified by Wolfensberger still hold currency in many quarters, there has undoubtedly been a shift towards a realization that people with disabilities should experience the same range of life chances as non-disabled people. In terms of mental illness, advances in the treatment of the symptoms of some mental health problems demonstrated that although 'cure' was not an option, the alleviation of the distressing symptoms amounted to the promotion of recovery. The Royal Commission's Report (1957) for the Mental Health Act 1959 acknowledged that the use of medication to suppress symptoms of mental illness meant that people no longer needed to be incarcerated for years in institutions. With the assistance of medication, these people could live satisfactorily in the community. However medication cannot be seen as the panacea in addressing mental health problems. The British Psychological Society warns that people with mental health problems are *routinely* prescribed medication despite its limitations and side effects whereas therapies such as counselling and cognitive behavioural therapy are undervalued despite evidence that they are effective. This reflects the historical perception that the medical model has primacy over social interventions. (Coleman, 1995) argues that because of this reductionist position, environmental and social factors have been ignored.

Political agendas that are influenced by perceptions of disability

Over the past few decades, disability has become increasingly politicized. There has been a growing awareness of human rights and how disabled people have been disadvantaged by social structures and provision particularly, although not exclusively in the areas of health and social care. This has been exacerbated by what Hudson (2002, p 11) refers to as 'the ideological issue: the respective merits of a free and universal (health) service versus one which is selective and means tested'. This has particular relevance for those who have become disabled by the ageing process either by physical frailty or organic mental health problems such as dementia. Being older does bring with it some significant difficulties. Incapacity increases markedly beyond the age of 70 and this increase does mean that there is a greater likelihood of disability.

The fact that the population of Britain is ageing is often seen as an indicator of increasing demand on health and social care provision. However a report by the Royal Commission on Long Term Care (Doh, 1999a, p xviii) concluded that: 'For the UK there is no "demographic timebomb" as far as long term care is concerned and as a result of this, cost of care will be affordable.'

As the NHS refocuses its aims and objectives through Government policy and legislation (DoH, 1998a,b, 1999a,b, 2000) the emphasis has been placed on acute care and brief intervention. Services that had historically been delivered free (free at point of delivery but funded by taxation) as part of health, such as personal care, have become means tested and re-framed as social care. However, the Royal Commission (DoH, 1999a) report recommends that the most efficient way of providing finance for long-term care is via services underwritten by general taxation based on need rather than wealth.

The notion that age equates to disability and therefore that the older person becomes a burden on the state is a commonly held, if false perception. This same perception is often extended to people who have mental health problems. Their economic viability and social usefulness is called into question which in turn, has implications for resource allocation. These perceptions impact on political agendas and sometimes come into conflict with the utilitarian objectives of Government – greatest good for the greatest number. This can mean that the prioritizing of need can be subject to populist pressure.

The promotion of anti-discriminatory practice

Anti-discriminatory practice lies at the heart of good care service delivery. Clients come into contact with services in the hope that they will be supported in countering the devaluing experiences of living in society at large. As has already been outlined in this chapter, people with disabilities and mental health problems face the impact of society's negative perceptions of their needs and abilities. Workers in health and social care need to accept people for their abilities rather than their disabilities. Workers have to transcend the historical perceptions in which they too have been entrenched. Prejudice is part of the human condition. Our attitudes are formulated as we progress towards adulthood and they inform our understanding of the world. It would therefore be unreasonable to expect care workers to be without negative thoughts. Workers in health and social care however need to be self-aware and gain insight into the attitudes that underpin their behaviour in order to challenge some of their historically derived perceptions. If this were easy, we wouldn't need legislation to protect people from prejudice and discrimination. For example, discrimination on the grounds of disability is now illegal and effort must be made to ensure that disabled people have access to the full range of services and opportunities. Legislation however is still required to safeguard people with disabilities, which indicates that as a philosophy, society does not readily embrace this principle but it is an acknowledgment of right.

Anti-discriminatory practice (ADP) is often seen in tandem with equal opportunity. It is important to emphasize that ADP is not the promotion of equality but of the promotion of equality of opportunity. The word equality could imply sameness, uniformity, a state of semblance. However this would deny diversity and the uniqueness of the individual therefore equality may be better defined in the context of disability as striving for equality in power, status and achievement.

Two words that have entered the helping discourse over the past 10 to 15 years are advocacy and empowerment. Ward and Mullender (1991, p 1) pointed out that these words imparted a rosy glow to anti-discriminatory practice but acted as a 'social aerosol' covering up the 'disturbing smell of conflict and conceptual division'. The promotion of advocacy and empowerment can be seen in pragmatic responses to service design. Many day and residential services have tenants or client meetings in which service-user representatives discuss current issues. This is certainly progress in terms of involvement but begs questions with regard to representation. For example, are the views of service users who do not communicate verbally taken into account: is representation dependant on the individual's skills and ability rather than the service-users' needs and concerns. The danger with any such scheme of user involvement in that it deteriorates into tokenism.

Person-centred approaches that put service users at the heart of designing their packages of care demonstrate respect for the individual's wishes, choices, beliefs and preferences. They acknowledge that fulfilment and quality of life revolve around a person's sense of power and control. Choices can only ever be made within the confines of available resources. The challenge in care services is the lack of resources to meet individual preferences and it is at this point that clients are in danger of losing control over their quality of life.

Assertiveness is another aspect of ADP. Unlike aggression, manipulation or passivity, assertiveness is respectful and honest. It acknowledges everyone's right to express preference. Being assertive is an essential life skill and by using it we keep our self-esteem. However, it is often difficult for people with a disability to be assertive or maintain assertiveness. ADP requires workers to respect the individual and encourage their sense of self worth.

Health and social care work can be brutalizing. Workers can come into contact with manifestations of the human condition which are incredibly distressing. Workers may wish to distance themselves from their clients' problems and lives to protect themselves from the stress of empathizing with their situations and circumstances. Sometimes, the culture in the workplace can contribute to this feeling of detachment. Bates (1993) explored how 16 to 18 year old young women adapted to care work as trainees on youth employment schemes. We would criticize why only young women were chosen as this in itself seems to be a stereotypical and sexist assumption but to some extent Bates' study decanted the gender element by identifying that those who were successful actually insulated themselves from the physical and emotional demands of the care task: 'Their adaptation to the occupational culture of "caring", as practiced in the workplace played a crucial role' (Bates, 1993, p 23). Central to this culture was the development of an impersonal and detached view of the work with alienated social relationships. College tutors emphasized the need for sensitivity, genuine caring and anti-discriminatory practice but this at times was overtly rejected by trainees, especially as they became more attuned to workplace practices.

Conclusions

Effective and sustainable performance in the field of health and social care appeared to Bates to depend as much on the absence of sensitivity as in its presence and this was recognized in the way that the trainees came to resist the meaning of caring. Resistance took the form of 'coping strategies' such as 'keeping busy' or 'switching off' or resisting their official work demands and thus gaining a measure of control over their labour. Bates' research was into the attitude of young care workers. However, it is important to note that the research subjects were responding to established practice culture presumably cultivated by mature and possibly qualified nurses or social workers. If oppressive practice is embedded in the workplace culture, there are potentially extremely serious consequences for service users. Workers need to evaluate constantly their responses and attitudes otherwise *discriminatory* practice is never far away. Practice experience provides use with a raft of knowledge that can be used to assess and meet the needs of service users. However, without careful consideration we can begin to ignore individual indicators and only respond to stereotypes. The consequences for the client are a denial of uniqueness and the receipt of a service that is homogenous and ultimately unresponsive.

References

Bates, I. (1993) A job which is right for me, in I. Bates & G. Risebrough *Youth and Inequality*, Buckingham: Open University Press.

Becker, S. (1997) *Responding to Poverty: The Politics of Cash and Care*, Longman: London.

Blaxter, M. (1990) *Health and Lifestyles*, London: Routledge & Kegan Paul.

Coleman, R. (1995) *Is the Writing on the Asylum Wall? Power to Partnership*, Gwynedd: Handsell Publications.

Department of Health (1959) *The Mental Health Act*, London: HMSO.

Department of Health (1998a) *Modernising Social Services*, White Paper, London: HMSO.

Department of Health (1998b) *Modern and Dependable: The New NHS*, London: HMSO.

Department of Health (1999a) *With Respect to Old Age: A Report by the Royal Commission on Long Term Care*, London: HMSO.

Department of Health (1999b) *Making a Difference*, London: HMSO.

Department of Health (2000) *A Quality Strategy for Social Care*, London: HMSO.

Department of Health (2001) *The Expert Patient: A New Approach to Chronic Disease Management for the 21st Century*, London: HMSO.

Drake, R. F. (1998) Professionals and the voluntary sector, in A. Symonds & A. Kelly (eds), *The Social Construction of Community Care*, Basingstoke: Macmillan Press, now Palgrave Macmillan.

Gendenning, C., Halliwell, S., Jacobs, S., Rummery, K. & Tryer, J. (2000) Bridging the gap: using direct payments to purchase integrated care, *Health and Social Care in the Community*, 8(3), 192–200.

Hudson, B. (2002) Interprofessionality in health and social care, *Journal of Interprofessional Care*, 16(1), 249.

Hughes, B. & Patterson, K. (1997) Labels can damage your health, *Community Care*, 6–12 July.

Kelly, A., Mabbett, G. & Thome, R. (1998) Professions and community nursing, in A. Symonds & A. Kelly (eds), *The Social Construction of Community Care*, Basingstoke: Macmillan Press, now Palgrave Macmillan.

Naidoo, J. (1984) *Evaluation of play it safe in Bristol*. Unpublished paper.

Oliver, M. (1996) *Understanding Disability*, Basingstoke: Macmillan, now Palgrave Macmillan.

Oliver, M. (1990) *The Politics of Disablement*, Basingstoke: Macmillan and St Martins Press, now Palgrave Macmillan.

Office of Population, Census and Surveys (OPCS) (1986) *National Survey of Disability in Great Britain*. OPCS Social Survey Division, London: HMSO.

Statham, M. & Timblick, D. (2001) Self concept and people who have learning disabilities, in J. Thompson & S. Pickering (eds), *Meeting the Health Needs of People who have a Learning Disability*, London: Balliere Tindall.

Townsend, P. (1979) *Poverty in the United Kingdom*, Harmondsworth: Penguin.

Ward, D. & Mullender, A. (1991) Empowerment and oppression: an indissoluble pairing for contemporary social work, *Critical Social Policy*, 32, 1–29.

Wolfensberger, W. (1972) *The Principle of Normalisation in Human Services*, Toronto: National Institute on Mental Retardation.

PART II

PREVENTION AND HEALTH PROMOTION

This Part deals with the need for primary health care nurses to promote mental health well being. Life produces many situations that generates stress and which, if left unaddressed, can lead to serious mental health problems. Road traffic accidents, bereavement, sexual attack or abuse, physical attack, witnessing a disaster are among many stressors experienced by people, which need to be recognized in their own right and responded to proactively.

This Part begins by identifying common mental health problems and then looks at prevention by assessing need and risk, recognizing when a social event is producing pathological responses and responding accordingly in a proactive manner.

CHAPTER 7

Common Mental Health Problems

DENIS A. HART

Indicative Benchmark Statements

▓ Recognition of the prodromal signs of mental illness

▓ Awareness of the effectiveness of early intervention

▓ A positive approach and optimism

▓ Identification of the main characteristics and needs of users and carers

▓ Participation in the assessment and management of factors of co-morbidity and precursors of mental illness

Introduction

To understand what may be meant by common mental health problems we must begin by locating the concept as a continuum of mental health conditions. Essentially, we begin by understanding what is 'normal' so we can then proceed to understand what is meant by 'abnormal'.

Psychology is defined as: 'The measurement of normal behaviour'. Attainment, intelligence and personality are key areas for psychological measurement or psychometric testing and enable the psychologist to determine whether there are, or are not, problems or deficits.

When individuals fall outside the expected or 'normal' range the psychologist may refer them to a psychiatrist who may consequently treat any abnormal behaviour by using a variety of techniques ranging from: *counselling* to *behavioural therapy* and from *medication* to *hospitalization*. Mental health conditions, we would argue, are quite normal and only become relevant when something happens which triggers them so they become pathological in degree or intensity.

Normality and abnormality

Everyone has a propensity for anxiety, mania, paranoia, schizophrenia and psychosis. Normal human behaviour is based upon instinctual mechanisms such as 'fight or flight' which invariably entails a heightened state of emotional arousal and an element of anxiety. We know that around 75 per cent of all visits to a General Practitioner concern a person's mental health rather than simple physical health issues and that many young people in their early 20s encounter psychiatric symptoms but recover quickly with or without treatment. Indeed, Lewis Carroll would never have written about Alice in Wonderland and the Mad Hatter without at least an element of fantasy, but who is to say whether or not his works crossed over into the territory of the psychotic.

Millar and Walsh (2000, p 4) point out: 'It is not possible to draw up a simple list of symptoms or do a test that will tell you whether someone is, or is not, mentally ill' and that: 'Most lay people would identify extreme mental illness as some fearful form of unsightly, uncontrollable, "madness" and blissful happiness and contentment as evidence of mental illness.' They quite rightly add that: 'in between these two hypothetical extremes there is a vast range of emotional and psychological experience that is much harder to describe and "classify" in mental health and illness terms.'

Mental Illness is probably best understood by reference to:

- the individual;
- the cultural context within which they live their lives; and
- what is 'normal' for them.

Mental disorder, anti-social behaviour and the law

A large body of legislation relates to general health services provided by doctors and other health professionals. Nowhere in the law, however, will you find a definition of 'health'.

> in the case of physical health, this may not be of great importance, as generally we know good physical health when we see it or enjoy it. A medical diagnosis, when we are unwell, is made by Doctors and other medical professionals rather than by a Court of Law. However, the situation is different in mental health, although 'mental illness' is the classification under which most patients are detained in hospital, it is not further defined by the Mental Health Act 1983. This raises the key issue of when and how a person becomes defined as being mentally ill. (Hart, 1998, p 12)

We, therefore, sometimes confuse mental disorder with anti-social behaviour. Mental disorder is defined under Section 1(2) as:

- Mental Illness;
- Arrested or incomplete development of mind;
- Psychopathic disorder; and
- Any other disorder or disability of mind.

The MHA (1983) divides mental disorder into 2 categories:

1 *Serious disorders*

- Mental illness; and
- Severe mental impairment.

2 *Minor disorders*

- Non severe mental impairment; and
- Psychopathic disorders.

'The main difference in terms of legal powers is that a patient suffering only minor disorders cannot be compulsorily admitted, or detained for treatment unless the treatment will benefit him or her' (Brayne & Martin, 2001, p 296).

The role of mental health nurses

Mental health nurses need be aware of the context of the individual within the assessment, the legal definition of metal illness and mental disorder but also need to be able to identify the patterns of symptoms that characterize and define specific disorders. So we need to be clear what these are and how they are clustered into definable problems.

The classification of mental and behavioural disorders

The International Classification of Disease, Version 10 (ICD-10) (World Health Organization, 1992) approach identifies 10 types of disorder and a residual category:

1 Organic mental disorders (dementia, delirium, organic amnesia);
2 Psychoactive substance use (Intoxication, harmful use, dependency, withdrawal);
3 Schizophrenia, schizotypal and delusional disorders;

4 Mood (affective disorders);
5 Neurotic, stress related and somatoform disorders (phobias, obsessive compulsive disorders, stress reactions);
6 Behavioural syndromes (eating disorders, sleep disorders, sexual dysfunctions);
7 Disorders of adult personality;
8 Mental retardation;
9 Disorders of psychological development (speech disorders, autism);
10 Childhood behavioural disorders (hyperkinesias, tics, conduct disorders and emotional disorders); and the residual category
11 Mental disorder not classified elsewhere – more frequently referred to as psychopathy.

Each disorder is accompanied by a set of diagnostic criteria to facilitate recognition, assessment and diagnosis.

● Lose their appetite; and
● Develop a pattern of sleep disturbance.

No single feature would warrant a diagnosis of depression but if all of these can be identified *and*:

● There is reduced concentration and attention;
● Ideas of guilt and unworthiness are expressed;
● The individual has a reduced concentration span;
● Ideas are expressed or acts occur of self-harm or suicide.

then the level of depression has moved from being a condition to a problem or illness.

   So, crossing from a normal response to a pathological one is usually identified according to the frequency and intensity of reactions and the number of symptoms manifested. But, Smith (2000) offers an alternative view that: mental disorder is made up of 3 elements:

1 a problems of *affect*; plus
2 a problem of *behaviour*; plus
3 a problem of *cognition*

We here argue this framework is a helpful test and suggest it be applied to all the common mental health problems presented in this chapter.

Common mental health problems

For our present purposes we have adapted the ICD-10 list to pinpoint the most common mental health problems encountered in primary health care, namely:

- Depression;
- Anxiety;
- Bipolar mood disorders;
- Schizophrenia;
- Psychoactive substance misuse;
- Self-harm and suicide;
- Eating disorders;
- Dementia.

Depression

We have already seen how it is normal to be 'fed up' and at the kinds of symptoms to watch out for that moves this into the territory of mental ill health. We need remind ourselves that depression has three core symptoms:

1 *Biological aspects*. Changes in sleep, appetite, weight, energy and physical activity;
2 *Cognitive aspects*. Reduced concentration and attention, increased negative thoughts and reduced decision-making abilities; and
3 *Emotional aspects*. A reduced emotional state, feelings of helplessness and futility and a loss of faith in the future, increased anxiety, agitation and irritability.

It has been estimated that the lifetime risk in the UK is around 10–24 per cent for women and 5–12 per cent for men.

Depression is essentially an over reaction to loss, whereas anxiety on the other hand is an over reaction to the *threat* of loss.

Anxiety

Smith (2000, p 177) explains that anxiety occurs when there is:

a preoccupation with areas of concern and therefore, inattention and poor concentration may be complaints. Thought blocks may be elicited and words are 'lost' within the explanatory dialogue. The individual's perceptual functions are in a state of high alert, and hyper-vigilance and hyper-attentiveness to environmental nuances are both observable.

However, we must not forget that anxiety is a quite normal response to stress. Were you anxious when you sat your last exams or if you have had to give evidence in court? We would be concerned if you replied that these events *did not* make you anxious. Anxiety only becomes a problem when it has a detrimental effect on an individuals *ability to function*.

Pathological anxiety may present in one of three forms:

1 Panic attacks;
2 Phobias; or
3 Obsessive compulsive disorders.

Anxiety is generally a fear reaction, the flight part of our instinctual response to threat or danger. So what is panic?

Millar and Walsh (2000, p 49) have defined panic attacks as: 'short bouts of overwhelming anxiety that occur suddenly and have no predictable pattern or trigger', and list a number of physical symptoms including palpitations, flushes or 'chills', hyperventilation, dizziness, chest pains, choking, nausea and stomach churning. Panic attacks have a neurotic base, for when we experience fear we are conscious of a threat from a conscious 'enemy'. The unpredictability of panic is located in the fact that: the subject *knows* there is something threatening them but isn't consciously aware as to what it is. In a nutshell, they want to run from something but they don't know what it is they want to run from as the object of their fear is known only subconsciously or subliminally. Otto and Gould (1996) see this leading to 'anticipatory anxiety'.

Patients who experience panic attacks will often 'map', as and when, they occurred to try to prepare themselves for the intense and distressing feelings that ensue. Anticipatory anxiety can be a helpful strategy so long as someone is engaged in parallel psycho counselling to help bring the unconscious fear from some long-past event into a conscious memory; without such support the patients can easily slip into developing phobias whereby entire situations are seen as the source of the threat as occurs, for example, in agoraphobia. Here the fear is no longer unconscious but rather has developed into an *unfound* fear of an object or situation.

Obsessional Compulsive Disorder is described by Smith (2000, p 177) as: 'obtrusive, repetitive thoughts and the physical manoeuvres instigated to eradicate, neutralise or prevent that thought context from occurring'. The patient recognizes that obsessive thoughts are generated from within themselves. They may see them as unreasonable and will attempt to resist them. However, the anxiety and tension created will need to be expressed and often this takes the form of stereotyped and ritualistic behaviour such as hand washing, touching, checking and counting procedures repeated repetitively.

Both depression and anxiety may occur as reactions (normal) or over reactions (pathological) to life stresses and the need to adjust or adapt to change. Ambelas (1987) ranked 16 life events in the order of perceived severity in producing stress, with 'death of a child' as the most significant followed by 'death of a parent', 'imprisonment', 'death of a close family member', and 'serious financial difficulty'.

Individual vulnerability, according to Zubin and Spring (1997) is determined by:

- Inborn vulnerability:
  - Genetic make up;
  - Consequent neuro-physiology of the organism; and
- Acquired vulnerability:
  - Life experience;
  - Development factors, such as disease, perinatal complications;
  - Family experience, peer interactions and social confidence.

In thinking about anxiety conditions we should remember the observation of Gamble and Brennan (2000, p 47) that:

> Many symptoms can easily be confused with obsession. For example, neglect of everyday tasks while brooding over unhappy events may be mistaken for obsessional incompleteness and hypochondriacal fears of contracting a disease may be confused with the obsessional fear of contamination though the former carries no subjective sense of resistance. The experience of the intrusion of the unwanted thoughts against conscious resistance, coupled with the awareness that the thoughts are their own are the key factors for distinguishing obsessional ruminations.

Bipolar mood disorders

Bipolar mood disorder is a psychotic mood disorder that affects mood, thinking and behaviour. It is characterized by recurrent swings between mania and depression. This is why it has often been referred to as 'manic depressive illness (or psychosis)'. While being 'fed up' can be confused with depression; being elated, excited or overjoyed can similarly be confused with mania. Millar and Walsh (2000) provide an important checklist as to the things to be watched for that indicate a manic response.

- Mood:
  - Elevated and expansive;
  - Irritable;
  - Labile (quickly changes).
- Thought:
  - Flight;
  - Grandiose delusions;
  - Jealous or persecutory delusions.
- Speech:
  - Rapid;
  - Loud;
  - Stringing together words which sound the same.

- Behaviour:
  - Disinhibited – sexually;
  - Aggressive;
  - Over familiar;
  - Over active;
  - Acts on wild plans or ideas, over spends.
- Bodily function:
  - Insomnia;
  - Increased libido;
  - Increased appetite;
  - Weight loss;
  - Inexhaustible.
- Perceptions:
  - Illusions;
  - Cues misinterpreted;
  - No insight;
  - Hallucinations;
  - Out of touch with reality.

People can suffer a single incidence of hypomania but it has been estimated that up to 95 per cent experience further episodes and the risk of suicide is high: 25–50 per cent attempt it and 15 per cent succeed. Millar and Walsh (2000) point out that it affects 1 per cent of the population and is most common between 20 and 30 years of age, but also in women aged 30 to 45 years.

Schizophrenia

Schizophrenia is most commonly associated with 'hearing voices' and has three phases:

- the prodromal;
- the acute; and
- the residual

The prodromal phase marks the beginning of the deterioration of the 'self' and is characterized by 'odd' or 'bizarre' behaviour, self-neglect, reduction in drive, vague or over elaborate speech content, detachment from previous relationships and of course the person may be seen to be talking to themselves in public as they 'reply' to the voices they hear. A minimum of two of these 'symptoms' must be present and evidenced for a minimum of six months before diagnosis is made.

The acute phase represents the illness at its most active state and for a diagnosis to be made, the ICD-10 classification requires any *one* of the following be evidenced for one month or more:

- thought echo, insertion, withdrawal or broadcasting;
- delusions of control influence or passivity, clearly referred to body or limb movements or specific thought, actions or sensations; delusional perception;
- third person auditory hallucinations, either running commentary on actions or discussing the patient among themselves;
- persistent delusions that are culturally inappropriate and completely impossible.

Or any two of the following:

- persistent hallucinations when accompanied by fleeting or half-formed delusions without clear affective content, or by persistent overvalued ideas or when occurring every day for weeks or months on end;
- breaks or interpolations in the train of thought, incoherence, irrelevant speech or neologisms;
- catatonic behaviour;
- negative symptoms of apathy, paucity of speech and blunting or incongruity of affect, resulting in social withdrawal that is not due to depression or neuroleptic medication.

None of these presenting 'symptoms' are eligible for inclusion in a diagnosis if organic brain disease or alcohol or drug intoxication, dependence or withdrawal are evident.

Craig (2000) pinpoints three commons sub-types:

1 Paranoid: characterized by persecutory delusions and hallucinations, the subject fits the 'stereotype' that 'they' are out to get him or her.
2 Hebephrenic: characterized by irresponsible and unpredictable behaviour, shallow mood, incoherent speech, aimlessness and self-absorbed smiling.
3 Catatonic: characterized by extremes of excitement and stupor and rigid symbolic thinking.

There are other forms or variations such as 'schizophreniform' and 'schizoaffective' disorders and 'induced psychotic disorders' but these are beyond the scope of this current chapter and we recommend that you consult appropriate detailed texts as and when this becomes necessary in your practice.

As we stated earlier schizophrenia is frequently characterized by 'hearing voices'. Blackman (2001) has produced an important text of the same title using a case study based upon the practices of the Hearing Voices Network: 'an international group of voice hearers who are challenging the notion that voices must be lived and experienced purely as signs of disease and illness' (Blackman, 2001, p 5).

Psychoactive substance misuse

Earlier in this chapter we introduced you to the ICD-10. We are now going to use an alternative framework, the *Diagnostic and Statistical Manual of Mental Disorders* (4th edn) or DSM IV (American Psychiatric Association, 1994) to examine psychoactive substance misuse.

We have already seen that most people have elements of most mental health conditions within their personalities, as part of normal, everyday responses. If we are burgled, we ask 'Why me?', but this doesn't mean we are paranoid. The DSM IV identifies 11 groups of substances that may be used to change mood or behaviour on a non-medical basis:

- Nicotine;
- Caffeine;
- Alcohol;
- Amphetamines and other similar acting sympathomimetics;
- Cannabis;
- Cocaine;
- Hallucinogens;
- Inhalants;
- Opioids;
- Phencyclidine (PCP);
- Sedatives, hypnotics and anxiolitics.

While psychoactive substance dependence is a diagnosable mental health problem we need to be clear that it is *not* regarded as a mental illness under the current the Mental Health Act legislation. As seen earlier we need to be careful how we link substance abuse to other formal mental illnesses which *do* have legal recognition. Craig (2000, p 183) helpfully explains: 'Whilst mood problems may be evident, particularly in relation to depression, anxiety, irritability, anger and lability, it is often unclear as to the degree to which this is induced by the substance used or was pre-existing, and in some instances, a precipitating factor in initial use'.

Psychoactive substance abuse is characterized by:

- a persistent desire which constitutes preoccupation;
- social withdrawal;
- activities to acquire the substance; and
- lack of control;

and a selection of moods ranging from anger to anxiety, frustration to depression and a general lack of tolerance.

Craig (2000, 183) adds: 'though cognizant of the problem and its detrimental effects on biopsychosocial functioning, individuals are unable to control this intake of the substance and are in fact aware of developing a tolerance for it, requiring increasing amounts to achieve the same desired effect'. Withdrawal presents its own set of problems most notable being autonomic nervous system hyperactivity.

Self-harm and suicide

About 1 per cent of all the deaths in Britain occur as a result of suicide with men being more likely to kill themselves and women more likely to attempt suicide. The peak age is 50 to 60, but there has been a rapid increase in young men aged between 15 and 25. Overt and covert self-harm is very different from attempting suicide as the primary aim is to inflict injury or suffering on the body rather than to die.

Millar and Walsh (2000) have identified a number of key indicators concerning self-harm:

- The behaviour is a way of dealing with emotional pain;
- Self-injury may be made obvious or disguised to look like an accident;
- Is used to relieve tension and express anger;
- Is used as a way to gain attention and help;
- Sufferers experience guilt;
- The behaviour can be repetitious and even 'addictive'

> A common pattern is to self injure, experience some relief for inner tension, but feel guilt and self loathing and vow to stop this behaviour in future, but then a build up of inner tension increases and, given certain entrenched triggers, such as stress, ultimately the self injurious behaviour is repeated (Millar & Walsh, 2000, p 74).

Treatment for self-harm is based upon getting the individual to recognize their need for inner hurt and then to find alternative ways of expressing it.

Furthermore, treatment and management needs to recognize physical safety, feelings, thoughts and behaviour. In extreme cases, where there is a high risk of suicide (intentional or accidental), the patient may need to be compulsorily admitted to a mental hospital under Section 2 (for assessment) or Section 4 (in an emergency, for treatment) of the MHA 1983. For less serious cases psychotherapy and counselling can produce obvious benefits especially cognitive behavioural counselling (Dryden, 2002) where the emphasis is on changing the person's sense of self-esteem.

Primary care nurses are most likely to play a key role when:

- identifying self-harm or suicidal behaviour;
- supporting the relatives; or
- supporting the patient later when discharged from hospital, if admission became necessary as a result of an accident.

Eating disorders

There are two main types of eating disorder: those caused by under eating – namely anorexia nervosa – and those caused by over eating – namely bulimia. Both concern a preoccupation with weight, body shape and image and frequently the two types overlap, for example, a person may consume a large amount of food (binge eating) and feel guilty and seek to purge their body by inducing vomiting, or by using slimming pills, diuretics or laxatives. The cause lies, to some extent, in pressures from contemporary society to be slim and beautiful but there is usually an underlying obsessional personality, who has low self-esteem.

The root of anorexia is often found in weight reducing diets that get out of control, and is found more often in women than men, indeed some authors have suggested 10 times more frequently. The age band most prone are the 15 to 35 year olds, again reflecting the cultural expectations and requirements to be one of the young, beautiful – and therefore – slim people.

Referrals to mental health practitioners regarding people suffering from eating disorders invariably come from relatives and friends rather than from the sufferer themselves. This indicates their lack of insight into the condition and a failure to recognize and acknowledge the problem even exists. Cook and Whitehouse (2002, p 65) add that, 'if untreated, eating disorders may result in a wide range of biopsychosocial morbidity, including severe malnutrition, amenorrhoea, osteoporosis, electrolyte imbalances, heart, kidney and liver damage, social isolation, depression, self harm, suicide and death'. They see eating disorders as warranting far more attention than they actually do receive as they create 'a deep well of misery, dysfunction and disability for sufferers and . . . those who are close to them' (p. 67). In particular the long term effects include:

> personality changes, relationship breakdown, loss of employment or education, social isolation . . . and even psychotic episodes. Many women with chronic eating disorders who have children may have their parenting ability compromised as a result of associated physical and psychological illness and the effects of unresolved psychological conflict on family and social relationships. Furthermore, there is a significant risk of intergenerational transmission of eating disordered attitudes and behaviour (p 67).

Dementia

Goldberg and Huxley (1992) estimated that 13 per cent of all referrals to community mental health teams are cases of dementia. While, Burns and Levy (1992) found that 8 out of 10 people aged 80 did *not* have any form of dementia. Older adults experience strong ageist attitudes from others where they are disempowered and regarded as 'senile', 'incapable' or as having little social worth. The question here for the primary health care worker is how do I sift out the genuinely pathological from the prejudice?

Smith (2000, p 182) assists here:

Primary problems relate to the impairment of short and long term memory functions and the implicit difficulties of vast gaps in personal and common knowledge . . . there may be a failure to recognise everyday objects, despite intact sensory pathways or agnosia and similarly an inability to perform motor activities despite intact understanding and motor functioning or apraxia.

The main symptoms are:

- self neglect;
- disregard for convention;
- social withdrawal;
- disinhibited hoarding;
- impaired abstract thinking;
- amnesia;
- paranoid ideation; and
- poor judgement.

Problems that:

develop insidiously and show a progressively deteriorating course may be diagnosed as a *primary degenerative dementia of the Alzheimer type*. Evidence to support such a diagnosis may be commonly observable after the age of 50, when it is termed presenile or after 65 years of age, when it is defined as senile in nature. (Smith, 2000, p 182)

Although women are more prone than men, this may simply be due to the fact that women generally outlive men. The key feature of dementia is a progressive and irreversible intellectual impairment in clear consciousness and the causes are: degenerative, vascular, infection, toxicity and metabolic and endocrine disorders.

The two most common forms are Alzheimer's Disease (senile dementia) and Multi Infarct Dementia (vascular in origin with sudden onset and rapid degeneration). Apart from the maintenance of physical health, medication and communication and memory aids, one of the most important things to ensure is that the carers are aware of the disease, its impact and feel supported in the care and support they give to the patient.

Standard Seven of the *National Service Framework for Older People* (DoH, 2001) states: 'Older people who have mental health problems should have access to integrated services, provided by the NHS and Councils to ensure effective diagnosis, treatment and support for them and their carers.' In practice, dementia is frequently misdiagnosed as a social problem and therefore intervention is delayed. Gunstone (1999) suggests that: 'the earlier nurses can be involved with patients, the more likely it is that crises will be averted.'

Early intervention can: 'reap untold benefits for carers, allowing for education and preparation and helping avert their depression which is at a much higher level than in the general population' (Bergman-Evans, 1994).

Conclusions

In this chapter we have provided you with a brief overview of some of the most common mental health problems likely to be encountered in primary health care, so you can begin to develop a framework for assessment, management and treatment.

Additionally we have begun to set the *context* in which diagnoses should be made:

- awareness of the legal definitions for mental disorder in case sectioning should become necessary. Remember that a diagnosis of mental disorder requires a problem of *affect* plus a problem of *behaviour* plus a problem of *cognition*;
- classification between what is 'normal' and 'abnormal' behaviour;
- involving the individual and their carers in assessment so as to become aware of what constitutes normal responding for that individual;
- awareness of demographic risk factors especially gender, age and culture attached to each mental health problem;
- the need to be aware of discrimination and how this can lead to a misdiagnosis such as confusing dementia with ageism; and
- awareness of the need for early intervention and an emphasis on prevention.

This context is carried forward in the National Service Frameworks, into the benchmark criteria, into the value base of good practice and is built upon in subsequent chapters in this text

References

Ambelas, A. (1987) Life events and mania: a special relationship?, *British Journal of Psychiatry*, 150, 135–240.

American Psychiatric Association (1994) *Diagnostic and Statistical Manual of Mental Disorders, 4th edn, Washington, DC: APA.*

Bergman-Evans, B. (1994) Loneliness, depression and social support of spousal care-givers, *Journal of Gerontological Nursing*, March, 6–16.

Blackman, L. (2001) *Hearing Voices*, London: Free Association Books.

Brayne, H. & Martin, G. (2001) *Law for Social Workers*, Oxford: Blackstone Press.

Brennan, G. (2000) Stress vulnerability model of serious mental illness, in C. Gamble & G. Brennan (eds), *Working with Serious Mental Health Illness: A Manual for Clinical Practice*, London: Balliere Tindall.

Burns, A. & Levy, R. (1992) *Clinical Diversity in Late Onset Alzheimer's Disease* (Maudsley Monographs), Oxford: Oxford University Press.

Cook, D. & Whitehouse, T. (2002) Food for thought: towards improving services for people with eating disorders, in P. Nolan & F. Badger (eds), *Promoting Collaboration in Primary Health Care*, Cheltenham: Nelson Thomas Ltd.

Craig, T. K. J. (2000) Severe mental illness: symptoms, signs and diagnosis, in C. Gamble & G. Brennan (eds), *Working with Serious Mental Health Illness: A Manual for Clinical Practice*, London: Balliere Tindall.

Department of Health (2001) *National Service Framework for Older People*, London: HMSO.

Dryden, W. (2002) *Handbook of Individual Therapy*, London: Sage.

Gamble, C. & Brennan, G. (eds) (2000) *Working with Serious Mental Health Illness: A Manual for Clinical Practice*, London: Balliere Tindall.

Goldberg, D. & Huxley, P. (1992) *Common Mental Health Disorders – A Bio-social Model*, London: Tavistock.

Gunstone, S. (1999) Expert practice: the interventions used by a community mental health nurse with the carers of dementia sufferers, *Journal of Advanced Nursing*, 30(4), 901–6.

Hart, D. A. (1998) *Using the Law in Mental Health*, London: Open Learning Foundation.

Marlow, J. & Smith, T. (2002) Collaboration and care of older adults with dementia, in P. Nolan & F. Badger (eds), *Promoting Collaboration in Primary Health Care*, Cheltenham: Nelson Thomas Ltd.

Millar, E. & Walsh, M. (2000) *Mental Health Matters in Primary Care*, Cheltenham: Stanley Thornes.

Nolan, P. & Badger, F. (eds) (2002) *Promoting Collaboration in Primary Health Care*, Cheltenham: Nelson Thomas Ltd.

Otto, M. & Gould, R. A. (1996) Maximising treatment outcome for panic disorder, cognitive behavioural strategies, in M. H. Pollack, M. W. Otto & J. F. Rosenbaum (eds), *Challenges on Clinical Practice: Pharmacologic and Psychosocial Strategies*, New York: Guildford Press.

Smith, L. D. (2000) The nature of health and the effects of disorder, in T. Thompson & P. Mathias (eds), *Lyttle's Mental Health and Disorder*, London: Balliere Tindall.

Thompson, T. & Mathias, P. (eds) (2000) *Lyttle's Mental Health and Disorder*, London: Balliere Tindall.

World Health Organization (1992) *ICD-10 Classification of Mental and Behavioural Disorders: Clinical Descriptions and Diagnostic Guidelines*, Geneva: WHO.

Zubin, J. & Spring, B. (1997) Vulnerability: a new view of schizophrenia, *Journal of Abnormal Psychology*, 86(2), 103–26.

CHAPTER 8

Mental Health Promotion

DENNIS CROSS

Indicative Benchmark Statements

▓ A commitment to health promotion for users and carers of mental health and social care services in accordance with the 'Public Health Strategy' and Health Improvement Programmes

▓ Education of users of mental health and social care services and their carers about preventative medicine and heath promotion

▓ Promotion of the understanding and acceptance of people with mental health problems in the wider community

▓ A commitment to promote mental health and well-being in local communities

▓ Participation in developing appropriate housing and vocational opportunities with users of mental health services and their carers

---

Introduction

This chapter provides a brief overview of mental health promotion and how a proactive stance can be beneficial to service users (by seeking appropriate help as symptoms emerge), carers (who can then offer better enhanced support) and the community (by assisting in changing negative stereotypical attitudes towards mentally ill people).

The urgent need to promote mental health has been highlighted by the World Health Organization (2001) Global Burden of Disease Study based upon the research of Murray and Lopez (1997). This research reported that mental health problems account for almost 11 per cent of the disease burden worldwide. It is also predicted that depression alone will be one of the greatest health problems worldwide by the year 2020. The author argues that there is increasing evidence to show that promotion, prevention and early intervention can reduce the level of mental health problems and thus have far-reaching consequences through improving mental health worldwide. In addition to achieving long-term cost savings this approach reflects a long-term investment in the emotional well-being of people as: 'the emotional well being of people influences how well their society functions' (Murray & Lopez, 1997).

Defining mental health

Seedhouse (1993) argues that defining health is no simple task and suggests that we must try to understand more about the complexity of the meaning of health, and of the various implications of the theories of health. He goes on to ask the following questions: 'If health is not to do with the quality of human life then what is it to do with?' and 'If health is properly and exclusively the concern of medicine and paramedicine, why is this so?'

The following statements about mental health have been endorsed by the World Health Organization's 192 member states:

- Mental health is a state of well being in which the individual realizes his or her own abilities, can cope with normal stresses of life, and is able to make a contribution to the community.
- Mental health promotion is an umbrella term that covers a variety of strategies; all aimed at having a positive effect on mental health. The encouragement of individual resources and skills, and improvements in the socio-economic environment, are among them.
- Most health care resources are spent on the specialized treatment and care of the mentally ill, and to a lesser extent on community treatment but little funding is available for promoting mental health.
- Mental health promotion requires multi-sectoral action, involving a number of government sectors such as health, employment/industry, education, environment, transport and social and community services as well as non-governmental or community-based organizations such as health support groups, churches, clubs and other bodies.
(World Health Organization, 2001)

What is meant by mental health promotion?

Wilson-Barnett and Macleod Clark (1993) argue that the broad term 'health promotion' refers to an approach and philosophy of care, which reflects awareness of the multiplicity of factors involved, and encourages everyone to value independence and individual choice. Such a philosophy rejects inequality in provision of resources to combat ill health and the imposition of one set of values, however beneficent, upon other people.

Standard One of the *National Service Framework for Mental Health* (DoH, 1999) is concerned with the promotion of mental health through a number of objectives. The report identifies the need to take steps to reduce the death rate from suicide and undetermined injury by at least one-fifth by 2010. We need to raise awareness of mental health issues with a view to reducing discrimination against people with mental health problems. We need to promote greater opportunities for people with mental health problems to access suitable employment, housing, education, welfare benefits, leisure and financial services. We need to promote mental health for people who are particularly vulnerable. We need to promote mental health in specific settings and encourage and support international co-operation in sharing good practice.

This first standard of the NSF should ensure health and social services promote mental health and reduce the discrimination and social exclusion associated with mental health problems. Health and social services should promote mental health for all, working with individuals and communities and combat discrimination against individuals and groups with mental health problems, and promote their social inclusion.

Mental health promotion is essentially concerned with how individuals, families, organizations and communities feel and the impact that this has on overall health and well being. To promote mental health means to carry out any action that enhances the mental well-being of individuals and groups, but it is also a set of principles that recognizes the impact on people according to how mental health services are planned, designed, delivered and evaluated. Many health-damaging behaviours are more prevalent among deprived groups, who lack strategies for coping with environmental, social and financial stress.

Mental health promotion, thereby, has the potential for the improvement of people's health overall. One major reason why some people break down is that they cannot cope with the stresses engendered by living in a constantly changing environment. First identified by Durkheim (1893) as *anomie*, and developed by Dubois (1980), rapid social change produces normlessness and leads to individuals being unable to cope. Sudden and profound changes in their way of life are likely to reduce the resistance of the body and mind to almost any kind of pressure. Dubois (1980) observed that the health of native people depends on the ability to reach and maintain some sort of equilibrium with the environment, and they fall prey to disease when ancestral conditions of existence suddenly break down. Nixon (1989) further observed that chronic degenerative diseases came to the forefront just when abundance replaced poverty in the heavily industrialized areas of the Western world.

Mental health promotion and the delivery of mental health services are often seen as separate tasks, in competition for scarce resources. This view may be based on the belief that mental health promotion is not relevant to people with long-term mental health problems. However, just as diagnosis is only one part of a person's life, so medical care is only one part of the support they need to cope, recover and avoid relapse. The other support will come from the family, friends, schools, employers, religious communities, and neighbourhoods and from opportunities to enjoy the same range of services and facilities within the community as everyone else. There is growing evidence that engaging with these wider issues improves physical and mental health and promotes recovery. Challenging discrimination and promoting opportunities for employment, housing, leisure and friendship are therefore central concerns for mental health promotion services.

Mental health promotion, therefore, involves any action to enhance the mental well being of individuals, families, organizations or communities and is described in depth in the Department of Health Document, *Making it Happen: a Guide to Delivering Mental Health Promotion* (DoH, 2001).

Mental health promotion and social exclusion

Mental health problems can result from a range of adverse factors associated with social exclusion and which can also be a cause of social exclusion. The World Health Organization (2001) has noted nine of particular relevance:

- Unemployed people are twice as likely to have depression as people in work.
- Children in the poorest households are three times more likely to have mental health problems than children in well off households.
- Half of all women and a quarter of all men will be affected by depression at some period during their lives.
- People who have been abused or been victims of domestic violence have higher rates of mental health problems.
- Between a quarter and a half of people using night shelters or sleeping rough may have a serious mental disorder, and up to half may be alcohol dependent.
- Some black and minority ethnic groups are diagnosed as having higher rates of mental disorder than the general population; refugees are especially vulnerable.
- There is a high rate of mental disorder in the prison population.
- People with drug and alcohol problems have higher rates of other mental health problems.
- People with physical illnesses have higher rates of mental health problems.

The relationship between mental health, wellness and mental illness

Dunn (1961) addressed the issue of wellness and his now classic definition of what he termed 'high-level wellness' was an integrated method of functioning. This state of 'wellness' is oriented toward maximizing the potential of that which the individual is capable within the environment where he/she is

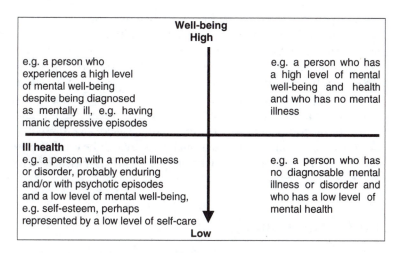

Figure 8.1 The links between well-being and ill-health
Source: Adapted from Tudor (1996)

functioning. He stressed that wellness was an ongoing process towards higher potential, not a static goal. High-level wellness is a feeling of being 'alive to the tips of the fingers, with energy to burn, and tingling with vitality'. He postulated that health professionals tend to focus on disease rather than wellness or prevention because it is easier to fight against sickness than to fight for a condition of greater wellness.

Whereas Tudor (1996) identifies a continuum between health and illness, he also argued that this could not simply be transferred to mental health. Adapting work by Downie et al (1990), Tudor sought to link well-being and ill-health by crossing two axes, as shown in Figure 8.1.

By using this framework, Tudor (1996) believes that it is possible to have a diagnosed mental illness and also to have a good level of mental health and well-being and goes on to demonstrate that it is possible and desirable to promote the mental health and well-being of people with mental illnesses and disorders.

Seedhouse (2002) reminds us of the difficulty in defining mental health and stresses that mental health is not simply the absence of disease. He states that disease is typically thought of as a deviation from a statistical norm whereas mental health is generally believed to be a positive state that enables people to do well in the social world. The problem is that different people; different cultures and different historical periods each define mental health and mental illness in different and conflicting ways. Seedhouse (2002) further states that physical health is continually affected by the mind and that positive thinking, learning to deal with anger and malice, and being part of creative, social networks can extend life and lessen our chances of becoming ill.

Seedhouse (2002) argues that despite overwhelming scientific evidence that mind and body are integrally related, health promotion is still split into separate specialisms: mental health promotion, exercise and nutrition, social health promotion, health education and many other categories. Therefore, he states that health promoters should spurn these artificial distinctions and instead aim to enhance the human experience, free from restrictive classifications and false images. He has thereby developed an interesting and new health promotion tool which he calls the 'rational field', to be used by any health care worker in any setting. Rational fields enable health promoters to plan and act in total honesty, using whatever methods are best suited to their quest to create autonomy.

Education and training

According to the Australian Commonwealth Department of Health and Aged Care (2000) mental health promotion requires different skills and approaches from those traditionally available in the health care sector, where the focus has been primarily upon treatment. These skills include ability to work with communities as well as individuals using strategies outside the mainstream health care setting, including policy development, community development and empowerment, and interventions focusing on improving physical and social environments.

The report further argues that without the development of these skills, it will be difficult to inaugurate and sustain mental health promotion interventions. It is, therefore, an important part of the strategy to educate and train the workforce appropriately. Mental health promotion involves programmes for individuals at risk, programmes for vulnerable groups, victims of child abuse and domestic violence. It also involves race and mental health, people who sleep rough, people in prison, and people with alcohol and drug problems.

In fact, combating discrimination and social exclusion involves action across whole populations. Mental health promotion is most effective when interventions build on social networks, intervene at crucial points in people's lives, and use a combination of methods to strengthen their effectiveness and coping skills.

A report by the Mental Health Foundation *Bright Futures – Promoting Children and Young People's Mental Health* (Kay, 1999) summarized the evidence on mental health promotion for children and young people. It highlighted the significance of supporting parents during pregnancy and after birth with home visits, high quality childcare, and helping through schools and community networks.

Psychosocial and cognitive development of babies and infants depends upon their interaction with parents. Programmes that enhance the quality of these relations can improve substantially the emotional, social, cognitive and physical development of children. These activities are particularly meaningful for mothers living in conditions of stress and social adversity. The World Health Organization (2001) has developed an international programme to stimulate mother–infant interaction that has been widely adopted.

Schools remain a crucial social institution for the education of children in preparation for later life. However, they do need to become more involved in a broader educational role to foster healthy social and emotional development of pupils. The WHO has developed a 'life skills' educational curriculum, which teaches a wide range of skills to school age children to improve their psychosocial competency. These skills include problem solving, critical thinking, communication, interpersonal skills, empathy and methods to cope with emotions. These skills enable children and adolescents to develop sound and positive mental health. Another WHO mental health initiative involves, 'Child-friendly schools', which promote a sound psychosocial environment to complete the life skills curriculum. A child-friendly school encourages tolerance and equality between boys and girls and different ethnic, religious and social groups. It promotes active involvement and co-operation, avoids the use of physical punishment, and does not tolerate bullying. It is also a supportive and nurturing environment, providing education that responds to the reality of children's lives. Finally, it helps to establish connections between school and family life, encourages creativity as well as academic abilities, and promotes the self-esteem and self-confidence of children. Exercise, relaxation and stress management also have a beneficial effect on mental health. Good social education programmes should address real issues faced by children such as illicit drugs, learning to consume alcohol in moderation, and reducing and refraining from smoking, and furthermore, teaching children interpersonal awareness, how to maintain social contacts and that greater control over self reduces emotional exhaustion and depression and pays dividends for them when they reach adult life.

A further report by the Mental Health Foundation underlined the need to consider the physical and spiritual facets of mental health and mental health problems, and to tailor individual programmes to individual circumstances. For example, the Health and Safety Executive (1995) *Survey of Self-Reported Work Related Illness* estimated that almost 300,000 people in Britain believed that they were suffering from work-related stress, anxiety or depression. Such recognition has contributed to the increase in the momentum, number and scope, of holistic practitioners. Keegan (1994) has explained how these practitioners, many of whom are nurses, are beginning to weave in the thread of living a wellness life-style as a major factor in the health process.

Programmes for individuals at risk

Programmes that target children with behavioural problems, can reduce the development of difficulties later on. Professional emotional support for pregnant women caring for their existing young children can decrease the rate of postnatal depression. Helping new parents to develop child-rearing skills is effective, and young, lone parents can be helped to cope better. High quality pre-school and nursery education have been shown to produce improvements in self-esteem, motivation and social behaviour. Pre-school education may substantially decrease the chances of drug abuse 20 years later.

The World Health Organization report (WHO, 2002) deals with health risks, where risk is defined as a probability of an adverse outcome, or a factor that raises this probability. As governments only have limited budgets they need to select the most cost-effective and affordable interventions that protect people, help them protect themselves, and prevent risks from occurring. Some risks have already been reduced, but changes in patterns of consumption, particularly of diet, alcohol, tobacco and other substances around the world are creating a 'risk transition'. Conditions such as cancers, heart disease, stroke, diabetes and mental health problems are increasing in prominence. This is particularly serious for many low and middle-income countries that are still suffering from the traditional problems of poverty, such as undernutrition and infectious diseases.

A study led by Brooker (1993) emphasized the value of health promotion for those already diagnosed as suffering from serious mental illness. This study examined families caring for a relative with schizophrenia, after community psychiatric nurses had been trained to deliver 'psychosocial interventions'. Brooker found that educating relatives about the nature of the illness was a crucial component, since providing information enabled families to cope better with the stress that such an illness produces. The research team explored two different educational approaches, one was based upon the 'deficit model' of education and the other based on an 'interactional model'. The 'deficit model' assumes that by providing general information about schizophrenia, families will be better able to cope. However, other educational researchers notably Barrowclough et al (1987) suggest that this 'deficit model' of education has a number of shortcomings, which in turn led to the development of the second model, the interactional model.

Brooker's (1993) study supported the 'interactional approach' with its emphasis upon understanding the reasons for people's beliefs about illness rather than focusing on pathology in general. While it is accepted that the interactional model will not necessarily lead to positive changes in behaviour, empirically it has been found to be more successful than the deficit model. Brooker goes further and encourages both managers and educators of community psychiatric nurses to establish educational programmes, which are underpinned by a psychosocial view of illness.

Post-qualification educational programmes in the use of psychosocial interventions have greatly increased during the past five years and many of them will soon be evaluated. Brooker (1993) also states that there is increasing recognition of the relationship between stress and illness and that the psychosocial intervention approach and the 'interaction model' of education will have even wider implications for mental health promotion.

Mental health promotion or mental health education?

Ewles and Simnet (1992) differentiated between *health promotion* and *health education*. They noted that a debate emerged in the 1980s because the range of activities undertaken in the pursuit of better health widened from traditional health education, which was about giving information, to a more proactive approach. With rising criticism, the traditional view was deemed to be too narrow and to focus too much on individual lifestyles and therefore be seen to be 'victim blaming'. New issues were emerging, which included political action to change social policies, putting employee health on the agenda of managers, and engaging in community development work for health. Cherniss (1988) and others noted how stress in the workplace can lead to severe mental and physical health problems usually taking the form of burn out whereby a previously committed professional develops a process of reification whereby they treat people as though they were objects. By contrast the creation of a healthy workplace can promote mental health. Learning to mobilize support at work and to participate in problem solving and decision making can improve mental health. Mental health problems associated with work include depression and anxiety, alcohol misuse, and sickness absence. Work overload, monotony, and pressure of work are key factors, as are lack of control over the work environment and exclusion from decision making. Special emphasis should be given to those aspects of work places, and the work process itself, that promote mental health. The World Health Organization (2001) has identified eight areas of action:

- increasing an employer's awareness of mental health issues;
- identifying common goals and positive aspects of the work process;
- creating a balance between job demands and occupational skills;
- training in social skills;
- developing the psychosocial climate of the workplace;
- providing counselling facilities;
- enhancement of working capacity; and
- early rehabilitation strategies.

High quality interventions for individuals who are unemployed can reduce the psychological impact of job loss, and promote re-employment, particularly for those at risk of mental ill health. Unemployment is a significant issue in mental health, in particular, youth unemployment. In this area, mental health promotion strategies seek to improve employment opportunities, for example, through programmes to create jobs, provide vocational training and social and job seeking skills. Research has shown that such programmes enhance self-confidence, increase motivation, reduce the negative feelings associated with unsuccessful job seeking and reduce depressive symptoms. Long term, the control group went on to achieve higher monthly earnings and had fewer job changes. Many local authorities and NHS trusts, often in partnership with the independent sector, have set up vocational training and employment support schemes for people with mental health problems. These need to be planned and integrated with other statutory employment services to ensure effective use is made of skills, resources and support systems. People who are vulnerable as a result of either divorce or unemployment can be helped to adjust, and shown how to build coping skills.

Research and evaluation

Evaluations of mental health promotion initiatives often make the mistake of targeting whole population groups and may not always include mental health or mental ill-health outcome measures, rather focusing on measures of the hypothesized risk and protective factors and processes involved. Effective research and evaluation are critical to the advancement of mental health promotion (Australian Commonwealth Department of Health and Aged Care, 2000). Measures to evaluate the impact of mental health promotion initiatives need to be able to assess processes operating at different levels, in different contexts and among different communities. Valid and reliable indicators of mental health outcomes, which permit the comparison of different projects across communities, are required to build a solid evidence base.

Mental health is not just the absence of mental disorder. The positive dimension of mental health is stressed in the World Health Organization's definition, 'Health is a state of complete physical, mental and social well being and not merely the absence of disease or infirmity.' Standard One in the *National Service Framework for Mental Health* (DoH, 1999) now puts mental health promotion at the centre-stage of mental health strategy. Health and Social Services have now been given a clear remit to promote mental health for all and to reduce the discrimination experienced by people with mental health problems. Health promotion not only contributes to health improvement, but can be used to challenge discrimination by improving the level of understanding of mental health issues within communities. For the individual, mental health promotion can help to improve physical health, increase emotional resilience, and enhance greater social inclusion and participation.

Making it Happen (DoH, 2001) requires all staff working in mental health services to address the needs of the 'whole person' which includes employment, occupation, housing and entitlement to benefits. This recognizes the fact that many of the factors that influence mental health lie outside health and social care, so mental health promotion is relevant to the implementation of a whole range of initiatives that relate to social inclusion, neighbourhood renewal and health at work.

Conclusion

This chapter has demonstrated to student mental health nurses that they should expect to see many changes during the course of their future careers. What they will be expected to do, where this will be done and with whom will need to be considered. The mental well being of our society is presently at risk from many influences and this will affect the future role of the mental health nurse. We must, as a professional group, react to the ever changing needs of the twenty-first century.

References

Australian Commonwealth Department of Health and Aged Care (2000) *Promotion, Prevention and Early Intervention for Mental Health – A Monograph*, Canberra: Mental Health and Special Programs Branch, Commonwealth Department of Health and Aged Care.

Barrowclough, C., Tarrier, N., Watts, S., Vaughan, C., Bamrah, J. & Freeman, H. (1987) Assessing the functional knowledge about schizophrenia: a preliminary report, *British Journal of Psychiatry*, 151, 1–8.

Brooker, C. (1993) Evaluating the impact of training community psychiatric nurses to educate relatives about schizophrenia: implications for health promotion at the secondary level, in J. Wilson-Barnett, and J. Macleod Clark, *Research in Health Promotion and Nursing*, Basingstoke: Macmillan, now Palgrave Macmillan.

Cherniss, C. (1988) Observed supervisory behaviour and teacher burnout in special education, *Exceptional Child*, 54(5), 449–54.

Department of Health (1999) *National Service Framework for Mental Health*, London: HMSO.

Department of Health (2001) *Making It Happen: a Guide to Delivering Mental Health Promotion*, London: HMSO.

Downie, R. S., Fyfe, C. & Tannahill, A. (1990) *Health Promotion: Models and Values*, Oxford: Oxford University Press.

Dubois, R. (1980) *Man Adapting*, Boston: Yale University Press.

Dunn, H. (1961) *High Level Wellness*, Arlington: R. W. Beatty.

Durkheim, E. (1983) 'The Division of Labour in Society', cited in Hewett (2002), *Durkheim's Anomie*, http://www.hewett.norfolk.sch.uk/curric/soc/crime/anomie.htm

Ewles, L. & Simnet, I. (1992) *Promoting Health: A Practical Guide*, London: Scutari Press.

Health and Safety Executive (1995) *Survey of Self-Reported Work Related Illness*, Oxford: Health and Safety Executive.

Kay, H. (1999) *Bright Futures: Promoting Children and Young Peoples' Mental Health*, London: The Mental Health Foundation.

Keegan, L. (1994) *The Nurse as Healer*, Albany: Delmar Publishers Inc.

Murray, C. J. L. & Lopez, A. D. (1997) Mortality by cause: foreign regions of the world: global burden of disease study, *The Lancet*, 349, 1269–76.

Nixon, P. G. F. (1989) Human functions and the heart, in D. Seedhouse & A. Cribb (eds), *Changing Ideas in Health Care*, Chichester: John Wiley and Sons.

Seedhouse, D. (1993) *Health: The Foundations for Achievement*, Chichester: John Wiley and Sons.

Seedhouse, D. (2002) *Total Health Promotion: Mental Health, Rational Fields and the Quest for Autonomy*, Chichester: John Wiley and Sons.

Tudor, K. (1996) *Mental Health Promotion: Paradigms and Practice*, London: Routledge.

Wilson-Barnett, J. & Macleod Clark, J. (1993) *Research in Health Promotion and Nursing*, Basingstoke: Macmillan, now Palgrave Macmillan.

World Health Organization (2001) *The World Health Report Mental Health: New Understanding, New Hope*, Geneva: World Health Organization.

World Health Organization (2002) *The World Health Report Reducing Risks, Promoting a Healthy Life*, Geneva: World Health Organization.

CHAPTER 9

A Positive Approach to Mental Health Nursing: Role, Values and Attitudes

DENNIS CROSS

Indicative Benchmark Statements

▦ Consideration of the power differential between users of services, carers and mental health and social care workers

▦ Skills in reflecting on the impact of own attitudes to mental health and social care

▦ The application of helping relationships as the cornerstone of their mental health nursing practice

▦ A caring and empathetic attitude to users of mental health and social care services and their carers

▦ Flexibility in the care of mental health service users, their families and carers to meet their changing needs and circumstances

---

In this chapter we will explore the attitudes and beliefs that are required in mental health nursing at a time of increasing and enduring change and attempt to conceptualize what contemporary mental health nurses do when they nurse. According to Shives (1998) attitudes are developed in various ways and may be the result of interaction with the environment, assimilation of other's attitudes, life experiences, intellectual processes, or a traumatic experience. The terms that are used to describe attitudes include accepting, caring, prejudice and judgmental. It will be argued that the values and attitudes prevalent within a traditional model of mental health nursing, underpinned by a biomedical approach, have often frustrated and failed us, although they are still extremely strong, entrenched and pervasive. However, with the arrival of evidence-based mental health care the opportunity for change appears to be upon us and with it, perhaps, the opportunity to enhance the quality of life for the whole community.

What are the outcomes of mental health/psychiatric nursing?

According to Peplau (1952), mental health nursing is primarily a practice-based discipline that values human beings, it rests on the assumption that each person is a unique individual whose needs may be physical, intellectual, emotional, social and spiritual. At its best it enables people to reach and maintain their mental health and social goals in order to achieve their optimum quality of life. Peplau goes on to say that mental health nursing is founded on the premise that human beings have dignity, are worthy of respect and have individual rights, responsibilities, needs and beliefs. However, mental health nursing is not just confined to boundaries of alleviating mental illness and mental suffering but is also concerned with the whole person and the promotion of mental health and wellness in individuals (Tudor, 1996).

Health and social care are rapidly evolving and expanding their traditional parameters, and mental health nurses need to take account of, and be responsive to, these changes and to the needs of users of mental health services. Therefore, the practice of mental health nursing involves complex partnerships with a variety of people and agencies, with carers, families and friends, and with members of other professions. However, what constitutes contemporary mental health is also difficult to define. Tilbury (2002) attempts such a definition around three elements.

- Mentally healthy people will be satisfied with and enjoying their lives. They will have a positive self-image but can accept their limitations and have the capacity to learn and develop throughout their lives.
- The second element relates to peoples' self-management in social relations. By this he means that the ability to make and sustain intimate social relationships is our most important capacity. The number and nature of such relationships may not be specified but we need close relationships with our parents, our children and at least one friend.
- Finally, it is only through a healthy capacity to relate that we could have a successful marriage or cohabitation with an ongoing relationship with a member of the opposite sex, which includes physical intimacy (although Tilbury specifies the opposite sex we believe that like-sex relationships need not be differently regarded).

Central to the core of mental health nursing is a strong emphasis on the development of interpersonal skills (Peplau, 1952), including self-awareness, which are essential to establish effective relationships with users, carers and colleagues in a multidisciplinary context. Mental health nurses need to be able to appraise critically their own performance, their skills, competencies, capabilities and techniques and their ability to give and receive appropriate supervision and support.

Many authors argue for the need for evidence-based mental health nursing practice (Newell & Gournay, 2000; Stetler et al, 1998). They state that evidence-based practice and clinical effectiveness are broadly similar terms, since both emphasize the importance of clinical practice which, when delivered to patients and clients, is effective in achieving health gain for them (Newell & Gournay, 2000). In this way Gournay (1995) calls for nurses to re-adopt a medical view of psychiatric disorder. However, Clarke (1999) refutes this contention by stating the simple counter-point that it is what nurses do with clients that matters rather than the rights or wrongs of any particular view. He refers to Laing who observed that you could learn all there is to know about schizophrenia and still not know anything about a particular schizophrenic. The focus of this chapter will be to try to identify the best way forward from these diverse views and to encourage mental health nurses to adopt a broader approach to their practice and beliefs that will benefit the person with mental health problems.

There are, however, some central issues that need to be considered in any exploration of the role of the mental health nurse. The first is that the relationship between health care professionals, patients and their families has frequently been described as frustrating, unsatisfying, noncollaborative and sometimes coercive (Ragins, 2003). People with mental health problems and their families are often waiting for their illnesses to go away or to be cured in order to get on with their lives. The result is that they are frequently angry with professionals for not helping them, or doing anything for them, since their lives do not seem to be improving at all. The problem according to Ragins (2003) is that ever since Kraepelin defined schizophrenia, or dementia praecox, one hundred years ago, as a chronic, unremitting, gradually deteriorating condition, it has been difficult to talk credibly about, or work towards, recovery with severe mental illness. Many people on all sides have abandoned the process of recovery out of despair and increasing numbers of people with mental health problems are described as 'treatment resistant'. In addition carers and families have become 'burnt out' and 'disengaged' resulting in abandonment, neglect and deterioration.

All this hopelessness exists despite clear evidence of the growing efficacy of treatment and greater success with people with serious mental health problems than traditionally had been thought possible. There is also evidence that people with schizophrenia who explain their condition spiritually, instead of medically, apparently fare better, for example people with schizophrenia in third world countries regularly report better outcomes than in the West. A recovery model of mental health nursing will take into account the recent sophisticated psychopharmacological research, the advances in psychological and psychosocial interventions, interpersonal therapy, behavioural family management and mental health care systems research.

The prevalent medical model tends to define recovery in quite negative terms. In this model symptoms and complaints need to be eliminated and illnesses need to be cured or removed. Patients need to be returned to their premorbid, healthy or non ill-health state. This is achieved through a comfortable relationship between powerful healing professionals and helpless patients complying with orders which they are not required to understand. However, most people with severe mental health problems are not permanently incapacitated, infantile, helpless beings who we need to protect and have the same dreams, hopes, and plans as the rest of us. Change frequently entails risk and structured change entails considering the options and a range of possible outcomes ensuing from them. Mentally ill people are frequently denied this on the grounds that patients lack awareness. What the medical model is preventing or protecting them from here is actually the opportunity for change, growth, experiencing reality, self-confidence and ultimately recovery itself.

To find a way out of this dilemma we need a broader perspective for mental health nursing, that can be obtained by examining other, established treatment/intervention models that conceptualize the recovery process and the helping relationship in very different ways to the medical model. Empowerment is the central concept, as people with mental health problems are enabled to help themselves. They can take responsibility for developing coping skills and adapting as part of the recovery process. The focus of this broader recovery perspective is on strengths rather than weaknesses and on people rather than illnesses. Psychosocial rehabilitation tends to conceptualize recovery more in terms of function than pathology. Here there is more of a concordance between the professional and the patient, than within the medical model, and people with mental health problems can experience active recovery regardless of the severity of their problems. These elements of recovery are:

- accepting having a chronic, incurable condition that is a permanent part of them, without guilt or shame, without fault or blame;
- avoiding complications of the condition;
- participating in an ongoing support system both as recipient and as provider; and
- changing many aspects of their lives including emotions, interpersonal relationships, and spirituality both to accommodate their problems and grow through overcoming them.

A 'recovery' perspective for mental health nursing

Recovery for people with mental health problems can relate to internal states, functions or external things. Internal states that can be recovered involve the person feeling good about themselves, having peace of mind, responsibility for themselves, a self-identity other than that of being mentally ill. Functions that may be recovered include the ability to sleep restfully, to read, to work, to have coherent conversations, to make love, to raise children, to drive a car. External things that can be recovered include a home, a job, friends, playing football, playing in a band, a spouse, a car, family relationships, television and participation in educational programmes.

On the other hand, Seedhouse (2000) thinks that there are practical difficulties involved with entering into a 'partnership' with people who are experiencing mental health problems. If the patient's view of life is badly distorted then how is the nurse to enter this world? How can the nurse advocate the interests of the patient if the patient's interests are damaging to himself and/or to others? Furthermore, if the mental health nurse thinks that the patient has certain basic needs but the patient thinks he/she has different ones, how can a partnership be established? Sayce (2000) describes an 'inclusion model' that works positively by redefining mental illness as disability and then goes out to form alliances by way of cross-disability support rather than waiting for other disability groups to address mental health issues. She believes that as the growing power of the mental health service user movement collides with pressures for increased social exclusion, we need robust, tested conceptual models to take the mental health world into a new phase of development. This can be achieved by developing therapeutic alliances between users of mental health services, their families and mental health professionals (Speedy, 1999).

The delivery of mental health and social care is changing rapidly and the treatment of mental disorders has gone through many stages of development during the past 100 years. The guiding principle throughout most of this time has been to move the mentally disordered person away from his or her normal family, social and community surroundings to a sheltered environment. During the past 20 years, the sheltered environment shifted from one that consisted of primarily custodial care in an institution to one that is dynamically oriented toward community-based rehabilitation of the person with a mental health problem. This shift in orientation and philosophical change in treatment is evident commencing with the role of primary health care team and throughout the active treatment and post-discharge phases of mental health and social care (Armstrong, 1995).

When an individual begins to experience mental health problems there is a profound effect not only upon them but also upon their family and friends. The role of the mental health nurse includes assisting the person, their family and friends with these problems and to understand their cause and nature as far as possible and also the means of restoring health and mental well being. These important nursing values can be expressed regardless of the setting or environment where mental health care is administered. The guiding principle of nursing care continues to be the nursing process (Barry, 2002), and the flexibility and openness of the nursing process allows it to be used in all care settings.

Many forces have shaped the changes in inpatient mental health care. The most significant influences include the economic forces that do not support long-term psychiatric care with funding arrangements shifting from chronic inpatient care to community models of outpatient care. It is argued that the development of new medications that claim to decrease the major symptoms of psychiatric disorders, psychosis, and depression when properly used, allow those who formerly required long-term institutional care to now be cared for in the community. More recently has been the advent of new training programmes, reports such as *Fitness for Practice* (UKCC, 1999) and *Making a Difference* (DoH, 1999) have enabled mental health professionals to work with different aspects of a mental health client's psychological and social functioning in both inpatient and community settings.

However, according to Brooker (2001), by the 1990s it had become clear that care in the community for people with serious mental health problems needed reconsideration. There have been many reports that indicate how it can be hazardous for people with serious mental health problems to live in the community (Philo et al, 1993; Ritchie et al, 1994). Brooker states that many frequent re-admissions were reported in times of crisis where people lived in poverty and isolation without work, where they had few social supports and networks and were at high risk of victimization, exploitation, homelessness or imprisonment. In addition, he speaks of the community tenure of this group by families who themselves have a range of problems and needs.

Nurses who were involved in the traditional care of people with mental health problems were primarily responsible for their physical well being. Their responsibilities included administering drugs prescribed by a psychiatrist and caring for people undergoing treatments such as insulin therapy or electroconvulsive therapy (ECT). This was nursing care that was provided under the disease (or biologic-medical) model (Tyrer and Steinberg, 1993) and is still the conceptual basis for the continued use of biologic therapies for those people with mental health problems. It is also the model that still sees the hospital as the setting for care, for research into genetic transmission of mental illness, for research on biochemical and metabolic variables among diagnosed 'psychiatric clients' and for the dominance of the medically trained psychiatrist in the mental health team. According to Wilson and Kneisl (1992) as long as people with mental health problems are admitted and treated according to medical diagnoses, knowledge of this framework is crucial. Furthermore, as long as knowledge expands, mental health nurses are responsible for translating that knowledge into care practices. Even mental health nurses who disagree with this approach must be generally familiar with it to communicate with peers within the mental health team. Knowledge of the disease model is also needed for identifying human responses associated with disorders so that the nurse can plan care.

The history of psychiatric/mental health nursing is slightly over a century old. Peplau (1994) writes that the history of psychiatric nursing is about the struggles, choices, and progress that nurses have made over the many years of its development. She considered that the whole history of psychiatric nursing has not yet been told but that the story is about beginnings and forward steps along a continuum of development. Before her death in 1999 she argued that one important lesson from history comes from the very courageous nurses, working in psychiatric hospitals, who were willing to take a stand on the unpopular issues of their day. At the turn of the twentieth century and earlier, psychiatric nursing was an unpopular field of work. It shared the general stigma attached to mental illness and to the institutions that cared for psychiatric patients. Peplau spoke of the changes in attitude towards the mentally ill following World War II when the nursing profession was able to rise to this challenge and oppose the oppression and work towards eroding the stigma. She stated that changes did not occur by design as much as by the persistence of a few psychiatric nursing leaders. In earlier years they had spoken out, persuaded and thereby shaped the general direction taken by the nursing profession. Their perspective, eventually adopted by the profession, was to include psychiatric nursing as an important component of the whole nursing profession.

Peplau (1952) described nursing as a significant, therapeutic, interpersonal process functioning co-operatively with other human processes that makes health possible for individuals in communities. When professional health teams offer health services, nurses help in the organization of conditions that facilitate natural ongoing tendencies in human organisms. She argued that nursing is an educative instrument, a maturing force that aims to promote forward movement of personality in the direction of creative, constructive, productive, personal and community living. According to Wilson and Kneisl (1992) to practice mental health nursing in this humanistic way, nurses must devote themselves to understanding what makes people human, how to express their joy of living, their sadness, their desire to love, their hopes for growth. Understanding these phenomena becomes even more crucial when mental health nurses must explain how the joy of living suddenly turns to the desire to die, how love of self and others turns to violence and hate, how the hope for growth turns to withdrawal and despair, and how alterations in the brain relate to these human experiences.

Barker (1999) states that he has been wondering about the nature of mental health nursing for as long as he has been a nurse. He considers that where psychiatric nursing came from and where it might be going, offers much potential for reflection. He states that psychiatric nursing has been transformed, almost overnight, into mental health nursing, suggesting that the focus of nursing has shifted (Barker, 1999). However, whether this shift is real or imaginary he is more concerned about whether nurses are offering the right kind of care, what is the most fitting form or context for such care and how we establish what is 'right' or 'fitting' anyway. He states that despite the efforts of many to suggest that the story is complete and that the formula for success is clear there is still much to be considered. Barker (2000) has developed a radically different model of mental health care, which he calls 'The

Tidal Model' (www.tidal-model.co.uk). The Tidal Model was constructed following a five year study of the need for mental health nursing (Barker et al, 1999a, b; Jackson & Stevenson, 2000). Fundamentally, Barker is saying that having mental health problems is inherently dis-empowering for the individual and that people's experience of their care and treatment within the psychiatric system emphasizes this sense of powerlessness. Mental health nurses should understand that people with mental health problems need to be heard and understood and that their interactions with them need to be empowering. There is now some evidence from evaluative studies with both users of mental health services and professionals such as that by Fletcher and Stevenson (2001) that there have been perceived gains from structuring care around this model.

The problem with mental health nursing according to McCabe (2002) is that while it was vibrant and applicable once, it is predicated on an approach to care and an understanding of mental illness that reflects an older time. Mental health nursing is now in the precarious position of having an ageing paradigm of practice, rooted in older knowledge and beliefs and recalcitrant to new knowledge and new realities of clinical practice. She makes reference to the importance of the 'giants' who helped shape the mental health nursing profession, such as Peplau (1952). Patients, who were once treated in inpatient settings with an emphasis on psychological, non-somatic treatment modalities, were in the care of mental health nurses for protracted periods of time, ranging from months to years. They were conceptualized as suffering from psychological problems rooted in adverse life events with subsequent development dysfunctions. She argues that mental health care is vastly different in today's managed care, and following a decade of research into genetics and brain function. She comments on the fact that clients are most often treated in outpatient not inpatient settings with somatically based treatment modalities such as medication, with increasingly less focus on therapy. Clients are only in the care of mental health nurses for discrete, brief, limited periods of time and are increasingly being conceptualized as suffering from brain-based disorders that are biological and genetic in origin. Although the concept of interpersonal interaction remains critical and central to mental health nursing, the manner in which this concept should be best expressed in our nursing practice has become increasingly confused and contentious.

The concurrence of an ageing paradigm that poorly matches current practice realities or research findings leaves mental health nursing with seemingly incompatible knowledge structures that increasingly divide the profession. Psychoanalytical, developmental theories coexist with neurobiological and humanistic theories with no clear connection between them. McCabe (2002) argues that these underpinning theories lead to distinctly different nursing care practices and that in the end this has led to the disempowerment of the mental health nursing profession. This state has also made it very difficult to construct national competencies for mental health nursing. However, the work of the Northern Centre for Mental Health (2000) *A Competence-Based 'Exit Profile' for Pre-Registration Mental Health Nursing* does seem to correspond to McCabe's (2002) list of assumptions underpinning a new paradigm for mental health nursing.

She goes on to state first that mental health nursing is a distinct and critical subspecialty of the profession of nursing. Mental health nursing has a distinct focus and body of knowledge that demarcates it from other subspecialties of nursing (McCabe, 2002). The focus of this nursing is health, and the focus of psychiatric mental health nursing is mental health. She argues that mental health and mental illness are different constructs, not opposite points on the same continuum. Mental health is manifested in behaviour, functional and dysfunctional, and that this behaviour is a complex, multifaceted construct consisting of factors including genetics and endocrine, environment and development, social, interpersonal, neurological and immunological. Mental health nursing is therefore, fundamentally concerned with behavioural change, and with the patient's response to health experiences. Mental illnesses are brain-based disorders with complex, multifaceted causative factors that include genetic, immunological, environmental and social components. Core mental health nursing competencies are derived from an understanding of the nursing role of behavioural change and the complex, multifaceted construct of behaviour. Mental health nursing interventions are based on scientific, theoretical knowledge, and are designed to address behavioural change and assist patients in their response to health experiences. Mental health nursing research that focuses on behavioural change is essential to develop and grow the scientific basis of our practice. Finally, individuals with mental illness, or at risk of mental illness, are the population of focus for psychiatric mental health nursing.

Conclusion

The role of the psychiatric mental health nurse is a controversial issue; different camps with different views bring about much thought for our development. Although we cannot foresee into the future, we can only expect changes to be made in accordance with the changing times. The length of stay in acute inpatient facilities will almost certainly reduce and we may not have the luxury of long-term therapy for clients in our care. We need to adapt and become cognizant of the major changes in the 'real' healthcare world.

Mental health nurses must, therefore, be prepared to work in an ever-changing health care system. According to Krauss (1995) they must have a blend of interpersonal theory, with a heavy emphasis on short-term approaches. They should be grounded in the latest neurobiology and psychopharmacology and knowledgeable of short-term family models of care. In addition the mental health nurse must develop awareness and skills in the physical assessment of patients with serious and enduring mental health problems and in the management of common medical diseases. The mental health nurse of the future will be able to carry out mental health/psychiatric therapy but will also be able to screen for diabetes or hypertension in the depressed client and to rule out somatic delusions or pain associated with tendonitis in the client suffering from schizophrenia.

Perhaps the most important dilemma, mental health nurses will face is that between the provision of care, support and treatment as opposed to their broader role in community safety.

References

Armstrong, E. (1995) *Mental Health Issues in Primary Care: A Practical Guide*, Basingstoke: Macmillan, now Palgrave Macmillan.

Baker, M. & Kleijnen, J. (2000) The drive towards evidence-based health care, in N. Rowland & R. Goss (eds), *Evidence-Based Counselling and Psychological Therapies*, London: Routledge.

Barker, P. J. (1999) *The Philosophy and Practice of Psychiatric Nursing*, London: Churchill Livingstone.

Barker, P. J. (2000) The Tidal Model: developing a person-centered approach to psychiatric and mental health nursing, *Perspectives in Psychiatric Care*, 37, 2.

Barker, P. J., Stevenson, C. & Jackson, S. (1999a) The need for psychiatric nursing: towards a multidimensional theory of nursing, *Nursing Inquiry*, 6(2), 104–12.

Barker, P. J., Stevenson, C. & Jackson, S. (1999b) What are psychiatric nurses needed for? Developing a theory of essential practice, *Journal of Psychiatric and Mental Health Nursing*, 6(4), 273–82.

Barry, P. D. (2002) *Mental Health and Mental Illness* (7th edn), New York: Lippincott.

Brooker, C. (2001) A decade of evidence-based training for work with people with serious mental health problems: progress in the development of psychosocial interventions, *Journal of Mental Health*, 10(1), 17–31.

Clarke, L. (1999) *Challenging Ideas in Psychiatric Nursing*, London: Routledge.

Department of Health (1998) *A First Class Service: Quality in the New NHS*, NHS Executive, http://www.open.gov.uk/doh/public/quality.htm

Department of Health (1999) *Making a Difference: Strengthening the Nursing, Midwifery and Health Visiting Contribution to Health and Health Care*, London: DoH.

Department of Health (2002) *Reforming the Mental Health Act, Part 1: The New Legal Framework 1(1.6)*, London: DoH.

Fletcher, E. & Stevenson, C. (2001) Launching the Tidal Model in an adult mental health programme, *Nursing Standard*, 15(49), 33–6.

Gournay, K. (1995) Schizophrenia: a review of the contemporary literature and implications for mental health nursing theory, practice and education, *Journal of Psychiatric and Mental Health Nursing*, 3, 7–12.

Hargreaves, S. et al (1977) Short versus long hospitalisation: a prospective controlled study, *Archives of General Psychiatry*, 34(3), 305–11.

Jackson, S. & Stevenson, C. (2000) What do people need psychiatric and mental health nurses for?, *Journal of Advanced Nursing*, 31(2), 378–88.

James, P. & Burns, T. (2002) The influence of evidence on mental health care developments in the UK since 1980, in S. Priebe & M. Slade (eds), *Evidence in Mental Health Care*, East-Sussex: Brunner-Routledge.

Krauss, J. (1995) Editorial. Managing costs and managing care: managing to make our systems humane, *Archives in Psychiatric Nursing*, 1(6), 309–10.

Mattes, J. A., Rosen, B. & Klien, D. F. (1997) Comparison of the clinical effectiveness of 'short' versus 'long' stay hospitalisation, *Journal of Nervous and Mental Disease*, 165(6), 387–94.

McCabe, S. (2002) The nature of psychiatric nursing: the intersection of paradigm, evolution and history, *Archives of Psychiatric Nursing*, XVI(2), 51–60.

Newell, R. & Gournay, K. (2000) *Mental Health Nursing: An Evidence-Based Approach*, London: Churchill Livingstone.

Northern Centre for Mental Health, Cross, D. J. & Readhead, K. E. (2000) *A Competence-based 'Exit Profile' for Pre-Registration Mental Health Nursing*, Durham: Northern Centre for Mental Health and The Northern and Yorkshire Regional Education and Workforce Development Sub-group for Mental Health.

Peplau, H. E. (1952) *Interpersonal Relations in Nursing*, New York: G P Putnam's Sons.

Peplau, H. E. (1994) Psychiatric mental health nursing: challenge and change, *Journal of Psychiatric and Mental Health Nursing*, 1(1), 3–7.

Philo, G., Henderson, I. & McLaughlin, G. (1993) *Mass Media Representation of Mental Health/Illness: Report for Health Education Board of Scotland*, Glasgow: Glasgow University Media Group.

Ragins, M. (Date accessed 06/02/2003), *Recovery*, online at:
http://home.att.net/~patrisser/helpingclients/recoverypsr.html

Ritchie, J. H., Dick, D. & Lingham, R. (1994) *The Report of the Inquiry into the Care and Treatment of Christopher Clunis*, London: HMSO.

Sayce, L. (2000) *From Psychiatric Patient to Citizen: Overcoming Discrimination and Social Exclusion*, Basingstoke: Macmillan, now Palgrave Macmillan.

Seedhouse, D. (2000) *Practical Nursing Philosophy: The Universal Ethical Code*, Chichester: John Wiley & Sons.

Shives, L. R. (1998) *Basic Concepts of Psychiatric-Mental Health Nursing* (4th edn), New York: Lippincott.

Speedy, S. (1999) The therapeutic alliance, in M. Clinton & S. Nelson (eds), *Advanced Practice in Mental Health Nursing*, Oxford: Blackwell Science.

Stetler, C. B., Brunell, M., Giuliano, K. K., Morsi, D., Prince, L. & Newell-Stokes, V. (1998) Evidence-based practice and the role of nursing leadership, *Journal of Nursing Administration*, 28(7), 45–53.

Thornley, B. & Adams, C. (1998) Content and quality of 2000 controlled trials in schizophrenia over 50 years, *British Medical Journal*, 317, 1181–4.

Tilbury, D. (2002) *Working with Mental Illness: A Community-Based Approach* (2nd edn), Basingstoke: Palgrave – now Palgrave Macmillan.

Tonelli, M. R. (1998) Philosophical limits of evidence-based medicine, *Academic Medicine*, 73(12), 1234–40.

Tudor, K. (1996) *Mental Health Promotion: Paradigms and Practice*, London: Routledge.

Tyrer, P. & Steinberg, D. (1993) *Models for Mental Disorder: Conceptual Models in Psychiatry*, Chichester: John Wiley & Sons.

United Kingdom Central Council for Nursing, Midwifery and Health Visiting (1999) *Fitness for Practice – The Report of the UKCC Commission for Nursing and Midwifery Education*, London: UKCC.

Wilson, H. S. & Kneisl, C. R. (1992) *Psychiatric Nursing* (4th edn), New York: Addison-Wesley.

CHAPTER 10

Risk Prevention

DENIS A. HART AND STEPHAN D. KIRBY

Indicative Benchmark Statements

▨ Utilization of appropriate research and relevant evidence to support decision-making relating to the selection and individualization of mental health nursing interventions

▨ Participation in therapeutic risk-taking in mental health and social care contexts

▨ Awareness of the need to share mental health nursing information with other agencies involved in maintaining public safety

▨ Assessment and management of risk in mental health and social care settings

▨ Recognition of the importance of identifying and removing environmental dangers within mental health and social care settings

Introduction

Mental health nurses have traditionally seen themselves involved in assessment, diagnosis and treatment of mental ill health; only recently have they become interested in the management of patients. Some of this new-found pressure has resulted from the hospitals closure programme of the mid 1980s and by the public perception of the failure of 'Care in the Community'. In this chapter we will explore the concept of risk, and your role in identifying risks early on in interventions both to prevent hospital admission becoming necessary and to reflect the duality of your role in ensuring community safety.

What is risk?

'Risk' is a term used regularly in every day-to-day practice with little thought being given to what it actually means. The *Oxford English Dictionary* (cited in Ryan, 1993, p 108) defines risk as: 'the possibility of an event occurring'. Here the word 'event' can be seen as an attempt to delimit the definition by placing an emphasis on a single aspect of a potential outcome rather than the entire set of possible consequences.

The Royal College of Psychiatrists (1998, p 1) acknowledge this to some extent when recognizing that: 'some risks are general, while others are more specific' . . . 'multi faceted, dynamic and contextual'. In practice, risk will mean different things to different people according to their own perception of the world based upon:

- their own upbringing and life experience;
- what they have seen happen in similar situations in the past; and
- the way they themselves balance the conflict between taking chances to help the patient and protecting the public.

Sadly, in mental health practice, Carson (1996), discovered that most definitions of risk nearly always emphasize the likelihood of harmful outcomes and only rarely recognize the potential benefits of risk taken. By adopting such a stance, practitioners are more likely to take the safest option, resulting in conservatism and containment rather than respond positively and proactively to patients allowing them to use opportunities to develop new insight and self understanding.

Risk is, thereby, most frequently likened to 'likelihood of violence' (Snowden, 1997) and to 'suicide, self harm and self neglect' (NHS Executive, 1994), rather than to adopting a changed approach to the individual patient to allow them to explore the possibility of changing themselves and their own behaviour.

Risk assessment

We have already recognized the need to balance the treatment of the patient against the possibility of harm to others and, by so doing, have begun to acknowledge the need to develop knowledge and skills in risk assessment.

Concerns about risk and how it is assessed and managed have always been important in mental health services. How we reach decisions as to which interventions are most appropriate to reduce or eliminate risk is a constant topic of discussion as factors regarding the harm and benefits associated with specific interventions need be carefully considered and balanced against each other.

In recent years, risk assessment has become even more significant as mental health practitioners have had to balance respecting and empowering patients and acknowledging additional rights as a result of the Human Rights Act 1998 against increasing concerns for public safety. Bean (2001, p 34) emphasizes the growing significance of the latter. In the past the public has been, 'asked to rely on clinical judgements about a patient's behaviour, rarely requiring the clinicians to state what "risk of serious harm", means. Might it not be time that we had answers to those questions?'

In practice, risk taking arises when decisions are to be made about furthering the independence of service users (Ryan, 1993) and thereby potentially exposing that patient to an increased risk of harm or injury to self or others. In a bid to minimize risk, increased attentions has been given to develop appropriate, valid and reliable assessment tools and to create new and more effective strategies to manage effectively the challenges that inevitably arise from increased risk taking.

Just as we have seen that 'risk' means different things to different people so too risk assessment will always be at best an inexact science. This can cause confusion for the novice practitioner who may be familiar with the natural sciences where predictability and consistency are norms. In risk assessment the problem arises because we are attempting to *apply* scientific methods and measures to human beings who have free will and are not compelled to do or act in deterministic ways.

Rudner (1968) argues that the natural sciences are inevitably deterministic, as a result of the universal law of gravity, for example, whenever an apple falls from a tree it will drop to the ground. On the other hand, the human sciences are inevitably probabilistic, for while universal laws may apply to people as much as they do to objects and substances, it is the consciousness and thought of human beings which give them 'free will', thereby resulting in the outcome of universal laws being variable. When working with people we therefore have to acknowledge free will and strive for the 'most probable' outcome rather than expect total consistency and uniformity.

Nevertheless, mental health practitioners do have an important role to play in developing assessment tools that minimize risk to the patient and others by enabling us to develop treatment strategies that are most likely to reduce harmful behaviours. To use such tools effectively practising nurses must have a sound understanding of the theories and issues which underpin the concept of risk in mental health practice.

Morgan and Priest (1991) identified four specific risk behaviours, namely:

1 *Aggression*: 'A hostile or offensive action or mental attitude, delivered within the controls of acceptable behavioural limits, in response to a perceived or real provocation.'
2 *Violence*: 'An expression of anger, fear or despair, through an extreme and forceful delivery of actions and emotions inflicting harmful or damaging effects.'

3 *Suicide or self-harm*: 'Inflicting damage, or injury, to self with an intention of relieving extreme tension or distress, or drawing attention to a need for help or causing death.'
4 *Severe self-neglect*: 'The act of disregarding care for self, with consequence of serious risk to personal health and well being.'

However, whenever we seek to assess risk behaviours, there are three underpinning considerations we ought to constantly keep in mind.

1 The assessment of risk should always be *a part of* a holistic assessment of the individual and never conducted as a stand-alone activity.
2 The person whom we are assessing will have strengths and positive qualities which should be recognized and incorporated into the care plan.
3 We must remain alert to our own prejudices and biases so as to prevent these from influencing our interpretation of the individual patient's behaviour.

It is important to remember that:

> the great majority of people with a psychiatric diagnosis are never violent and most of the violence in society is not committed by people with a psychiatric diagnosis. Variables such as low social class, young age, male gender, and substance or alcohol abuse are much better predictors of violence than mental state. Despite this, a disproportionate amount of media attention and public fear is focused on those patients who *do* commit violent acts! (Pilgrim & Rogers, 1999, p 181).

Bearing this in mind, we can see that not all risk behaviours are 'concerns' and that much will depend upon the context in which they are displayed. For example, aggression can be seen as beneficial as well as detrimental, acting as a safety valve to keep others at distance or to force long-overdue decisions or actions to be taken. On the other hand violence, whether actual physical assault on another, damage to property or extreme outbursts of verbal and/or written threats can only be regarded as detrimental.

Having attempted to define and contextualize risk it is now helpful to explore some of the principles that underpin risk assessment.

Principles of risk assessment

Risk assessment and management are approaches found in a variety of disciplines notably the:

- financial and insurance industry (Institute of Chartered Accountants, 1997);

- criminal justice system (Kemshall, 1996); and
- health and safety (Health and Safety Executive [NHSE], 1995).

Actuarial risk

Derived from the financial and insurance industry, actuarial risk assessment may be seen as the measurement of risk behaviours that is based upon the calculation of probability.

Remember earlier, Rudner's (1968) concept of the human sciences as probabilistic sciences. Here this notion is adapted in an attempt to predict the future behaviour of an individual patient by looking at: 'the behaviour of others in similar circumstances' (Kemshall, 1996, p 10). Such a model relies on the 'calculation of probability based upon statistics and population studies' and will therefore inevitably emphasize 'general trends' rather than be 'person specific'.

We know from insurers that we are twice as likely to be burgled if we live in an end terrace house but this doesn't help us to know *which* end terraces are more likely to be burgled than others nor does it encourage us to explore this further. In practice, such a statement is frequently interpreted as we should avoid buying an end terrace house at all costs. The same problem applies in assessing the risk posed by patients. If we know that diagnosed schizophrenics are far more likely to revert to violent behaviour than neurotics, does this mean we will release all neurotic patients regardless of their behaviour and never release anyone diagnosed as schizophrenic?.

Vinestock (1996, p 8), for example, has argued that: 'dangerousness is a perception by observers, that on the basis of what the subject has done or said in the past, there is a given probability of violent behaviour or harm in the future'. In many ways this is most unhelpful as it implies that people can never change, and would appear to make therapeutic intervention a total waste of time as predictors of *future* risk are to be based solely on evidence of *past* behaviour. If Vinestock were right we should always be able to predict accurately, yet in reality, empirical data on the performance of professional risk assessors does not inspire confidence. Monahan (1984) reviewed five major studies and found (pp 47–9) that: 'psychiatrists and psychologists are accurate in no more than one out of three predictions of violent behaviour over a several year period among institutional populations that had committed violence in the past (and thus had high base rates for it) and who were diagnosed as mentally ill'.

Risk assessment in criminal justice

Several years ago the Home Office spent several hundred thousands of pounds attempting to develop a predictive tool as to which offenders were most likely to reoffend. In spite of extensive investigation the Home Office concluded that nothing appeared to be more effective than: 'the judgement of the individual Probation Officer writing the Pre-Sentence Report or the Report for the Parole Board review'. Essentially the 'what works' factor was the: 'intimate knowledge that the individual Probation Officer has about the behavioural and attitude of the individual offender'.

In other words the assessment was based upon knowledge of the whole person and not about the behaviour alone. This has been carried forward by the Youth Justice Board (Roberts et al, 2001) with the development of ASSET (the standard assessment tool used by youth offending workers to appraise the risks posed by individuals to themselves and to the general public).

Before proceeding to explore the issues of clinical assessment it is important to pause and pull together some general principles for risk assessment. Kemshall (1996) reminds us when assessing risk, practitioners and managers should consider:

- the appropriate assessment methods to be used; and
- the likelihood of the risk management strategy being proposed leading to benefits for the individual while reducing the likelihood of risk to others.

As we have seen so far in this chapter, these considerations should be based upon a number of principles.

- Do not rely on clinical instruments alone to determine risks.
- Risk assessment is an interpersonal process.
- Focus on probability rather than certainty.
- Ground assessments in theory.

Ryrie (2000) added a number of other principles to our list, perhaps the most relevant to be added now is that:

- Risk assessment is an ongoing process.

Clinical assessment

Clinical assessment is designed to develop a 'balanced judgement and informed opinion that seeks to explain and understand risk behaviour' (Ryan, 1993, p 109). It invites a wide range of factors related to the person, the situation and their interaction and uses information based on interviewing, observation and reviewing service users' social history including previous clinical notes and the result of psychological and psychometric testing.

Those undertaking the assessment should be aware of the various models devised to explain violent and destructive behaviour, for example:

- *biological explanations* based on analysis of instinct or drive (ethological theories) or based upon neurological, hormonal or genetic factors;
- *psychological explanations* based upon social learning theory, motivation, cognition and the resultant psychopathy which can occur when social learning fails; and
- *transactional explanations,* which include considerations for the age, gender, sexuality, race and cultural backgrounds of the individual and how much individual characteristics have been regarded by others negatively in the past and with what consequences.

For example, Fernando (1998) writing about black people explained that the crisis for them:

> is not one of large numbers of black people breaking down with psychiatric disorders, but one of large numbers of black people coming to psychiatry forcibly, receiving more serious diagnoses compared to other groups and receiving greater doses of medication and greater restraint in settings of greater security.

Mason (1998) maintains that clinical risk assessment and prediction should be based upon:

- current offence (if known);
- behavioural cues;
- criminal history (if relevant);
- medical/psychiatric history;
- childhood development; and
- social and family circumstances;

to which we would add:

- previous responses to treatment;
- personal qualities and strengths;
- capacity to cope under pressure;
- sources of support available (internal and external);
- level of understanding;
- attitude towards treatment; and
- attitude towards self and others.

Here we use the concept of attitude towards self and others to gain a better understanding of the patients' motivation and their level of concern and empathy for others.

Ryan (1993) adopts a similar conclusion arguing that decisions about risk assessment should be based on an effective combination of both empirical evidence and clinical experience with actuarial adjuncts being made only to supplement clinical judgement. Harris et al (1993) prefer to see actuarial measures as the anchor point upon which to build 'structuring discretion' as clinical experience and holistic assessment are used to make an evaluation of the risk the *individual* patient poses to themselves and others.

Models of clinical risk assessment and predication

Limandi and Sheridan (1995) present three models based on material devised earlier by Ryan (1993) (see Table 10.1).

Risk management

Once the risk assessment has been completed, the next stage is to formulate effective risk management plans, which focus on the probability of a given outcome or several outcomes occurring. The risk management plan should clearly state precisely and specifically the nature or level of the risk. Doyle (1999) specifies seven key questions that help us when estimating the level of risk:

- What is the likelihood of harm occurring?
- How often is it likely to occur?

Table 10.1   Three models of clinical risk assessment

The Linear Model	This can be ideally suited to forensic settings where there are significant legal implications for all involved. Such models typically follow a series of clearly stated, logical steps, which are then followed by decision making regarding the most appropriate management methods. A caveat needs to accompany the use of this model and method in that the practitioner needs to be aware that for it to work logically or objectively, contextual factors are largely ignored. In essence the method of managing the threat can become more important then the content.
The Hypothetic-Inductive Model	This 'personal' approach relies more on the nurse's previous experience and knowledge of the service user while looking for patterns of behaviour and particular cues to the risk behaviour. A drawback with this approach is that this method of prediction can be (and is) limited by the nurse's previous experience and favoured methods of intervention. Consequently it is least effective with inexperienced nurses.
The Risk Benefit Model	Here the nurse should assume that all potential outcomes are possible but that some are identified and then placed into the current context. Nurses can then rate the likelihood of each outcome given the current and future contexts that may be available for the service user. This is done by balancing the identified risks with perceived benefits. The principal drawback with this method is that it can be time consuming, leaving the nurse weighed down by all the possibilities especially as the number and range of outcomes are potentially infinite.

Source: Limandi and Sheridan (1995)

- What possible outcomes may there be?
- Who is at risk?
- What is the immediacy of the risk?
- What is the time scale for assessment?
- What are the circumstances that are likely to increase or decrease the risk?

Woods (2001) has explained that for risk management to be effective clear statements of anticipated risk, and how these can be avoided, need to be made; thereby the impact of any risk is minimized.

This means that further questions need to be asked, such as:

- Do we have the personal and professional experience and resources to manage the risk?
- Is our working environment conducive to managing the risk?
- Particularly within the community are the carers, friends or neighbours likely to hinder the risk management plan?

Ryrie (2000) has developed this further, explaining that clinical risk management is the intended purpose of the assessment process. It involves the development of treatment strategies to reduce both the severity and frequency of identified risks (Snowden, 1997).

The areas shown in Table 10.2 are those that are deemed to be necessary for an effective risk management plan:

Practitioners should clearly understand and remember that the risk management plan does not constitute the end to the risk assessment process. We must remember that risks are contextual and situational and vary over time. The risk management plan is only a short-term strategy and should be constantly and methodically reviewed by all the individuals responsible for and involved in the service user's care (Ryrie, 2000). The most important message to stress to all practitioners and other people involved in risk assessment and management is the need for regular and effective communication and the establishment of up-to-date records. Through these channels the service users' progress, any changes to their mental state, any changes to the risk management plan, any changes to their treatment/management regime must be

Table 10.2 The areas deemed necessary for an effective risk management plan

The circumstances associated with previous risk behaviours
Any early warning signs that immediately precede risk behaviours
A description of what must change to reduce risk
The presentation of possible strategies to enable change to occur
An assessment of the service user's likely collaboration with each strategy
The roles and responsibilities of those involved in the service user's care
Responsibilities for responding to emergency situations
Dates for routine review and circumstances that would necessitate an immediate review

Source: Ryrie (2000)

communicated. It is the care co-ordinator within this risk management scenario who has the prime responsibility for ensuring that effective and dynamic lines of communication are established and maintained between all parties concerned.

Early warning signs

No risk assessment and risk management programme would be complete without a comprehensive analysis along relapse prevention lines which will have identified High Risk Factors as part of the process. High Risk Factors or early warning signs are: 'those internal or external events which increase the probability of behaviour happening' (Moore, 1996, p 116). Moore believes the best person to alert others to increased risk are patients themselves, but accepts this is not always possible and so it will frequently be down to others to trigger the warning process. To do this the case manager needs to:

● know what to look for; and
● be confident that the reporting of the warning signs is in the patient's best interests.

Understanding of *significant* warning signs is essential:

Most will be identified during assessment and added to during the monitoring phase as new situations arise. Others can often be suggested through relevant research into the specific conditions or behaviour. Pioneering work into early signs of relapse in schizophrenia, for example, has provided a checklist of commonly experienced phenomena and encourages the person concerned (and those closest to them) to identify other, more idiosyncratic signs too. The procedure then tests out the predictive accuracy of the signs and the ability of those involved in the next relapse. Through this process, recurrence of illness is detected at the earliest possible stage. (Moore, 1996, p 117)

There are obviously great benefits from this, for example the illness can: 'be treated far more quickly, often through a minimal increase in anti-psychotic medication, rather than deterioration to the point where drastic measures like hospitalisation are necessary' (Moore, 1996, p 117), but of course there is the other obvious benefit that the individual receives appropriate support and treatment *before* they pose a threat to others in the community.

The community safety agenda

As the Government is poised to review the Mental Health Act and has established Multiple Agency Public Protection Panels (MAPPPs) the need to have

reliable assessment tools and effective treatment strategies becomes imperative for everyone working in mental health. The general advice must be 'to
avoid making a prediction of No Risk', for, as Moore (1996, p 114) explains:
'everyone represents a risk, in the sense that they are theoretically capable of
causing harm'.

A 'No Risk' prediction is also unhelpful at the practical level leaving 'the
professional open to scathing and quite avoidable condemnation if proved
wrong' (Moore, 1996, p 141). Moore (1996, p 143) offers a strategy for
report writing and concludes: 'above all let the evidence drive the conclusion'.

The Community Safety Agenda dictates that we consider victims, especially
likely future victims in our assessments and in our plans. This adds an important new dimensions namely: How available does a victim need to be?

Sex Offender Orders introduced by the Crime and Disorder Act 1998
require paedophiles not only to be registered but also to stay away from places
frequented by children such as school grounds, swimming pools and play-
grounds. Here the concept of availability is being addressed as part of the calculation of the risk the paedophile presents to children in general.

Regardless of the presenting problem we need to appreciate that there
needs to be an available victim in any event which involves actual or potential harm to another and address this in our evaluation.

Moore (1996, p 106) has produced key questions to be addressed:

> What opportunity does the individual have to exercise a normal drive? How active
> has the individual been in seeking out victims? What characteristics are sufficient,
> or necessary, for a person to be selected as a victim? What would disqualify then
> from selection? Has any action of the individual increased the likelihood of trig-
> gering behaviour in a potential victim?

Conclusion

Assessment of individual risk begins with a holistic appraisal of the person
themselves, their background, family and personal history, the problems posed
and their attitude towards themselves, treatment and other people. Within the
diagnosed illness we need to be clear of the behaviour and triggers likely to
lead to recurrence and base decisions to increase self-accountability upon a
calculation of the benefit to the patient against the potential risks or costs to
others.

The assessment should look at motivational drive and aetiology and identify the controls and disinhibitors that have the greatest impact on the patient.
The result is an assessment based on evidence, which thereby offers the greatest possible probability of non-recurrence in a world governed by individual
whims.

The identification of early warning signs and of potential victims are both
vital components of the process and as community safety is even more

emphasized and Multiple Agency Public Protection Panels (MAPPPs) established, mental health practitioners are likely to be held more and more accountable for both their actions and their predictions.

References

Bean, P. (2001) *Mental Disorder and Community Safety*, Basingstoke: Palgrave – now Palgrave Macmillan.

Carson, D. (1996) Structural problems, perspectives and solution, in J. Peay (ed.), *Inquiries after Homicide*, London: Duckworth, 120–46.

Doyle, M. (1999) Organisational response to crisis and risk: issues and implications for mental health nurses, in T. Ryan (ed.), *Managing Crisis and Risk in Mental Health Nursing*, Cheltenham: Stanley Thornes, Ch 4, 40–56.

Fernando, S. (1998) *Mental Health Race and Culture*, London: MIND.

Harris, G. T., Rice, M. E. & Quinsey, V. L. (1993) Violent recidivism of mentally disordered offenders: the development of a statistical prediction instrument, *Criminal Justice and Behaviour*, 20, 315–35.

Health and Safety Executive (1995) *Five Steps to Risk Assessment*, London: HMSO.

Institute of Chartered Accountants (1997) *Business Risk Management*, London: ICAEW.

Kemshall, H. (1996) *Reviewing Risk: A Review of The Assessment and Management of Risk and Dangerousness: Implications for Policy and Practice in the Probation Service*, London: Home Office.

Limandi, B. J. & Sheridan, D. J. (1995) Prediction of intentional interpersonal violence: an introduction, in J. C. Campbell (ed.), *Assessing Dangerousness: Violence by Sexual Offenders, Batterers and Child Abusers*, London: Sage, 1–19.

Mason, T. (1998) Models of risk assessment in mental health practice: a critical examination, *Mental Health Care*, 11(12), 405–7.

Monahan, J. (1984) The prediction of violent behaviour: towards a second generation of theory and policy, *American Journal of Psychiatry*, 141, 10–15.

Moore, B. (1996) *Risk Assessment: A Practitioners Guide to Predicting Harmful Behaviour*, London: Whiting and Birch.

Morgan, H. & Priest, P. (1991) Suicide and other unexpected deaths among psychiatric inpatients: generalising useful knowledge, *International Journal of Law and Psychiatry*, 11, 249–57.

NHS Executive (1994) *Guidance on the Discharge of Mentally Disordered People and their Continuing Care in the Community (HSG994)27*, London: Department of Health.

Pilgrim, D. & Rogers, A. (1999) *A Sociology of Mental Health and Illness*, Milton Keynes: Open University Press.

Roberts, C., Baker, K., Merrington, S. & Jones, S. (2001) *Validity and Reliability of ASSET: Interim Report to the Youth Justice Board*, Oxford: Centre for Criminological Research University of Oxford, online at: http://www.youth-justice-board.gov.uk/policy/assetprn.pdf

Royal College of Psychiatrists (1998) *Management of Imminent Violence: Clinical Practice Guidelines: Quick Reference Guide*, London: Royal College of Psychiatrists.

Rudner, R. (1968) *Philosophy of Social Sciences*, Chicago: University of Chicago Press.

Ryan, T. (1993) *Good Practice in Risk Assessment and Risk Management*, London: Jessica Kingsley Publishers.

Ryrie, I. (2000) Assessing Risk, in C. Gamble & G. Brennan (eds), *Working with Serious Mental Illness: A Manual for Clinical Practice*, Ch 7, 97–111.

Snowden, P. (1997) Practical aspects of clinical risk assessment and management, *British Journal of Psychiatry*, 170(supp 32), 32–4.

Vinestock, M. (1996) Risk assessment: 'A word to the wise', *Advances in Psychiatric Treatment*, 2, 3–10.

Woods, P. (2001) Risk assessment and management, in C. Dale, T. Thompson & P. Woods (eds), *Forensic Mental Health: Issues in Practice*, Edinburgh: Ballier Tindall, Ch 9, 85–97.

CHAPTER 11

Creating and Maintaining a Safe Environment

NEIL WOODWARD, LYN WILLIAMS AND PETER MELIA

Indicative Benchmark Statements

- Participation in negotiation, formulation and communication of therapeutic interventions with users of mental health and social care services and their carers

- Awareness of the need to share mental health nursing information with other agencies involved in maintaining public safety

- Assessment and management of risk in mental health and social care settings

- Participation in the management of violent and aggressive behaviour

- Recognition of the importance of identifying and removing environmental dangers within mental health and social care settings

---

There has been much debate as to the influence of environment on incidences of self-harm, suicide and homicide and it is not our purpose to reiterate or re-rehearse these arguments. We would however, like to give some attention to environment and the extent to which we as mental health professionals contribute to its impact on our clients. In this, the authors feel it imperative that we accept from the outset, the considerable and significant role nurses play in creating an impression of the (physical and human) environment on the patient. For the sake of brevity and to fully exploit the unique contributions of the authors to the various dimensions of this chapter we shall consider the risk to self (suicide and self-injuriousness) and the risk to others (dangerousness) as separate entities.

It is our over-arching belief, however, that safety (not just being safe but feeling safe) is an imperative, which cannot be compromised if we are to deliver effective and comprehensive mental health services. In this we deliberately make no separation between staff, patients or carers but apply this principle to all who have contact with mental health services. Our proposition is that staff cannot effectively deliver effective therapeutic services unless they feel safe in so doing and patients cannot benefit from therapeutic interventions unless they feel safe enough to so do.

Dimensions of risk to self (suicide and self-injuriousness): what the boffins tell us

A task force was set up in the latter half of the 1990s and charged with undertaking a national confidential inquiry into homicides and suicides (DoH, 1999). An important lesson from history here is that in this case the inclusion of the term 'confidential' in the title referred to the manner in which the group dealt with information from those giving evidence. Most especially here it was the case that their priority was to gather full and accurate information and the group had no responsibility for establishing fault or blame. It was their stated opinion that when the focus was shifted from a 'blame culture' to one of establishing facts, learning lessons and changing practice the willingness of others to offer evidence increased manifold.

Of the national figures for deaths recorded by the Coroners' office as being suicide, 24 per cent (more than 1000 cases) had had contact with mental health services in the year prior to death. Half of this number had in fact had contact with mental health services in the week prior to death.

The figures below refer only to the 24 per cent of recorded deaths by suicide where there had been contact with mental health services in the year prior to death (n = circa 1000).

The most common method of suicide among men in the mental health population was hanging, and among women in that same population was self-poisoning by overdose, usually using the psychotropic medications prescribed for their mental health problems. More than half (63 per cent) had a history of self-harm and almost a fifth (19 per cent) had a history of violence towards others. There was a high prevalence of drug and alcohol abuse and again almost a fifth (17 per cent) had a history of abusing both alcohol and drugs.

The most commonly recorded diagnoses were depression, schizophrenia, personality disorder and drug or alcohol dependence with half having co-morbid states and dual diagnoses.

Suicide by mental health service users which occurred on the ward while the individual was receiving in-patient treatment were invariably by hanging and most frequently occurred during the evening and night. A significant number of in-patient suicides (25 per cent) occurred while the individual was under a 'special observations' regime and many staff contributing to this inquiry stated difficulties in maintaining observation were largely due to ward design and layout.

Of suicides by mental health service users who were not currently receiving in-patient treatments, 41 per cent occurred shortly after discharge and before the first follow up appointment. This number was at its peak in the week following discharge and was highest on the day after discharge.

A significant factor here appeared to be related to treatment optimism (on the part of the patient) as many such suicides occurred following the patient discharging him- or herself within seven days of admission for treatment.

Other high risk factors (statistically speaking) included non-compliance with treatment, disengagement from services and limited or poor social inclusion (often unemployed, single and living alone).

A synopsis of factors that increase the risk of suicide and serious self-harm would, then, include:

- a history of mental health problems;
- a history of self-harm;
- a history of drug and/or alcohol abuse;
- complex mental health needs (co-morbidity and dual diagnosis);
- non-compliance with treatment;
- disengagement from services;
- single and living alone;
- unemployment;
- recent discharge from mental health services; and
- pessimistic about treatment efficacy and recovery.

An environmental response

The group published its findings in 1999 (DoH, 1999) and made a total of 31 recommendations to reduce suicide among the mental health population in a number of ways by focusing on the human, physical and procedural environment. All of these areas deserve (if not demand) some consideration, albeit brief.

The human environment

The main aim here was to improve the skills of 'front line' staff in the recognition, assessment and management of suicide risk. This included attention to motivational skills training and multi-agency working to facilitate better maintenance of contact with disengaged patients and particularly the homeless; to legitimately link treatments for drug and alcohol dependence to mainstream psychiatric services; to increase the treatment potential and outcomes for patients with dual diagnoses; and to reduce non-compliance and treatment pessimism by improving both the acceptability and acceptance of effective treatments.

It should be noted here that the term 'disengagement' refers to the patient's unwillingness to go along with what we (the clinicians) feel is right and proper for him or her and is, therefore, a far more complex dynamic than might be suggested by the immediate impact of the term. This demands a more collaborative approach from the clinician and one in which the patient feels empathically understood and validated by his or her clinical team.

It is the experience of the authors that an essential factor in the disengagement of many patients is the fact that the experience of admission for psychiatric treatment can be particularly unpleasant. In the report '*Acute Problems, A Comprehensive Study of The Quality of Care in Acute Psychiatric Wards*' (Sainsbury Centre for Mental Health, 1998), many patients reported feeling particularly unsafe and vulnerable with little sense of privacy or cleanliness. Women are particularly concerned about their personal safety. It is difficult to imagine that psychiatric intervention can be really effective if the basic safety needs of our patients is poorly met.

The physical environment

Major factors here relate to means and opportunity and are most acutely focused on (i) observation and engagement and (ii) the prevention of suicide by removing the physical means by which an individual may secure a ligature.

An essential starting point for the physical environment is therefore to ensure there are no readily made anchor points for securing ligatures as this is the most common method used for suicide in in-patient services. The removal of load bearing curtain rails, showerheads, door and window hinges and coat hooks and their replacement with collapsible alternatives are an essential factor in making safe the physical environment. Adequate levels of staffing to ensure sound and timely levels of observation and engagement of patients, particularly during the evening and night, are similarly essential as is the minimization of 'blind spots' and the more open design of wards to ensure the environment does not hinder observation of patients.

The procedural environment

It will come as no surprise that the passage of information was yet again identified as a major issue in the failure to pick up and prevent suicides later considered to have been predictable and there is again a recommendation that there should be a single set of notes in which all disciplines record entries to aid communication. A somewhat more creative recommendation here, however, was that these should be a simplified version of a universal system of documentation (in effect a patient passport) which should follow the patient throughout his or her health career to include:

- clinical risk assessment recording key indicators and triggers;
- allocation to care under the CPA according to the evidence of risk and subsequent monitoring, review and re-evaluation; and
- transfer of information between services.

It was also felt essential that there was full information on previous convictions for violence available to mental health practitioners and that patients with a history of violence in the context of mental illness should receive the highest level of care under CPA.

In a similar vein it was also considered essential that family and psychological interventions should be available to high-risk clients, that there should be robust procedures for following up patients who disengage or are non-compliant and that there is a procedure for intensive post-discharge support and crisis intervention/resolution.

Dimensions of risk to others (dangerousness)

Similarly, the issue of staff safety has been one of increasing responsibility for many years and there has been a number of tragic, high profile cases, outlined with forceful impact by Braithwaite (2003):

1984   Isabel Schwartz, Social Worker
        Stabbed to death in Bexley Psychiatric Hospital
        Isabel's father said 'I hope this tragic event will never happen again'
        It has. Repeatedly
1985   Norma Morris, Social Worker
        Killed in Haringey
1986   Francis Betteridge, Social Worker
        Strangled in Birmingham
1988   Audrey Johnson, Social Worker
        Killed in London
1992   Katie Sullivan, Voluntary Worker
        Stabbed to death in MIND hostel in the Royal Borough of
        Kingston-upon-Thames
1993   Georgina Robinson, Therapist
        Stabbed to death
1993   Jonathan Newby, Voluntary Worker
        Stabbed to death
1998   Jenny Morrison, Social Worker
        Stabbed to death

Similarly the Health and Safety Act (1974) makes it incumbent that it is the responsibility of both the employer and employee to ensure all steps are taken to ensure the well being of individuals within the workplace. This is further edified in the Health Service Circular, HC 76(11), which outlines that it is the responsibility of every individual in the workplace to offer assistance to any person in need. The principle here being that it is a duty to use personal judgement and always act in good faith in the best interest of all.

In clinical practice, the potential for things to go wrong are closely related to the relationship between the health care practitioner and the client and good assessment is always the underpinning principle to risk and needs identification. In particular there is a need for mental health professionals to have appropriate training and supervision to ensure they are competent and confident in assessing the mental health needs of individuals and identifying any relationship between an individual's mental health deficit and potential for offending behaviour. From this there needs to be clear account given to the risks presented by any individual to the safety of staff or other clients.

There are steps we can take, however, to ensure that the environment supports the health care practitioner when things go wrong and broadly these can be overviewed under the headings of:

- Preparation of health care professionals;
- Professional practice; and
- Environment and support systems.

It is the experience of the authors that while in practice these areas are inextricably linked, thought can be given to each area independently.

Preparation of health care professionals

Training and preparation of staff is a key factor underpinning any approach to working with clients who may present particular dangers, either directly as a result of mental health deficit or incidentally (for example working in prisons and secure services). Such training needs to be focused, however, to acutely meet the particular needs of the clients in that particular service and should build upon the repertoire of core skills developed by psychiatric nurses. In particular the UKCC's document, '*The Recognition, Prevention and Therapeutic Management of Violence In Mental Health Care*' provides an outline framework for such and offers an excellent baseline of theoretical aspects, de-escalation strategies, breakaway techniques and restraint techniques that could form the basis of training programmes for nurses working with this client group. The same document also has comprehensive guidance on what trusts should include in their relevant policies, procedures, protocols and guidelines to support staff working with vulnerable clients and ensure good levels of care.

Similarly it is equally essential that nurses and other health care professionals are trained in identifying behavioural indications of increased risk of violence, can recognize the indicators and dynamics of a violence cycle and take steps to de-escalate potentially violent situations. Some early work in this area was outlined by Kaplan and Wheeler (1983) and further developed by Breakwell (1997) to offer an excellent model for recognizing, understanding and intervening in situations that are becoming potentially hostile.

In particular the need for training here is on the use of talking skills, body posture and relationship (de-escalation skills). The aim of training is to enable mental health staff to act to prevent high-risk situations getting out of control and similarly this demands the mental health practitioner giving thought to environmental hazards and the potential for the environment to contribute towards the situation. A core feature of risk management for mental health professionals is having a clear idea of the individual's capacity for high-risk behaviours (what may loosely be termed 'dangerousness') and the conditions under which that potential is likely to be recognized.

Melia and Kirby (2003) asserts that neither personality disorder nor mental illness in isolation will cause an individual to become dangerous towards others but notes that there must be some additional motivation. They outline, by example, that an individual maintaining aberrant sexual predilections will not necessarily act on those predilections unless there is some disinhibiting factor, causing him or her to so do. Disinhibiting factors in relation to violent impulses are predominantly determined by anger and processes of moral reasoning. An important point here is that the mental health professional does not respond to provocation with reciprocity as this can cause the individual to feel justified in acting out on some perceived moral outrage.

Certainly many reports relating to personal safety highlight the need for staff to receive appropriate training regarding personal safety, recognizing danger, de-escalation skills and physical intervention skills when working with clients who may become agitated or aggressive. In particular the improved confidence of staff that can be achieved by adequate training can itself have a considerable impact in the prevention of incidents of aggression and the reduction of associated incidents. Infantino and Musingo (1985) carried out a research-based approach to the evaluation of the impact of training in a mental health environment. Similarly McDonnell (1997) demonstrated that the introduction of training programmes for staff working with challenging behaviours considerably increased the confidence of staff and concomitantly reduced the number of incidents.

In particular this highlighted the value of de-escalation skills and Breakwell (1997) commented on the need to train staff in an awareness of an aggression cycle and to give particular attention to the various stages of the model (see Figure 11.1), in particular an awareness of triggers that can cause the client to act on feelings of being angry or upset and the resultant process of escalation.

In this it is argued that we all have a baseline of behaviour which for most people is non-aggressive. When a behaviour changes it emerges from that baseline to the trigger phase and this is a particularly high risk time. In this phase anything other than careful intervention by the practitioner can cause considerable escalation, possibly to actual aggression. In clinical practice the trigger can be any action or statement that could be perceived by the client as provocative and staff need to have a good assessment of their individual clients and the factors likely to trigger any one individual.

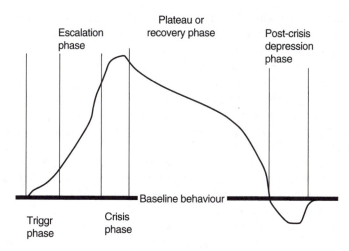

Figure 11.1 The aggression cycle

In such situations, however, a good knowledge of the client and the appropriate use of de-escalation skills can be extremely useful in preventing activation of trigger factors or preventing the client moving from the trigger phase into the escalation phase. Where this is not possible it is important to have a good knowledge of what works with the client to minimize vulnerability at such times and help the individual through the plateau or recovery and post-incident depression phases and back to baseline behaviours.

Important to note here that while in the plateau or recovery phase the client is still in a heightened state of sensitivity and this is a high risk time for further incidents of violence. Similarly as the client moves into the post-crisis depression phase there is an increased risk of self-harm and suicide.

Professional practice

Again in this area a crucial factor is the mental health professional's knowledge of the client and capacity or ability to recognize when the client is suffering psychiatric distress or has an impaired cognitive capacity to solve problems or make sense of a given situation. It is relatively frequent and common, particularly when working with psychotic patients, for the cognitive capacity to be so severely impaired that the individual is unable to make good judgements, even with an appropriate level of information. Consequently the potential for the individual to misperceive behaviours on the part of the mental health practitioner is considerably increased.

Similarly there is a wealth of information around the adverse effects of high expressed emotion working with clients who suffer psychiatric disorders and it is particularly important that mental health practitioners maintain professional relationships with their clients which are emotionally unchallenging and using low expressed emotion techniques, in particular avoiding moral judgements and blame or censureship.

Similarly it is imperative that individual practitioners have good knowledge and understanding of the individual's history of high-risk behaviours and, particularly working with forensic clients, knowledge and understanding of past history of offences and the circumstances in which they occurred. This can reveal valid information on the likely targets (for example men, women, children or such) and the processes by which individual clients may groom an environment to enable an assault to take place. It can also give a good indication of the likely trigger factors that can lead to clients presenting high risk behaviours and more importantly can inform the practitioner how to prevent or manage an out of control situation.

Again, we would reiterate that it is essential to have a good understanding of the impact of your own presence in terms of body language on the client and to use that presence in a collaborative, communicative manner, to help develop a therapeutic relationship with the client and to prevent the relationship becoming hostile.

Demonstrating good knowledge and understanding of your client's problems can contribute significantly to the development of therapeutic relationships. Many clients will actually feel significantly reassured and impressed by the fact that the mental health practitioner has taken time to compile a good understanding of the client's past problems and mental health history. This can be further enhanced by utilizing such knowledge to demonstrate that you are there to offer help and encouragement and that you are concerned about the wellbeing of the client.

Body posture is particularly important when you actually approach a client who may already be agitated, aggressive or particularly anxious. It is important not to reflect the client's own state of agitation in your behaviour as this can further inflame a situation. Caraulia and Steiger (1997) suggest the following tips to maintain a safe stance when dealing with clients who may be agitated, aggressive or anxious.

- Maintain a distance of 2–3 feet from the individual, so that you do not give any indication that you may be invading their personal space.
- Keep the hands open and in a neutral position, so that the client does not misperceive you to be making a fist or concealing some weapon.
- Keep the feet apart slightly, in an L shape, and stand slightly sideways towards the patient so that he does not feel that you are 'squaring up'.

This body posture will appear less threatening to the patient and potentially less challenging but is also a good position for protecting yourself if the client does make any attempt to assault. Another particularly important factor in the preparation for the role is giving good consideration to the nurse's attire and the impact this may have in terms of the gaze of the patient. The nurse needs to ensure they are dressed in a manner that facilitates the discharge of the responsibilities in a timely and appropriate fashion and this was to some extent considered by the guidance issued by the Royal College of Nursing publication in 1998 and in particular focused on the need for the nurse to be dressed in a manner that exhibits a professional demeanour. Some obvious and easily identifiable safety features here are to avoid wearing excessive jewellery, in particular items such as large earrings which can be dragged or pulled, and neck ties (other than the clip on type) as these increase the risk of strangulation and are an easy target for a disturbed client. Keeping long hair tied back and wearing footwear that would not inhibit the individual if they needed to respond to, or escape from, an incident or situation is also advisable. Obviously the general clothing of the nurse should similarly ensure they are able to discharge their duties without impedance.

Similarly nurses need to be aware that their clothing does not contain any imagery which may be construed as aligning them to a particular political or social order that may cause offence to a client. This can include wearing football tops, or military style clothing imbuing politically based connotations (Frude and Davies, 1999). Staff working in forensic situations or with forensic patients also need to be mindful of the style of clothing worn as many clients, particularly those with a history of sexual offending and known to have impaired or distorted cognitive processes, can misperceive styles of dress as sexually provocative or sexually alluring. This can be a trigger factor in contributing to patients' disturbed behaviour.

Again in this it is not only a mindfulness about your own physical appearance but the need to have a good understanding of your patients' mental health deficit and history of offending behaviours. The rule of thumb is that the style of clothing worn for work should highlight your role as a professional person working in a client-centred way rather than as a sexual being.

Environment and routines

Again there are some essential and basic routines and systems staff can employ to minimize the potential for their personal safety to become jeopardized. These are particularly important for individuals who work in the community but remembering that all health professionals travel to and from the place of work and can become targeted at such times and so are equally important in such circumstances.

Some basic approaches that have been adopted include issues such as car security and these can be summarized as:

- Park your car park in a well-lit area, away from bushes or potential hiding places.

- Ensure the car is parked facing your intended exit and that there are no obstructions that may need careful manoeuvring.
- If parking on a hill, park with the car facing down the hill as the chances of stalling if attempting to drive away in a state of heightened anxiety are far greater moving up the hill and if parking is in a cul-de-sac, ensure the car is facing the exit to the cul-de-sac and does not need turning around at a later point.
- Have your keys in your hand when approaching your car so you do not have to fumble around a bag or pockets to locate your keys.
- While in your car, ensure all doors remain locked and if a car alarm is fitted familiarize yourself with how the 'personal attack' system is operated.
- Always be aware of property within the car and how this may be viewed by others (especially where hospital or health service insignia are visible as this can indicate the possible presence of medical equipment and medications).
- Be particularly aware at potential stopping points (such as traffic lights and major road junctions) as it has become more common for individuals to make 'quick grab' attacks. This can be a particular danger to nursing staff who are known to carry bags containing medical equipment and medications in the course of their duties (for example community psychiatric nurses).
- Do not leave hospital parking permits displayed in the window of the car as displaying the parking permits for hospitals can be an attraction to individuals seeking medical equipment or medications.

The authors would recommend that Trusts adopt a system of identification by hand held badges, similar to those worn by staff while on duty, and is entirely in line with the Patient's Charter which requires all health care staff to be identifiable by name. Such systems are more desirable for health care staff than the permit system (visible in the windscreen) as it does not immediately identify the cars of health care staff as being such.

In a similar vein it is considered fairly essential that all staff employ some system for ensuring that colleagues know their whereabouts and have a mechanism for regular reporting in. In this way if things do go wrong the gap before the alarm is raised is minimal. Simple mechanisms here can be employed to ensure that when leaving an area colleagues know where you are going and how long you are likely to be and to employ an agreed check in time. The NHS Executive (1998) recommended that in all community teams there should be a routine and properly managed system of ensuring there is good knowledge of where staff are working in the community at any given time.

A simple system such as an appointments board and phone contact systems can be employed to routinely monitor the whereabouts and well being of individual staff. In addition the RCN (1998) advised the adoption of a 'check in' system for staff, particularly when working with clients who are considered to present a particular risk. In this there is a routine expectation that the staff will phone in both at agreed times during the course of the contact and when leaving the client or finishing a shift.

A common and useful system often employed to ensure this works effectively is to identify one individual with responsibility for ensuring that the whereabouts of all staff within the team was known and that each member was safe. In particular there is a need to ensure a robust mechanism for ensuring each member of the team has safely finished their duties and had left the work environment for home (and that no one was left incapacitated or held against their will in a client's home or some other area).

Many community mental health teams also ensure up to date records of all staff details are immediately available in case any individual staff became uncontactable and there were fears about their well being. As a minimum these should include name, address, contact telephone numbers and car registration and description. This system is particular valuable if it becomes necessary to bring in the Police as having this essential information to hand will greatly aid their search efforts (and reduce the time taken to ensure the police have all available information to expedite their searches).

Similarly, when working with a client it is essential to keep a good knowledge of the environment and be aware of exit points. In this regard the rule remains the same irrespective of whether working in the community with clients in their own homes or within inpatient services. It is essential that when working alone with clients there is an easily accessible exit point that can be used by the nurse if a threatening situation arises and one that cannot easily be impeded by the client. In this case it is essential to ensure that the nurse remains in a position where they can not be backed into an isolated situation by the client. Ideally the nurse should be positioned between the client and the door and a little forethought before entering a room will enable the nurse to position the seats for this to take place as a matter of apparent routine.

Walker et al (2002) highlight the need to take care when advancing into a room particularly if moving away from the door, to be aware of the increased risk to safety and to try and keep an exit from a room clear in case there is need to escape. In particular the experience of the authors is that it is similarly important when walking with the client, to walk at the side or slightly behind the client and always maintain a position where the client is in full view. If you find yourself in a position where you are slightly in front of the client it is difficult to observe what is happening and it can facilitate an opportunity for the client to make an unobserved attack if they are so motivated.

These basic techniques are of particular value and are highlighted in Healey (2003) who reported a situation where a Health Visitor became isolated in a house, being threatened by the relative of a client wielding a claw hammer. It was only her ability to adopt good interpersonal and de-escalation skills and her management of the environment which enabled her to reach an exit point that allowed her to leave the situation unharmed and raise the alarm.

Many forensic institutions similarly take steps to design rooms having two juxtaposed exit points. This makes it difficult for any individual to barricade him or herself in the room in the first place but also makes it easier for staff to enter from different points should the worst case scenario happen and people become hostages within the room. Similarly, forensic environments ensure the fitting of doors that open outwards to prevent doors being barricaded or jammed shut to prevent entry by other staff.

There has also been an increasing use of personal alarms and these seem to be well received and valued by staff though as Mason and Chandley (1999) point out the use of the alarm is only as effective as the response it attracts. It is the experience of the authors, however, that there is value in the use of personal alarms as staff are more confident if they feel they have some mechanism for attracting help should things go wrong. Due to the diverse number of alarms available, and the lack of clarity about who is responsible for responding to them we feel it is essential that training is given to staff both in the use of alarms and their responsibilities when becoming aware of an alarm being activated by a colleague or some other individual within that area. Training should include the awareness of protocols and operational procedures for the use of personal attack alarms in specific clinical areas.

Walker et al (2002) note that nurses do often jeopardize their own personal safety to the promotion of therapeutic alliance and their caring demeanour and while this must always be applauded in its intent it needs to be carefully balanced in its value to the client. In particular we must note here that alarms are only as effective as the use of the voice and are entirely dependent upon the individual's whereabouts and whether either the voice or the alarm is audible to other staff within the vicinity. This again requires planning and careful consideration of the environment and the systems put in place to support staff.

Braithewaite (2001) agrees that issuing alarms to staff is good practice, but comments that these are only properly effective where good training is given as many staff are not aware of what they should do when one is activated and may not have the skills to de-escalate or control a situation of physical violence in any case. In our experience personal alarms are very effective for attracting attention when things go wrong, for giving nurses the sense of security in their routine practice and for attracting attention if it is felt necessary. The effectiveness, therefore, is entirely dependent on managers providing a well planned and agreed response mechanism to be actioned in the event of an alarm being activated. This view is supported by Frude and Davies (1999).

Clearly then there is much overlap in the procedural, environmental and human factors associated with risk to self and others and there needs to be clear attention given to an awareness of the impact of the individual's contribution to the environment at any given time. As mental health professionals we do our clients, our families, our peers and ourselves a gross disservice when we take unwitting and unacceptable risks with the safety of ourselves or others.

Conclusion

It has long been a truism in mental health services that there is a balance between safety (security) and therapy and we as experienced mental health professionals would like to challenge this antiquated notion as we believe there is no such balance. It is our opinion that a balance suggests compromise (the view that either we do not offer too much therapy as we have to maintain security or conversely that we have to take major risks as we are here to offer therapy) and we do not accept this. If we offer security without therapy we are affording our clients little more than asylum and incarceration. If we offer therapy without security we are whistling in the wind and there is little hope of truly engaging our clients unless they and we feel safe.

Only when there is security *and* therapy do we truly achieve efficacy of effort.

References

Braithewaite, R. (2001) *Managing Aggression*, London: Routledge.

Braithewaite, R. (2003) *Turning Down the Heat*, London: Pavilion.

Breakwell, G. M. (1997) *Coping with Aggressive Behaviour*, British Psychological Society, University of Surrey.

Caraulia, A. & Steiger, L. K. (1997) *Non violent crisis intervention: Learning to defuse explosive behavior*, Brookfield WI: CPI Publications, 139.

Consterdine, P. (1997) *Streetwise: The Complete Manual of Personal Security and Self Defence*, Trowbridge: Redwood Books.

Department of Health (1999) *Safer Services: National Confidential Inquiry into Suicide and Homicide by People with Mental Illness*, London: HMSO.

Department of Health & Social Security (1976) *The Management of Violent or Potentially Violent Hospital Patients*, London: DHSS.

Frude, N. & Davies, W. (1999) *Preventing Face to Face Violence. Dealing with Anger and Aggression at Work*, (3re edn), London: Association of Psychological Therapies.

Garnham, P. (2001) Understanding and dealing with anger, aggression and violence, *Nursing Standard*, 16(6), 37–42.

Health and Safety Executive (1974) *Health and Safety at Work Act*, London: HMSO.

Healy, P. (2003) Risky business, *Nursing Standard*, 17(17), 15–16.

Infantino, J. & Musingo, S. Y. (1985) Assaults and injuries amongst staff with and without training in aggression and control techniques, *Journal of Hospital and Community Psychiatry*, 32, 497–8.

Kaplan, S. G. & Wheeler, E. G. (1983) Survival skills for working with potentially violent clients, *Social Casework*, 64, 339–45.

McDonnell, A. (1997) Training care staff to manage challenging behaviour: an evaluation of a three day training course, *The British Journal of Developmental Disabilities*, 43(85), 156–62.

Mason, T. & Chandley, M. (1999) Management of Violence and Aggression for Healthcare Workers, Edinburgh: Churchill Livingstone.

Melia, P. & Kirby, S. D. (2003) Assessing and engaging people with personality disorder, in S. Kirby, D. A. Hart, D. Cross & G. Mitchell (eds), *Mental Health Nursing: Competencies for Practice*, Basingstoke: Palgrave Macmillan, Ch 18.

NHS Executive (1998) *We Don't Have to Take This: NHS Zero Tolerance Campaign*, London: HMSO.

Royal College of Nursing & NHS Executive (1998) *Safer Working In The Community*, London: RCN Publishing.

Sainsbury Centre for Mental Health (1998) *Acute Problems: A Survey of the Quality of Care in Acute Psychiatric Wards*, London: Sainsbury Centre for Mental Health.

United Kingdom Central Council for Nursing, Midwifery and Health Visiting (2001) *The Recognition, Prevention and Therapeutic Management of Violence in Mental Health Care*, London: UKCC.

Walker, J., Wren, J. & Skalycz, A. (2002) Safety first, *Nursing Times*, 98(9), 20–1.

PART III

CONTINUUM OF TREATMENT

By now we have reached the core of the text namely what can be done once the person has been assessed as being mentally ill and in need of treatment. We will thus explore the treatment continuum beginning with community-based services then at the importance of mental health hospitals and specialist secure facilities and finally go on to explore the need for a continuity of care upon discharge.

CHAPTER 12

Interdisciplinary Approaches to Community Mental Health Practice

DENIS A. HART AND ANGELA HALL

Indicative Benchmark Statements

■ Application of the mental health policies and frameworks for service delivery

■ Identification of the scope and range of comprehensive, integrated mental health and social care services

■ Contribution to the current systems of care, e.g.: Care Co-ordination

■ Awareness of the relationships between NHS Direct, Primary Health Care Trusts and Specialist Mental Health Services

■ Ability to contribute to multidisciplinary Care Co-ordination

Introduction

This chapter aims to provide an insight into the development of Integrated Community Care Policy in Mental Health and the Models of Service Provision that have been developed. It will also identify the relationships between Primary and Secondary Services and explore how this has led to an Integrated Care Co-ordination Framework for Health and Social Care in Mental Health.

In the past four decades Government policy has driven the location of mental health care from the large institutions into the community. Many socio-economic and political factors provided the impetus for change and are considered well in other texts (e.g., Means & Smithm, 1994; Rogers & Pilgrim, 2001).

The Mental Health Act 1983 accelerated the hospital closures programme by recognizing that any admission to hospital should be encouraged under Section 131 on a Voluntary basis although provisions for compulsory admissions were carried forward, under Sections 2, 3 and 4 respectively. The Government introduced the Mental Illness Specific Grant (MISG) to establish community mental health teams and to ring fence money for the after care of patients. Furthermore Section 117 of the MHA 1983 provided for free aftercare for all patients who had been previously compulsorily detained under Section 3.

The MISG therefore led to mental health being seen as outside of the National Health Service and Community Care Act (NHSCCA) (1990) and this worked effectively while budget levels remained high even long after most hospitals had closed. During the late 1990s a number of local authorities were taken to judicial review as budgets became reduced and they sought to means test all discharged patients voluntary and compulsory alike. In essence CMHTs had failed to recognize their connectedness to adult teams and community care legislation. Discharged informal patients should receive services from the main community care budget and pay for them subject to means (Health and Social Services And Social Security Adjudication Act, 1983) while formally detained patients whether under Section 3 or Section 37 of the MHA 1983 should receive services free as part of their after care plan. This has been further complicated in 2002 by the abolition of the MISG but local authorities have been instructed by Government for the foreseeable future to top slice 30 per cent of the community care budget for the provision and development of multi-disciplinary community mental health services.

The need to recognize the importance of the NHSCCA (1990) is further evidenced by the fact that GPs became fund holders which, essentially, gave them the power to employ their own mental health workers or to pay for those already established. This led to many GPs employing counsellors and encouraging practice nurses to become more involved in mental health work, who quickly realized that they were unable to meet effectively the needs of these patients and simply passed them back to the CMHTs.

With 'New Labour' came strong directives being made in relation to how mental health services should be developed in the form of *Modernising Mental Health Services* (DoH, 1998) and the *National Service Framework for Mental Health* (DoH, 1999a), *A First Class Service* (DoH, 1999c) and the *NHS Plan* (DoH, 2000). The essence of this policy direction is to ensure effective services are put in place, which can:

- use the established evidence base available; and
- manage patients safely in the community, minimizing risk by offering support and assisting in recovery (adapted from Sainsbury Centre, 2001).

The once contemporary reference to the 'internal market' has now disappeared and has been replaced by an expectation of co-operation and collaboration within and across services. The Government's emphasis has been on 'joined upness' and this is reflected in the way mental health care should be delivered according to the NSF standards (DoH, 1999a). The monitoring and auditing of mental health services, through clinical audit can be a valuable method of evaluating the quality of service provided. Rather than having an audit imposed by management, the clinical team can be proactive, establishing their own criteria. Multi-disciplinary auditing is seen as the best way forward (Ash, 1997) and should incorporate organizational reflective learning. While then, the CMHT provides a focus for clinical and organizational interventions it should nevertheless respond to feedback from auditing to ensure a more responsive service, which ultimately meets the needs of the mentally ill and their carers.

Despite the agreed standards (DoH, 1999a) and the policy directives, there continues to be variation in how these are implemented, if at all, and there exist diverse models of services delivery. We will now briefly outline the main models of community mental health care.

Models of service provision

Caplan's (1964) theory of preventative psychiatry provides a framework for practitioners in locating the principles and aims of mental health services. The boundaries shown in Table 12.1 distinguish primary, secondary and tertiary

Table 12.1 Theory of preventative psychiatry

Stages of preventative psychiatry	Aim of interventions	Main services involved
Primary prevention	To intervene with people at risk of mental illness, i.e. people in crisis to offer help and coping to reduce likelihood of mental illness developing.	Helplines i.e. Childline, Samaritans, NHS Direct Support Groups i.e. Gingerbread, Homestart UK, Compassionate Friends, Cruse Primary Care Groups
Secondary prevention	To ensure early detection and treatment for people experiencing mental illness. It includes early diagnosis and intervention.	Primary Care Groups including, Counsellors, Primary Care Link Workers, Psychological Services, Liaison Psychiatry and Community Mental Health Teams, Acute In-patient, Partial Hospitalization and Day services.
Tertiary prevention	To promote the person's quality of life and minimize the degree of distress and disability caused by the mental illness	Community Mental Health Teams, Day Services, Crisis Resolution Teams, Assertive Outreach Teams, Community Units (extended care, rehabilitation)

Source: Caplan (1964)

levels of prevention but you should note that these may not be so clear cut in actual practice.

In mental health it is often difficult to locate or identify the point where illness begins, as mental health problems can be linked to learned processes, developmental changes or difficult psychological and social situations. Pivotal to Caplan's (1964) theory is the belief that mental illness develops from negative adjustment and poor coping responses to life 'crises'. Caplan's theory is essentially an optimistic one in so far as he sees people in crisis as being at both their most vulnerable and in their most receptive state to receive help and make lasting change. Within this model, community mental health services may be seen as not only supporting the individual but also as improving the interaction between the person and their environment and to promote timely intervention to encourage positive adjustment and coping strategies.

Primary care trusts (PCTs)

The NSF stresses that health and social care agencies should seize the initiative for change in local communities The development of PCTs and the *Shifting the Balance of Power* (Department of Health, 2001a) have continued a policy driven towards a primary care led NHS. The population served by any particular PCT usually forms the basis around which partnership working, planning and co-ordinated service delivery takes place. With the creation of PCTs, the boundaries between primary and secondary or specialist care shift, and accepted definitions of care are eroded as more specialist work is undertaken both in primary care settings and people's homes (Onyett, 2003).

Despite conflicting views as to their role, there is evidence to show that PCTs have the potential to produce better working relationships between primary and secondary services that consequently show CPNs working effectively in the area of primary care (Lee et al, 2002). Changed practice inevitably will require a similar change in the kinds of people required to deliver services. *The NHS Plan* (DoH, 2000) recognizes the need to build further capacity within primary care and sets out to recruit 1000 graduate primary care workers who will receive training in providing brief solution-focused therapies of proven effectiveness for people of all ages. Many secondary mental health services have employed, and attached, primary link workers to improve the interface between primary and secondary services and to act as gatekeepers to the more specialist mental health services. *The NHS Plan* (DoH, 2000) also proposes the appointment of 500 new 'Gateway' workers by 2003/4. They will be employed to work with primary care, A&E Departments, NHS Direct and Crisis Teams to help respond to those needing immediate help.

Helplines

One recent innovative approach that has been set up are telephone help lines, designed to help people cope with the psychological and social problems that can impact on their mental health. The major new national service set up is NHS Direct where people can receive expert advice from trained professionals. Other National Helplines have been available for some time, for instance The Samaritans who provide 24 hour counselling for people in need of help, not just for those who are suicidal (Wright and Giddey, 1993). Many other voluntary helplines are available for people with more specific psychological or social difficulties and their numbers are available from directory enquiries.

Liaison mental health nursing

Liaison mental health nursing is a term used to cover the provision of mental health services to people working in a wide range of medical settings. It recognizes the psychosocial problems that can co-exist with any physical illness or disease. Similar to other models of provision, like crisis intervention and assertive outreach, it developed from the USA with its predecessor being psychiatric consultation liaison nursing. There was limited research into the effectiveness of the role and what research that has been conducted has tended to focus on the system and process of referrals (Davis & Nelson, 1980; Fincannon, 1995; Newton & Wilson, 1990).

In the UK the role of liaison developed in response to the increasing numbers of people attempting suicide, particularly self-poisoning, during the 1980s. The nurse's role in carrying out a mental health assessment was found to be effective (Catalan et al, 1980), and the expansion of liaison mental health nurses based in A&E Departments began. Other areas that are supported with liaison mental health nursing are cancer care, HIV and AIDS, cardiac rehabilitation, Chronic Fatigue Syndrome, Post-traumatic Stress and body image disorders (Regel & Roberts, 2002). According to Regel and Roberts (2002), the aims of liaison mental health, therefore, are seen to be:

- to provide an in reach to a diverse range of medical services;
- to identify and assess mental health problems in people with a physical illness;
- to recognize the impact of any mental illness on the person's physical health;
- to intervene to reduce the impact and effects of mental health problems on a person with a physical illness; and
- to educate non-mental health colleagues as part of their role in mental health promotion.

Secondary mental health services

Secondary specialist services aim to provide both secondary and tertiary care to people experiencing mental illness. Secondary prevention (Caplan, 1964) is focused on early detection and intervention. Screening of, and working with, 'at risk' groups can also be considered an aim of secondary care, although it is more difficult to evaluate the effectiveness of this, in comparison with other screening programmes, for example, cervical cancer. Tertiary prevention (Caplan, 1964) aims to reduce the impact of the illness on the person's functioning and quality of life and in mental health those with a serious and complex mental illness are most likely to experience the most disabling effects. It is the responsibility of all secondary services to ensure that adequate secondary and tertiary care is planned and provided in collaboration with service users and others involved in their care.

Primary mental health workers

There appears to be three identifiable models of working in primary care for the mental health worker. One is a facilitator of mental health services (Armstrong, 1995), occupying a diverse role with the expectations of delivering education and training to non-mental health personnel, promoting mental health awareness and providing access to other services. A second model is that of collaboration (Nolan & Badger, 2002; Tummey, 2001), whereby the Primary Mental Health Worker (PMHW) establishes a link between primary and secondary care offering brief intervention and also acting as a 'gatekeeper' for services. The third model, identified in the work of Gask et al (1997) and supported by Roberts (2002), is that of consultation/liaison which involves the PMHW working closely in collaboration with the GP and the primary care team. The main aim of this is to ensure that the care of patients with neurotic illnesses remains in primary care settings.

In 1995 the HAS report (NHS Health Advisory Service, 1995) stated that the PMHW role should be undertaken by a senior mental health clinician who should have autonomy, accountability and the ability to utilize specialist knowledge to assist other professionals in making decisions or in working with people with mental health problems. Nolan and Badger (2002, p 145) stated that the core attributes of a PMHW are:

- specialist knowledge of specialist mental health (dependant upon their own particular specialist field);
- experience of working in a community setting with people with mental health problems and their families;
- a senior level within their profession, with the ability to take responsibility for decision making;
- assessment skills;

- an ability to provide clinical supervision and consultation to other professionals on a variety of levels;
- excellent communication and networking skills; and
- a range of direct work/therapeutic skills.

As PCTs continue to evolve, Badger and Nolan (1999), claim that CPNs will be the largest professional group involved and have a significant part to play in the organization, management and delivery of mental health services in primary care, essentially they will be the major source of PMHWs.

Community mental health teams

Originally set up under the MHA 1983, CMHTs are multi disciplinary usually consisting of community psychiatric nurses, social workers and a consultant psychiatrist although there are many variations as to which other professionals are involved with the team such as occupational therapists and psychologists.

Some CMHTs have traditionally aimed to provide a wide range of services to the population, which ultimately has led to the reported neglect of people with severe mental health needs. *The Third Quinquennial National Community Psychiatric Nursing Survey* (University of Manchester, 1991) found that 80 per cent of people with schizophrenia were not on a CPN caseload. It is the role of the CMHT to liaise with primary care and other referring agencies to ensure that appropriate referrals are presented to the team. Many teams have redefined the client group to which they will respond, referring to their clients as people with serious or enduring mental illness, which has led to a gap in services for those considered to have more common mental health problems (DoH, 1999a). CMHTs have been viewed by some as the cornerstone of community care (Ovretveit, 1993) as they provide a focal point for all other service provision.

Where CMHTs continue to accept a range of service user referrals, a system for gatekeeping is required, to ensure those with greatest need are prioritized. The person receiving the referral initially deals with the information, however another worker may be allocated to carry out the assessment following a weekly team meeting. Any urgent referrals are dealt with by the team member receiving the initial enquiry, or the one on duty that day. Following a comprehensive assessment the team member will either accept the role of care co-ordinator for ongoing provision, refer to another member of the team or refer back to the referring agency with advice. The ongoing intervention and plan of care will be agreed between the care co-ordinator, the service user and any others significant to the client's care. The need for assessment of any carer shall also be explored and when necessary provided in keeping with provision outlined by the Community Care (Patient in the Community) Act (1995).

On-going intervention should be informed by the current mental health evidence base identifying best practice, including the service user's perception (DoH, 2001b). Findings have shown that CPNs are in a strong position to carry out psychosocial interventions providing that they have the appropriate training and supervision (Haddock & Slade, 1996; Rogers & Pilgrim, 2001). The NSF (DoH, 1999a) and the Mental Health Policy Implementation Guide for CMHTs (DoH, 2002) set out to ensure clients receive a better and more efficient service. It is clear that one service is less likely to be able to respond to people with a range of needs, relating to their mental health and therefore if services providers are integrated and adopt a truly evidence-based approach, in their approach then service users are more likely to receive an effective co-ordinated response. A seamless service can be achieved through the care co-ordination process which promotes:

- a single point of referral to secondary mental health services;
- a unified health and social care assessment;
- co-ordination of the respective roles and responsibilities of each agency in the system; and
- access through a single process, to the support and resources of both health and social care (adapted from DoH, 1999b).

The same policy document summarizes the key roles and functions of the Community Mental Health Team as follows:

- dealing with referrals and enquiries to the team;
- providing comprehensive assessments including assessment of any risk;
- applying criteria based responses, Critical (respond within 4 hours), Substantial (respond within 2 days), Moderate (respond within 10 days), Routine (respond within 21 days);
- screening for mental health problems in the general population;
- acting as a gatekeeper to other secondary mental health services;
- acting as care co-ordinator – Assessment – goal setting – planning interventions – produce care plans, crisis plans – review and evaluate effectiveness. Use of standardized tools for monitoring user outcomes;
- working within a professional, legal and ethical framework for practice;
- engagement and disengagement, developing working alliances;
- recognizing factors influencing relapse and providing early intervention;
- providing information and education to service users and their carers;
- developing vocational, occupational and financial opportunities to improve the person's quality of life;
- monitoring the side effects of psychotropic drugs, and negotiating medication plans and advanced directives with service users and their families;
- brokering for other services required;
- inter-professional working with others involved in meeting service user needs; and

- engaging in clinical supervision and clinical audit to ensure quality of care and value for money.

Interdisciplinary working is generally accepted as the ideal, as it is thought to improve the quality and diversity of care offered. Gamble and Brennan (2000) suggest that for this to happen several areas would need to be addressed including a shared understanding of each others' roles, and the contribution they can make to a clients care (Gijbels, 1995). Power is an important factor in team working, medical staff are traditionally viewed as having more power and this can lead to conflicts and non-cooperation. This then leads to ineffective negotiation of care packages and also inappropriate delegation of work.

The interface between primary care and secondary mental health services is crucial and Brooker and Repper (1998) identify several models that exist to manage this. The 'replacement approach' involves the CMHT replacing the GP in providing care. The 'shifted out-patient approach' involves mental health practitioners being relocated to primary care settings, however where this model is used CMHTs were found to have the lowest numbers of people with a severe mental illness on their caseload (Onyett et al, 1994). The 'liaison attachment' model is where there is a named link worker who undertakes the initial screening and acts as a gatekeeper who refers, where appropriate, to secondary services and, if that is not appropriate, then on to other services. There is support from GPs in relation to this approach (Hughes et al, 1992), which appears to have been adopted by many secondary services to enable them to refocus on those people with a serious mental illness.

Crisis intervention/intensive home treatment

Crisis intervention as a model of care began in the US with the essential aim of preventing unnecessary admission to hospital. This is primarily based on the work of Lindemann (1944) and Caplan (1964) who both realized that the point of 'crisis' is a critical stage when appropriate intervention can lead to more positive outcomes for the individual.

Following successful 'crisis' services in Denver in the USA (Langsley et al, 1971) a few similar services were set up in the UK, namely in Barnet, Coventry, Tower Hamlets, Lewisham and Tunbridge Wells. These have now been superseded by intensive home treatment teams (IHTT) or crisis resolution teams (CRT). These relatively new services are predominantly for people with a serious mental illness who are subject to care co-ordination rather than those at risk of *developing* mental illness who are engaged by the crisis intervention team. The IHTTs and CRTs offer 24 hour, 7 days a week, flexible, home-based care, which aims to replace, or at least, reduce the number of admissions to hospital. The response should be rapid and the contact intensive, so much so that in some cases it may require several visits each day. The service is available until the crisis is under control and then the client is referred on to more appropriate services for on-going care.

The provision of crisis resolution services however is developing slowly, the NHS Plan (DoH, 1997) set a target for 335 teams by 2004. However, by October 2001 there were only 35 such teams.

Assertive outreach

Several substantial reviews of assertive community treatment (ACT) have been undertaken. The most recent Cochrane Review (Marshall & Lockwood, 2001) concluded that compared to standard community care, people allocated to ACT, were more likely to remain in contact with services and be living independently. They were also more likely to have found employment and be more satisfied with the service they receive. This method of treatment was found to be a more attractive way of working for professionals as clients were less likely to be admitted to hospital and when they were admitted they spent less time there.

In essence, assertive outreach is a way of engaging services with clients that cannot, or do not wish to, engage with services. Assertive outreach is not a treatment in its own right; it is a vehicle by which evidence-informed treatment packages can be offered to clients. Models of case management are generally considered to be effective for people with a severe mental illness yet much of this is based on the original positive results of the assertive outreach model by Stein and Test (1980). In the UK however the research has been mixed (UK 700 Group, 2000) and the Cochrane Review (Marshall & Lockwood, 2001) on general case management found no difference in outcomes to standard care. The results for the assertive outreach model are more positive (Marshall & Lockwood, 2001) and from this evidence the introduction of assertive outreach teams within all communities is part of Government policy (DoH, 1999a). The NHS Plan (DoH, 1997) target of having 220 teams by 2004 to meet the needs of an estimated 20,000 people is progressing well as there are currently 170 teams established, catering for the needs of 9000.

A framework for the delivery of secondary mental health care

With the implementation of Care in the Community came the introduction of care management as the framework for ensuring that service users' needs would be met. Care management was the UK version of case management, which had been introduced in the USA by Stein & Test (1980) and had showed positive outcomes for service users. Case management and care management both emerged in social care, while health developed an equivalent framework termed Care Programme Approach (DoH, 1990). However in April 2001 following guidance from the *National Service Frameworks for Mental Health* (DoH, 1999) care management and care programme approach were combined to produce care co-ordination (DoH, 1999c). This move was to provide a more integrated whole-systems approach to the provision of mental health care. Care co-ordination is presented as a framework to meet the modernization agenda for the NHS and Social Services. It demands the effective provision of integrated health and social care services to adult service users, particularly for those with complex and enduring mental illness, and their carers. Service users themselves provide the focus for care planning and care delivery across services, to include the full range of community resources they need in order to promote their recovery and social inclusion (DoH, 1999c). So care co-ordination would follow the service user across statutory services, for example criminal justice service and drug and alcohol services. Care co-ordination is the framework for all care delivery to adults of working age in contact with secondary mental health services, either health or social care. While essentially aimed at ensuring effective care for people with complex needs, even those receiving input from one practitioner are included as it provides a framework for good professional mental health and social care practice.

There are two levels of care co-ordination, which are detailed in Table 12.2.

Table 12.2   The two levels of care co-ordination

Level of care co-ordination	Characteristics of people to include some of the following
Standard	They require the support or intervention of one agency or discipline or they require only low-key support from more than one agency or discipline
	They are able to self-manage their mental health problems
	They have an active informal support network
	They pose little danger to themselves or others
	They are more likely to maintain appropriate contact with services
Enhanced	They have multiple care needs, including housing, employment etc. requiring inter-agency co-ordination
	They are only willing to co-operate with one professional or agency but they have multiple care needs
	They may be in contact with a number of agencies (including the criminal justice system)
	They are likely to require more frequent and intensive interventions, perhaps medication management
	They are more likely to have mental health problems co-existing with other problems such as substance misuse
	They are more likely to be at risk of harming themselves or others
	They are more likely to disengage with services

Source: Adapted from DoH (1999b)

Managing risk

The management of risk has become more prominent in community care policy, following high profile media coverage of inquiries into mental health care (Blom-Cooper et al, 1995; Ritchie et al, 1994; Ryan, 1999). Risk assessment and management are integral parts of the case management process. Those with a severe mental illness must be followed up within one week after discharge from hospital and as part of the enhanced care co-ordination are required to have a crisis and contingency plan. Other policy initiatives to manage risk have been the previous use of Supervision Registers and the introduction of supervised discharge legislation (DoH, 1995). The provision of good quality risk management falls within the remit of clinical governance (DoH, 1998). People with severe mental illness are prone to many risks: stigma and discrimination; abuse and exploitation; loss of human rights. However, the risks given most attention are suicide, violence, aggression and self-neglect. This is particularly so if the person has a co-existent drug use problem. The responsibility for assessing risk should not be delegated solely to the care co-ordinator, rather, the assessment of risk in a community setting must be based on a comprehensive, multidisciplinary assessment of the clients 'clinical' (individual) and 'actuarial' (statistical) risk factors (Ryan, 1999). Balancing the potential risks with the need for user autonomy is a tightrope all mental health professionals must walk.

Conclusion

Many changes in how community mental health care has developed and how services have changed or re-emerged with a different purpose have been mainly in response to an increasing evidence base. When this has been supported by Government funding and directives, change has been evident, for example in the development of assertive outreach teams. The pace of expansion of services has also been reflected in non-statutory agencies and in terms of resources. Mental health and social care professionals now have a varied and extensive range of support services they can utilize in promoting community mental health. A knowledge and understanding of local services is essential in order to be able to direct and secure appropriate interventions to meet the needs of service users and their families.

Community mental health teams are central providers and as such must develop close collaboration with the range of services, ensuring that communication, liaison, transfer and documentation procedures are mutually agreed (DoH, 1999a). The integration of CMHTs is an attempt to provide a seamless service for people with mental health needs and to ensure a collaborative approach that gives service users choice and responsibility in meeting their needs. The approach also encourages mental health promotion and prevention encouraging a variety of approaches.

As Millar and Walsh (2000, p 100) conclude:

you can help in the development of a healthy lifestyle and increase awareness of unhealthy coping strategies, which might lead to future mental health problems . . . You can teach problem solving techniques which empower the patient to take back control in a step-by-step approach to solving difficulties. You can play an important role in educating people about the facts rather than the fears of mental illness and aim to reduce its negative impact when it does occur.

In the chapters that now follow we will be exploring a range of techniques that can be used to enable effective treatment.

References

Armstrong, E. (1995) *Mental Health Issues in Primary Care: A Practical Guide*, London: Macmillan Press – now Palgrave Macmillan.

Ash, J. (1997) Multi-disciplinary audit and the mental health nurse, *Mental Health Care*, 1(2), 58–60.

Audit Commission (1986) *Making a Reality of Community Care*, London: Audit Commission.

Badger, F. & Nolan, P. (1999) General practitioners' perceptions of community psychiatric nurses in primary care, *Journal of Psychiatric and Mental Health Nursing*, 6, 453–9.

Blom-Cooper, L., Hally, H. & Murphy, E. (1995) *The Falling Shadow: One Patient's Mental Health Care 1978–1993*, London: Duckworth.

Brooker, C. & Repper, J. (eds) (1998) *Serious Mental Health Problems in the Community Policy, Practice & Research*, London: Balliere Tindall.

Caplan, G. (1964) *Principles of Preventative Psychiatry*, New York: Basic Books.

Catalan, J., Hewitt, J., Kennard, C. & McPherson, J. (1980) The role of the nurse in the management of self-poisoning in the general hospital, *International Journal of Nursing Studies*, 17, 275–82.

Davis, D. & Nelson, J. (1980) Referrals to psychiatric liaison nurses: changes in characteristics over a limited time period, *General Hospital Psychiatry*, 2, 41–5.

Department of Health and Social Security (1975) *Better Services for the Mentally Ill*, London: HMSO.

Department of Health (1988) *Community Care: Agenda for Action (The Griffiths Report)*, London: HMSO.

Department of Health (1989) *Caring for People: Community Care in the Next Decade and Beyond*, London: HMSO.

Department of Health (1990) *The Care Programme Approach for People with a Mental Illness*, London: HMSO.

Department of Health (1995) *Mental Health (Patients in the Community) Act*, London: HMSO.

Department of Health (1997) *The New NHS: Modern and Dependable*, London: HMSO.

Department of Health (1998) *Modernising Mental Health Services: Safe, Sound and Supportive*, London: HMSO.

Department of Health (1999a) *National Service Framework for Mental Health*, London: HMSO.

Department of Health (1999b) *Effective Care Co-ordination in Mental Health Services: Modernising Care Programme Approach*, London: HMSO.

Department of Health (1999c) *A First Class Service*, London: HMSO.

Department of Health (2000) *The NHS Plan*, London: HMSO.

Department of Health (2001a) *Shifting the Balance of Power within the NHS*, London: DoH.

Department of Health (2001b) *The Expert Patient: A New Approach to Chronic Disease Management for the 21st Century*, London: HMSO.

Department of Health (2002) *Mental Health Policy Implementation Guide: Community Mental Health Teams*, London: HMSO.

Fincannon, J. L. (1995) Analysis of psychiatric referrals and interventions in an oncology population, *Oncology Nursing Forum*, 22(1), 87–92.

Gamble, C. & Brennan, G. (2000) *Working with Serious Mental Illness: A Manual for Clinical Practice*, London: Balliere Tindall & RCN.

Gask, L., Sibbald, B. & Creed, F. (1997) Evaluating models of working at the interface between mental health services and primary care, *The British Journal of Psychiatry*, 170, 6–11.

Gijbels, H. (1995) Mental health nursing skills in an acute admission environment: perceptions of mental health nurses and other mental health professionals, *Journal of Advanced Nursing*, 21, 460–5.

Haddock, G. & Slade, P. D. (1996) *Cognitive-Behavioural Interventions for Psychotic Disorders*, London: Routledge.

Hughes, I., Kidd, R., Cantor, R. & Killick, S. (1992) Do GP's want community mental health facilities?, *Psychiatric Bulletin*, 16, 413–15.

Langsley, D. G., Matchotka, P. & Flomenhaft, K. (1971) Avoiding mental hospital admission: a follow-up study, *American Journal of Psychiatry*, 127(10), 127–30.

Lee, J., Gask, L., Roland, M. & Donnan, S. (2002) Primary care led commissioning of mental health services: lessons from total purchasing, *Journal of Mental Health*, 11(4), 431–9.

Lindemann, E. (1944) Symptomatology and management of acute grief, *American Journal of Psychiatry*, 101, 141–8.

Marshall, M. & Lockwood, A. (2001) *Assertive Community Treatment for People with Severe Mental Disorders (Cochrane Review)*, Oxford: The Cochrane Library 4.

Martin, J. P. (1985) *Hospitals in Trouble,* Oxford: Blackwell.

Means, R. & Smith, R. (1994) *Community Care: Policy and Practice*, Basingstoke: Macmillan, now Palgrave Macmillan.

Millar, E. & Walsh, M. (2000) *Mental Health Matter in Primary Care*, Cheltenham: Stanley Thornes Publishers.

Newton, L. & Wilson, K. G. (1990) Consultee satisfaction with a psychiatric consultation-liaison nursing service, *Archives of Psychiatric Nursing*, 4(4), 264–70.

NHS Health Advisory Service (1995) *Child and Adolescent Mental Health Service: Together We Stand: The Commissioning, Role and Management of Child and Adolescent Mental Health Services*, London: HMSO.

Nolan, P. & Badger, F. (2002) In search of collaboration and partnership, in P. Nolan & F. Badger (eds), *Promoting Collaboration in Primary Mental Health Care*, London: Nelson Thornes.

Onyett, S. (2003) *Teamworking in Mental Health*, Basingstoke: Palgrave Macmillan.

Onyett, S., Heppleston, T. & Bushnell, D. (1994) A national survey of community mental health teams, *Journal of Mental Health*, 3, 175–94.

Ovretveit, J. (1993) *Co-ordinating Community Care: Multidisciplinary Teams and Care Management*, Buckingham: Open University Press.

Regel, S. & Roberts, D. (2002) *Mental Health Liaison: A Handbook for Nurses and Health Professionals*, Edinburgh: Harcourt Publishers Ltd.

Ritchie, J., Dick, D. & Lingham, R. (1994) *The Report of the Inquiry into the Care and Treatment of Christopher Clunis*, London: HMSO.

Roberts, D. (2002) Working models for practice, in S. Regel & D. Roberts (eds), *Mental Health Liaison – A Handbook for Nurses and Health Professionals*, Edinburgh: Bailliere Tindall, Ch 2, 23–42.

Rogers, A. & Pilgrim, D. (eds) (2001) *Mental Health Policy in Britain*, (2nd edn), Basingstoke: Palgrave – now Palgrave Macmillan.

Ryan, T. (1999) *Managing Crisis and Risk in Mental Health Nursing*, Cheltenham: Stanley Thornes.

Sainsbury Centre for Mental Health (2001) *Mental Health Policy: The Challenges Facing the Government*, London: Sainsbury Centre for Mental Health.

Stein, L. & Test, M. (1980) Alternative to mental hospital treatment, *Archives of General Hospital Psychiatry*, 37, 392–7.

Tummey, R. (2001) A collaborative approach to urgent mental health referrals, *Nursing Standard*, 15(52), 39–42.

UK 700 Group (2000) Cost-effectiveness of intensive v standard case management for severe psychotic illness, *The British Journal of Psychiatry*, 176, 537–43.

University of Manchester (1991) *The Third Quinquennial National Community Psychiatric Nursing Survey*, Manchester: University of Manchester.

Wright, H. & Giddey, M. (1993) *Mental Health Nursing: From First Principles to Professional Practice*, Cheltenham: Stanley Thornes.

CHAPTER 13

Supporting People and their Families During Psychopharmacotherapy

MIKE FLEET

Indicative Benchmark Statements

- Education of users of mental health and social care services and their carers about preventative medicine and health promotion

- Application of the fundamental knowledge of psychopharmacology

- Contribution to the management of mental health medication, including prevention, detection and alleviation of side-effects

- Practice in accordance with an ethical and legal framework which ensures the primacy of patient and client interest and well-being, and respects confidentiality

- The application of helping relationships as the cornerstone of their mental health nursing practice

Introduction

Since the 1950s antipsychotic medication (hereafter referred to as neuroleptic), has played an important role in the field of mental health care. Owing to the ability of pharmaceutical companies to produce high quality, standardized units of medication it has been possible to undertake double-blind random controlled trials with medication. Therefore, there is a plethora of evidence supporting the efficacy of varying types of medication.

This chapter will explore the principles and practices underpinning psychopharmacotherapy as a component of a biopsychosocial approach to nursing care. This will include examination of Peplau's (1952) interpersonal relations model to examine the structures and processes of relationships involved in supporting clients and their families. Communication and interpersonal strategies including psychoeducation, relationship maintenance and engagement, negotiation, empowerment, collaboration, partnership, motivational interviewing and advocacy skills will be examined.

The challenge of serious mental illness

Ever since the advent of neuroleptic medication as a means of treatment in serious mental illness, clients have experienced several challenges from mental health professionals. One of these challenges has come from cure-focused approaches. The major problem with these approaches are that people with enduring problems have often experienced cure-focused strategies but their problems remain (Curson et al, 1988). The focus in general psychiatry is now on the concept of 'maintenance therapy', however, maintenance is a service-led goal, clients want to recover their lives (Coleman, 2003). Continuing attempts to effect a cure demoralize both clients and staff, potentially leading to hopelessness. There can be a natural devaluing of support and care (Perkins & Repper, 1996).

Given the nature of mental health problems one major feature of life that clients experience is their relationship with mental health professionals (Perkins & Dilks, 1992). While this relationship can be positive there is a potential for abuse. Sometimes the opinions of people with a serious mental illness are dismissed as a reflection of psychopathology. Sometimes there can be humouring of the person, listening politely and then taking no notice. In the worst cases there can be a use of professional power to assert that the nurse knows best, limiting information about the options available. Even limiting the person's choice(s) by making support dependent on doing what the nurse thinks is best, making one form of help contingent upon another.

Modern mental health care is based on a needs-led approach whereby needs are defined more broadly than just at the physiological level (Maslow, 1970). Under this approach people with serious mental illness differ from others as a result of their lack of ability to meet their needs with a normal social skills framework. The primary role of the nurse is to assist people to access the ordinary activities, facilities and relationships (Perkins & Repper, 1996). Sometimes people's needs are not necessarily the same as their wants. This can at times be frustrating from a professional viewpoint, the need to intervene with practices that professionals know to be effective may not be acceptable to clients.

Informed consent and autonomy

The meaning of informed consent appears to vary depending on the context in which it is used (Skegg, 1999). Informed consent has no current clear definition yet everyone one of us has the right to accept or decline the suggestions of others. Autonomy could be considered as having the capability to think and make decisions, acting freely on these decisions without negative interference or hindrance by others (Gillon, 1985).

Respect for autonomy and the right to consent to or refuse treatment is a widely accepted value in health care. Clients have the right to have any proposed treatment including risks and alternatives clearly explained to them. Respect for autonomy involves regarding clients as persons entitled to the same basic rights as everyone else; the right to know, the right to privacy and the right to receive care and treatment (Thompson et al, 1994). Autonomy refers to an individual's ability to reach his or her own decisions and requires practitioners to respect those decisions. However, this respect can come into conflict when considering the roles and duties that society expects and demands of mental health professionals.

Beneficence implies the duty to do good and maximize good. It obliges that professionals help clients by promoting and safeguarding their health and welfare. Therefore, placing a burden on professionals to utilize evidence-informed interventions to decrease the harm that mental illness can cause. Non-maleficence imposes the duty to do no harm or to minimize harm. This requires that the professional refrains from doing anything that could be detrimental to others. How then can we marry this concept with the fact that, sometimes, toxic medications are given to clients against their express wishes?

Although there is no general consensus as to the essential elements of consent it would seem to involve such elements as communication, information giving and capacity. Communication is the single most important way of securing co-operation and concordance with treatment (Thompson et al, 1994). Communication involves listening to clients, using a language that is both familiar and jargon-free so that understanding is shared (Rumbold, 1999).

Without accurate information clients cannot make informed choices and so cannot act autonomously. The Nursing & Midwifery Council Code of Professional Conduct (NMC, 2002) demands that all clients have a right to receive information about their condition. But there is little guidance on what information a client should be told. The Department of Health (1990) issued some fairly detailed guidelines in a Health Circular. These guidelines state that clients should be made aware of the nature of their condition and what would happen to them if no treatment is provided; what the treatment options and respective benefits are, with awareness of any substantial or usual inherent risks and side effects associated with each option. In particular, the client must be made aware of any dangers that may be special in kind or magnitude or special to a particular client.

The main professional problem relates to this risk disclosure. Should every risk however unlikely be disclosed? If not, where should the line be drawn? In order for consent to be truly informed it has been suggested that professionals disclose whatever information a reasonable person would want to know, plus whatever else the actual client wants to know (Brook, 1993).

Would a reasonable person want to know every possible negative effect of a medication? Would this lead to undue anxiety? Would not being told about a negative effect and then experiencing that effect be damaging to the trust formed in the working alliance? As we have seen, limiting information about treatment options can be an abuse of the power of the health professional. The disclosure of risk information must be made on an individual basis. There needs to be an adequate balance between autonomy and information overload.

Psychopharmacology and psychopharmacotherpy

Special types of cells called *neurones* enable the brain to function. The neurone is made up of the cell body from which an *axon* gives off several branches or terminates in a *dendrite*. This branching enables the neurone to communicate with many others. Communication is via electrical impulses passing from one neurone to another across the gap between each cell, the *synapse*. This transmission of the electrical impulse across the synapse is done by the release of *neurotransmitters*, stored in *vesicles*, at the terminal of one neurone (the *presynaptic neurone*) and the uptake of these transmitters at the next neurone (the *postsynaptic neurone*). See Figure 13.1.

At the moment there are about 40 known transmitters, but there may be others not yet identified.

These neurotransmitters pass across the synapse and attach themselves to specific *receptors* on the next neurone. This then alters the biochemistry of the

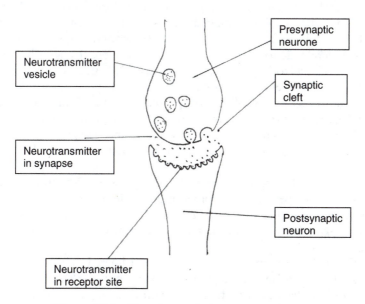

Figure 13.1 Neurotransmission across synapse

receptor, this alteration can result in a change in function such as a change in mood or level of alertness. Apart from stimulating the receptor, the function of the neurotransmitter may be to actually inhibit the receptor cell. The neurotransmitters are affected by the environment in the synapse. The electrochemical nature of the synapse changes almost constantly. Neurotransmitters can enter the synapse but not connect to receptors owing to the receptors being fully occupied, the environment of the synapse may destroy the neurotransmitter before it passes its message to the receptor or the presynaptic neurone may reuptake the neurotransmitter making it unavailable to the postsynaptic neurone. The reuptake of the neurotransmitter serotonin may be relevant in depression or the negative symptoms of schizophrenia (University of York, 1999).

One other neurotransmitter thought to be of relevance in schizophrenia is dopamine. The 'dopamine hypothesis' considers that dopamine transmission in people with schizophrenia is overactive. Therefore the blocking of the uptake of dopamine is thought to be helpful, resulting in a reduction of activity in the postsynaptic neurone. This is thought to be therapeutic if this blockage occurs in the mesolimbic and mesocortical areas of the brain, but can lead to parkinsonism, dystonia and tardive dyskinesia when it occurs in the nigostriatal tract, or endocrine effects such as enlarged breasts, weight gain, lactorrhoea, amenorrhoea and impotence when it occurs in the tuberoinfundibular tract (Brennan et al, 2000).

The older neuroleptics, the so-called typical antipsychotics include Chlorpromazine, Trifluoperazine, Thioridazine, Haloperidol and Flupentixol. While very good at reducing the positive symptoms of schizophrenia, these medications also produce negative effects in the majority of clients. The newer medications, the atypical antipsychotics include Clozapine, Olanzapine, Amisulpride, Olanzapine, Sertindole and Resperidone. These medications have less severe negative effects and treat both the positive and the negative symptoms of schizophrenia. These are usually effective at low doses producing positive effects without incurring negative effects. At higher doses extrapyramidal effects can be problematic and some cause serious haematological problems, agranulocytosis can be a problem with clozapine, hence the need for regular blood monitoring (Kane, 1987).

The potential negative effects of neuroleptic medication include:

- *Parkinsonism*: slowing of movement and expression. Rigidity and tremor;
- *Acute dystonias*: persistent pathological change in muscle tone, such as neck muscle spasms or fixed upwards gaze;
- *Acute dyskinesia*: such as involuntary movements of the head and neck and resting tremor;
- *Tardive dyskinesia*: involuntary or unco-ordinated movements of the orofacial and tongue muscles, limbs. Tics, grunting or vocalization;
- *Akathisia*: restlessness, agitation, leg shifting or tapping of feet;

- *Neuroleptic malignant syndrome*: rigidity, hyperpyrexia, tachycardia, fluctuating levels of consciousness;
- *Anticholinergic effects*: such as dry mouth, blurred vision, urinary retention, erectile dysfunction, constipation;
- *Antihistamine effects*: sedation;
- *α-adrenergic blockade*: dizziness, postural hypotension, tachycardia

Symptom monitoring and management tools

Evidence for the efficacy of neuroleptic medication is widespread (Kane, 1996). However, the efficacy ranges from very good to no beneficial effect at all (Curson et al, 1988). At times the dosages of neuroleptic medication used have appeared excessive. The non-response of clients has been viewed as owing to poor absorption and hence the need to increase dosages (Thompson, 1994). There is overwhelming evidence (Aubree & Lader, 1980; Harrington et al, 2002; Hirsch & Barnes, 1994) that there is no advantage in prescribing higher doses. However, initially high doses that appear to benefit clients in reducing symptoms are sometimes needlessly maintained, increasing the risk of negative side effects. One way to counter this is to undertake regular symptom monitoring. Monitoring has several functions. One function is to develop a *baseline* against which changes can be discerned and measured. This baseline then allows the *discrimination* of changed perceptual, cognitive and affective processes.

Using tools such as for example, the Brief Psychiatric Rating Scale, (BPRS) (Overall & Gorham, 1962) it is possible to monitor the severity of a client's symptoms on a regular basis. The BPRS could be applied routinely as it takes little of the client and the nurse's time. The symptom severity, either globally or for each symptom, can provide evidence of the efficacy of current treatment whether medication or psychological therapies. The regular use of monitoring therefore allows clients not only the opportunity to assess the efficacy of the medication and other interventions but also enables them to take responsibility for their illness and undertake targeted medication if their illness relapses. However, targeted medication may not be enough. In one study (Jolley et al, 1990) after one year the relapse rate for clients taking only targeted medication was four times higher than for those taking maintenance medication and increasing as necessary. It would appear, therefore, that the taking of regular medication is more effective on relapse rates than the use of targeted medication.

Monitoring negative effects

The use of the term 'side-effects' can be misleading. 'Side-effects' implies that these effects, while potentially devastating for the client, may be considered as trivial. For the purposes of this chapter 'side-effects' will be referred to as 'the negative effects of the medication'. As we have seen, neuroleptic medication has both positive and negative effects, some effects are general to the medication group and some are peculiar to each medication. The major source of information for nurses regarding the negative effects of medication is the *British National Formulary* (BMA & RPSGB, 2002). Unfortunately effects are frequently grouped together and the reader is referred to those of one medication, usually Chlorpromazine. The negative effects of individual medications are not given. Most neuroleptics produce a similar range of negative effects but differ in the severity of one effect over another.

As we have seen neuroleptics are not the 'smart bombs' of pharmacology, they cannot target accurately precise areas of the brain: even if the precise area concerned (with, for example, schizophrenia) were identified accurately. Once absorbed the drug will act on various sites in the body. While it is possible to control some of these negative effects by the use of other medications these too have their negative effects, in addition to a potential for abuse in some cases. Treatments should be used with respect to the balance of costs and benefits: the balance between the negative effects and the beneficial effects. If the benefits outweigh the costs then it would appear to be ethical to maintain the treatment. When the costs outweigh the benefits then other considerations must be taken into account. Respecting the autonomy of the client, does the client want to continue with treatment that has many negative effects but enables him to maintain his social and family roles? If so what is the moral justification in denying him treatment, especially if no alternative can be found?

The concept of informed consent requires that the benefits of treatment, the risks of treatment and the risks of non-treatment should be made clear to the client. Knowing the potential risks of neuroleptic treatment how can the nurse use the working alliance to help the client to monitor for and hopefully minimize these risks? There are several systems for assessing and monitoring negative effects; these can be tools utilized by the clinician only such as the Abnormal Involuntary Movements Scale (Guy, 1976) to detect tardive dyskinesia; the Simpson and Angus (1970) scale to detect extrapyramidal effects and a scale to detect akathisia (Barnes, 1989). The necessity with these scales is that the clinician is trained in their use, as routine clinical examination by even experienced psychiatrists can miss important negative effects that can be detected by systematic screening (Weiden et al, 1987).

However, clients themselves are capable of monitoring for negative effects, in fact probably more so as they are with themselves for 24 hours a day and more aware of their own bodies than the clinicians can ever be. A useful self-monitoring scale is the Liverpool University Neuroleptic Side-effects Rating Scale, (the LUNSERS) (Day et al, 1995). Covering 51 'effects', the scale includes 10, such as weak fingernails, that are 'red herrings'. The rationale for the red herrings is not so much to 'catch out' the client but rather to provide a subscale for those people who naturally overrate themselves on such questionnaires. The major advantage of using these tools is not merely to detect and assess the severity of the negative effects. The major advantage is that it proves to the client that nurses are aware of these effects and are collaboratively working with clients to provide a detailed pattern of the problems the client is experiencing. The only effective way to deal with a problem is to assess it accurately. The use of rating scales, again, provides evidence for the nurse in their role as client advocate. As we have seen the power of the mental health worker can be abused to dismiss the opinions of people experiencing mental health problems, while the use of objective and validated rating scales provides empirical evidence that the client's experiences are real.

The working alliance

It is evident that a major feature of a client's life, especially where social networks have been damaged, is the nurse–client relationship, the working alliance. Peplau (1952) identified several influences on this working alliance. The influences affect both aspects of the relationship. Society has certain expectations of nurses and their role, the expectation that a nurse will provide effective care and support. Hence the nurse needs to develop and mature as an individual understanding their own feelings, needs and attitudes, developing an appropriate knowledge and skills base. The nurse needs to be aware of the client's feelings, needs and attitudes to enhance the partnership.

On the other hand the illness can be a potential learning experience for clients. The client needs to understand his or her own feelings, needs and attitudes and those of the nurse to enhance the partnership. There is an influence of health promotion and the health care setting on the client and his or her family. Both the client and the nurse are influenced by family, society, education and community agencies. All these influences are impinging on the nurse to effect a professional working alliance.

Peplau (1952) identified four phases of the relationship; *orientation, identification, exploitation* and *resolution*. Whenever a client becomes ill the nurse has to help him to meet his needs in the new situation. The nurse needs to be empathetic to the client's need to be orientated to the new situation, the need to be orientated to new people and to his or her ill health.

During the *orientation* phase the client may very well be anxious and forget some of the information given. The task of the nurse is to provide repetition of information. The client who has not totally understood their condition will need space and time. The client needs to be able to ask questions, the answers to which provide the client with information and a greater insight into the situation. If this is taken into account, orientation can become more complete for the client; the client becomes better informed about their condition, therefore assessing the situation more proficiently. There are two main models of information giving: the *deficit model* and the *interaction model*. In the deficit model the premise is that lack of information plays a causative role in producing attitudes and behaviours that have a detrimental effect on the client. Therefore by providing relevant information the knowledge deficit will be eliminated with the result of more beneficial attitudes and behaviours. In the interaction model the difference between 'disease' and 'illness' is highlighted: disease being a medical concept referring to 'objective' pathology; while 'illness' refers to the 'subjective' effects on the client having a disease.

In general lay people develop their own subjective models of illness in order to make sense of ill health, and this model will influence the assimilation of any new information offered to them. These models help the client to cope with, and control, the negative and distressing consequences of the illness. Information given by professionals will be assimilated, organized and possibly rejected on the basis of the client's model. To change the client's model requires us to give detailed help as to how a new way of looking at the illness translates into more effective management strategies for the client, enabling the client to achieve some degree of control in a difficult situation. As Peplau states, the nurse and the client learn to work in a co-operative manner to resolve difficulties.

The *identification* phase begins when the client becomes clearer in mind about their problem. The client identifies with those nurses experienced as being useful to the client. The client engages with, and places trust in, staff who then do the things they say they will do. The goal of engagement is to form a trusting relationship or working alliance that will enable the nurse to support the client through treatment. Voluntary engagement in treatment will only take place if the client sees that affiliation with a treatment agency can be of benefit. The relationship is initially built on helping the client to achieve ends that he or she identifies as important. Clients identify with nurses who are open and honest in their approach and who provide information for them (Simpson, 1991). At this point the relationship can take one of several different directions. The client can become more involved in his care and enhance the relationship along productive lines. Or he could avoid involvement, requiring the nurse to reflect on possible associated anxiety. Or he can become passive and let the nurse do everything for him, including making decisions that can be far-reaching and vital, such as taking or refusing medication. The direction the relationship takes will depend on the client's previous experience, his present condition and the relationship he has established with the nurse.

The *exploitation* phase is the main 'working' phase for both the client and the nurse. As the informed client gains a clearer picture of the situation, identification of needs begins. This phase is characterized by the client making full use of the resources available, both physical and human resources. The working alliance is the chief way that the client uses the situation and the nurse for benefit. The client seeks more information about health problems and discusses things with other users to see whether the information received is correct. The relationship is at a potentially meaningful level. In this phase care planning and implementation can be a co-operative process. Ideally this is a dynamic phase of growth from dependency to a situation in which both the nurse and the client identify and exploit areas of independence and interdependence. The nurse who can see this change in behaviour and adjusts to this need for independence is less likely to encounter resistance, as the client benefits from these efforts to become healthy.

The *resolution* phase is one in which the client begins to take steps to live a healthy life in their own environment. The termination or handover of care needs to be planned carefully, the client prepared for the next situation. What Peplau (1952) describes as a 'freeing process'.

Psychoeducation

Psychoeducation is a major component of supporting people through psychopharmacotherapy. Education is not only about the types and dosages of the medication: not only about the negative effects of the medication and how to monitor for and overcome the negative effects, but education must be about the risks that can be owed to the illness itself and the role that abstinence from medication plays. Education plays an important role in the development of motivation to change one's behaviour; if one is unaware of the potential risks of one's current behaviour why bother to change?

As we have seen from Peplau's (1952) model the client identifies with nurses whom the client experiences as being useful to him. One way of being useful to the client is to provide answers to the client's questions, which often include 'why should I take these drugs?' or 'what will happen if I do not take these drugs?' Obviously precise answers cannot be given to specific clients, after all, nobody can accurately predict the future. However, looking at the evidence each relapse brings with it an increased probability of future relapses (McGlashan, 1988) while each relapse increases the potential for social debility (Hogarty et al, 1991).

Therefore, it is vital for the sake of respect for the autonomy of the client that they are fully aware not only of the risks of taking the medication, but the risks of not taking the medication. The concept of informed consent must, therefore, tacitly contain the concept of informed refusal, the responsibility for one's health is a shared goal, not simply the province of the professional.

Strategies for improving medication compliance

What is compliance? There is debate concerning the terminology. Compliance would appear to imply that a treatment regime is dictated by one individual for another. A more collaborative term could be concordance between the client and the mental health professionals' prescribed treatment. Is anyone really 100 per cent concordant with their medication, taking the prescribed medication at the prescribed time, every time? The current problems with antibiotic resistant bacteria owes much to those millions of people who stop taking their antibiotics when they start feeling well rather than finishing the prescribed course. People with long-term illnesses are frequently non-compliant with their treatment regime, ask any diabetes or asthma sufferer. This non-compliance is wide spread and costs the NHS somewhere in the region of £100 million per year.

There are many reasons why people do not adhere fully to their treatment regime. These reasons could include the negative side effects, which can impact on many aspects of life in the physical dimension and the social dimension leading to stigma and social debility. There can be an impact on lifestyle and social relationships, taking regular medication can restrict alcohol intake, causing some people miserable nights at the pub, which in many adults is a (if not *the*) major venue for social interaction. Cultural influences, whether familial or societal can lead to refusal to take types of medication or the medium in which they are provided.

In order for anyone to allow any intervention, whether pharmaceutical or psychological they have to fulfil all the factors of the health belief model (Janz & Becker, 1984): the influence of the perceived severity of the illness – the illness must be worthy of treatment; the influence of the perceived vulnerability of the person to the illness in question; the influence of the perceived efficacy of the treatment on offer and whether there are any perceived barriers to the use of the treatment; and finally the influence of environmental prompts to take any prescribed treatment.

Although it has been subject to criticism (Perkins & Repper, 1998), compliance therapy (Kemp et al, 1997) has been found to be having positive effect on client outcomes. Compliance therapy is a cognitive psychoeducational approach to enhancing the client's motivation to adhere to a prescribed drug regime. It is a three-phase structure looking at eliciting the client's stance towards medication, exploring ambivalence towards treatment and working towards maintenance. The basis of compliance therapy is a modification of motivational interviewing (Miller & Rollnick, 1991) emphasizing personal choice and responsibility in a non-blaming atmosphere – the very essence of respect for the client's autonomy.

Motivation is a state of readiness to change rather than a personality trait. The task of the therapist is to help the client move to a greater readiness to change. This is achieved by respecting the principles of motivational interviewing. These principles include a non-judgemental acceptance of the whole client including the non-adherence, the illness and all its associated problems. The main psychoeducational component is the development of the discrepancy between the client's current behaviour and their desired goals. The client has the perception that non-adherence benefits outweigh the costs. The positive consequences of no negative effects outweigh the negative consequences of relapse and/or hospitalization. It is the task of the nurse to tip this balance in favour of greater perceived costs than benefits. Increasing awareness of the perceived costs and benefits can be done in several ways. These include providing new information about problems that can be abstinence-related, such as voices being worse and increased risk of debility and reframing past events, highlighting the role unmedicated symptoms played.

In order to maximize the working alliance, it is vital that the nurse avoids arguing that a problem exists, as this is likely to cause psychological reactance – the tendency to take the opposite position in order to assert one's freedom. It is important to roll with resistance, offering but not forcing new perspectives while looking for opportunities to reframe or reinforce accurate perceptions and supporting self-efficacy, to enhance the client's confidence in their ability to cope with the task of recovery. Belief in the potential for change is an important prerequisite for motivation.

Conclusion

Despite developments in mental health legislation, adherence to medication is a matter of choice. Legislation requiring clients to be fully compliant with medication is not only open to criticism on an ethical level but a practical level. Enforcing medication compliance has a very-short-term gain, the fact remains that most serious mental illnesses are long-term conditions. The need, therefore, is for the client to choose to adhere to a psychopharmacotherapy regime.

The role of the nurse is to enable the client to make this an informed choice: by respecting the client's autonomy; their right to decide; providing information that the client needs to make the decision; supporting the client in their choice, whether by providing support with, and monitoring of, medication administration, symptom management and negative effects or supporting the client and maintaining the working alliance when the choice the client makes is not the one that professionals consider the right choice.

The benefits and costs of neuroleptic medication are well documented. With increased access to information from the World Wide Web and other media, society in general is becoming more aware of these issues. In order to develop, maintain and improve the working alliance with their clients the burden is now on nurses to ensure that their clients have their autonomy respected.

References

Aubree, J. C. & Lader, M. H. (1980) High and very high dosage antipsychotics: a critical review, *Journal of Clinical Psychiatry*, 41(10), 341–50.

Barnes, T. R. E. (1989) A rating scale for drug induced akathisia, *British Journal of Psychiatry*, 154, 672–6.

Brennan, G., Roberts, C., Gamble, C. & Chan, T. F. (2000) Chemical management of psychotic symptoms, in C. Gamble & G. Brennan (eds), *Working with Serious Mental Illness: a Manual for Clinical Practice*, Edinburgh: Bailliere Tindall, Ch 15, 265–87.

British Medical Association & Royal Pharmaceutical Society of Great Britain (2002) *British National Formulary No 44*, London: BMA & RPSGB.

Brook, D. W. (1993) *Life and Death: Philosophical Essays in Biomedical Ethics*, Cambridge: Cambridge University Press.

Coleman, R. (2003) The stepping stones to recovery, online at: http://www.samh.org.uk/thepoint/spring2003/stepping_stones.html

Curson, D. A., Patel, M. & Liddle, P. F. et al (1988) Psychiatric morbidity of a long-stay hospital population with chronic schizophrenia and implications for future community care, *British Medical Journal*, 297, 819–22.

Day, J. C., Wood, G., Dewey, M. & Bentall, P. A. (1995) Self-rating scale for measuring neuroleptic side effects validated in a group of schizophrenic patients, *British Journal of Psychiatry*, 166, 650–3.

Department of Health (1990) *Patient Consent to Examination and Treatment*, HC(90)22, London: HMSO.

Gillon, R. (1985) *Philosophical Medical Ethics*, Chichester: John Wiley.

Guy, W. (1976) *Assessment Manual for Psychopharmacology, Revised Version*, Bethesda: US Department of Health, Education and Welfare.

Harrington, M., Lelliot, P., Paton, C., Konsolaki, M., Sensky, T. & Okocha, C. (2002) Variation between services in polypharmacy and combined high dose of antipsychotic drugs prescribed for inpatients, *Psychiatric Bulletin*, 26, 418–20.

Hirsch, S. R. & Barnes, T. R. E. (1995) The clinical treatment of schizophrenia with antipsychotic medication, in S. R. Hirsch & D. R. Weinberger (eds), *Schizophrenia*, Oxford: Blackwell Science, 443–68.

Hogarty, G. E., Anderson, C. M., Reiss, D. J. & Kornblith, S. J. et al (1991) Family psychoeducational, social skills training and maintenance chemotherapy in the aftercare of schizophrenia. II Two year effects of a controlled study on relapse and adjustment, *Archives of General Psychiatry*, 48, 340–7.

Janz, N. K. & Becker, M. H. (1984) The health belief model: a decade later, *Health Education Quarterly*, 11(1), 1–47.

Jolley, A. G., Hirsch, S. T., McRink, A. & Wilson, L. (1990) Trial of brief intermittent neuroleptic prophylaxis for selected schizophrenia outpatients: clinical and social outcome at two years, *British Medical Journal*, 301, 837–42.

Kane, J. M. (1987) Treatment of schizophrenia, *Schizophrenia Bulletin*, 13(1), 133–56.

Kane, J. M. (1996) Schizophrenia, *New England Journal of Medicine*, 334, 34–41.

Kemp, R., Hayward, P. & David, A. (1997) *Compliance Therapy Manual*, London: Maudsley Hospital.

Maslow, A. (1970) *Motivation and Personality*, (2nd edn) New York: Harper & Row.

McGlashan, T. H. (1988) A selective review of North American long-term follow-up studies of schizophrenia, *Schizophrenia Bulletin*, 14, 515–42.

Miller, W. & Rollnick, S. (1991) *Motivational Interviewing: Preparing People to Change Addictive Behavior*, New York: Guilford Press.

Nursing & Midwifery Council (2002) *Code of Professional Conduct*, London: NMC.

Overall, J. E. & Gorham, D. R. (1962) The Brief Psychiatric Rating Scale, *Psychological Reports*, 10, 799–812.

Peplau, H. E. (1952) *Interpersonal Relations in Nursing*, New York: Putnam.

Perkins, R. & Dilks, S. (1992) Worlds apart: working with severely socially disabled people, *Journal of Mental Health*, 1, 3–17.

Perkins, R. & Repper, J. (1996) *Working Alongside People with Long-term Mental Health Problems*, London: Chapman & Hall.

Perkins, R. & Repper, J. (1998) Softly, softly, *Mental Health Care*, 2(2), 70.

Rumbold, G. (1999) *Ethics in Nursing Practice*, (3rd edn), London: Bailliere Tindall.

Simpson, G. M. & Angus, J. W. S. (1970) A rating scale for extrapyramidal side effects, *Acta Psychiatrica Scandinavica*, 45(supp 212), 1–19.

Simpson, H. (1991) *Peplau's Model in Action*, Basingstoke: Macmillan, now Palgrare Macmillan.

Skegg, P. D. G. (1999) English medical law and 'informed consent', *Medical Law Review*, 7(2), 135–65.

Thompson, C. (1994) The use of high dose antipsychotic medication, *British Journal of Psychiatry*, 164, 448–58.

Thompson, I. E., Melia, K. M. & Boyd, K. M. (1994) *Nursing Ethics*, (3rd edn), Edinburgh: Churchill Livingstone.

University of York (1999) Drug treatments for schizophrenia, *Effective Health Care*, 5(6), York: University of York.

Weiden, P. J., Mann, J. J. & Hass, G. (1987) Clinical non-recognition of neuroleptic induced movement disorders: a cautionary study, *American Journal of Psychiatry*, 144, 1148–53.

CHAPTER 14

Using Counselling in Mental Health Practice

MAGGIE HADLAND

Indicative Benchmark Statements

▨ The application of helping relationships as the cornerstone of their mental health nursing practice

▨ Facilitation of therapeutic co-operation with mental health service users and their carers, taking account of those who nurses find difficult to engage

▨ Maintenance of therapeutic alliances with users of mental health and social care services through partnership, intimacy and reciprocity

▨ Participation in negotiation, formulation and communication of therapeutic interventions with users of mental health and social care services and their carers

▨ Application of the basic principles of person-centred counselling interventions

Introduction

Counselling is one of a range of helping skills available to the mental health nurse. This chapter will introduce the reader to the different counselling approaches, and the importance of the core conditions as the pre-requisite to successful client work. The development of the therapeutic relationship is looked at in detail, with examples of interventions. Guidance is included on how to work ethically and to recognize limits to competence and how to refer.

Mental health nursing is essentially about the therapeutic relationship between nurse and patient, and that is also what counselling is. An awareness of counselling theories and skills is an invaluable part of the mental health nurses' role. Counselling skills can enhance the quality of the relationship with all the patients or clients with whom mental health nurses work. There is some debate about whether counselling per se is appropriate for everyone, but clients with diverse mental health problems such as personality disorder and psychosis have been helped by counselling (Lambers, 1994a, b).

What is counselling – just tea and sympathy?

Counselling is a word that is used frequently, although not always strictly correctly! 'He'll have to be counselled about his lateness . . .' or 'She was counselled about her attitude . . .' are often heard in the workplace. In both these examples, counselling is linked with, and is sometimes synonymous with, disciplinary process. It is often mistakenly assumed to be about giving advice, as many dictionary definitions suggest: 'Counsel (verb): Advise (person to do); Counsellor (noun): advisor, especially of students' (*Oxford Handy Dictionary*, 1986) and has passed into popular usage in this way, as in 'debt counselling' for instance. People often have an image of counsellors as well-meaning but amateurish 'do-gooders', sometimes scathingly described as 'the tea and sympathy brigade'!

What these definitions have in common is that they are based on communication, listening and interpersonal skills (Woolfe, 1997), and these skills form the basis of most social encounters, friendship and helping interventions. The difference is that counselling is not about advice giving, friendship, or disciplining someone, but is an intentional and carefully constructed encounter. It is essentially a helping skill that puts the emphasis on the relationship between the counsellor (the person offering the help) and the client (the person in need of help), and offers a relationship in which the client is enabled to grow (Rogers, 1961).

There are as many definitions of counselling as there are writers on the subject.

> a relationship which a person may use for his own personal growth. (Rogers, 1961, 19)

> people become engaged in counselling when a person, occupying regularly or temporarily the role of counsellor, offers or agrees explicitly to offer time, attention and respect to another person or persons temporarily in the role of client. (BAC, 1985, cited in Palmer et al 1996)

There are three elements to the counselling relationship; the client who is seeking help (Rogers, 1959); the counsellor, who has the necessary personal qualities and skills to help the client; and the relationship itself, which will provide the client with the conditions necessary for personal growth to take place. These are the core conditions and evidence suggests that they are not only important in a counselling relationship, but in almost all successful human interactions (Truax and Carkhuff, 1967). The core conditions are therefore essential in any helping relationship.

The core conditions

Congruence (genuineness)

Congruence has been defined as a state of being in which how the counsellor feels and how he or she behaves is the same – there are no defences or pretences (Mearns & Thorne, 1999). Counsellors themselves identified a number of themes as describing what congruence means, and these include being oneself, being open to experience, being focused in the moment, and willingness to be known (Adomaitis, 1992 cited in Grafanaki, 2001). Congruence is fundamental to the therapeutic process, in that the other core conditions are impossible if the therapist is not 'real' (Truax & Mitchell, 1971). It is closely linked to consistency between verbal and non-verbal behaviours (Graves & Robinson, 1976; Haase & Tepper, 1972), and eye contact, leaning forward and smiling were all perceived as important predictors of congruence (Seay & Altekruse, 1979).

Developing congruence involves progressing from what Mearns (2000) calls 'portrayal', in which the counselling student will try to present themselves as the perfect counsellor, no matter how testing the client may be. Congruence comes when the counsellor stops trying to portray some ideal self and behaves more naturally in the therapeutic encounter. This in turn increases the counsellor's capacity for self-acceptance, therefore reducing the need for defensive behaviour. Congruence is not a constant state, however, and even experienced counsellors report that boredom, tiredness, preoccupation with other things and negative feelings towards the client get in the way of being genuine (Grafanaki, 1997).

Acceptance – (unconditional positive regard, non-possessive warmth)

Both clients and counsellors bring personal characteristics and individual differences with them to the counselling relationship. Clients may have very different lifestyles and values to our own, some of which we find it hard to accept or approve of. Acceptance however is not about approval or disapproval, but is offering the client space to be themselves without conditions. Rogers (1957) describes unconditional positive regard as acceptance for the client's negative feelings as well as the positive ones, caring for the client as a separate person with permission to have his or her own feelings and experiences. There is no expectation that the client will do or become what we want. Mearns and Thorne (1999, p 59) consider it to be: 'the fundamental attitude of the . . . counsellor towards the client', demonstrated by consistent warmth and acceptance. It is not the same as liking (ibid, p 3) and neither is the effective counsellor someone who simply smiles and nods whatever the client says (Wilkins, 2001).

But how easy is it to be accepting? We will all meet a client that we find difficult to accept – they may be prejudiced, have very different views or lifestyle to ours, or have committed a crime we cannot accept (most students say that they would find clients who have abused children the most difficult to make a therapeutic relationship with). So what do we do? Accept the client and not the behaviour? Wilkins (2001) believes that the key to acceptance is trying to understand the person behind the behaviour – understanding how the experiences in the client's life influence his or her beliefs and behaviours means that we no longer need to either judge or tolerate, but we can truly offer unconditional positive regard.

Empathy

Empathy was originally a German word '*einfuhlung*', or 'in-feeling', and translated as 'empathy' became a term used to describe the feelings captured by a work of art (for instance, an artist who had successfully translated the essence of an individual or object onto canvas could be said to have 'empathy' with the subject). The term was not used to describe a therapeutic intervention until much later. In the counselling setting, empathy can be defined as being willing to enter into the personal world of the client, and communicating that empathic understanding so that the client feels understood (Haugh & Merry, 2001). Empathy is not sympathy, which is more about how the counsellor would feel in that situation: nor is it identification, in which the counsellor's own sense of self becomes lost. Rogers (1951) describes it clearly:

> the counsellor is perceiving the hates and hopes and fears of the client through immersion in an empathic process, but without himself, as counsellor, experiencing those hates and hopes and fears. (p 29)

> empathy . . . is to perceive the internal frame of reference of another with accuracy and with the emotional components and meanings which pertain thereto as if one were the person, but without ever losing the 'as if' condition. (pp 210–11).

Empathy is not enough without being able to communicate empathic understanding to the client, as Rogers (1959) pointed out in his statement of the characteristics of the therapeutic relationship. In practice, the core conditions are difficult to separate from one another, as congruence and acceptance are communicated to the client by empathy (Wilkins, 2001).

Counselling approaches

There are three main theoretical approaches to counselling practice: psychodynamic; humanistic; and cognitive behavioural. All three are characterized

by a basic assumption about human nature, a theory of personality development, clinical theory which underpins the therapeutic work with the client,
and related skills and techniques (Feltham & Horton, 2000). All perceive the
client as a unique individual with the potential for change, and all place
the therapeutic relationship at the centre.

Psychodynamic counselling

Psychodynamic counselling developed out of the psychoanalytical theories of
Freud and has as its central assumption the existence of a dynamic unconscious mind that exerts influence on our conscious behaviour. Psychodynamic
counselling tends to focus on unresolved emotional conflicts, and the goal of
therapy therefore is to make the contents of the unconscious conscious. This
is done using a technique called 'free association', in which the client expresses
whatever comes to mind, and the role of the therapist is to observe and interpret the content of the free association (Gilliland et al, 1994). Dreams,
described by Freud (1900 cited in Brown, 1972) as 'the royal road to the
unconscious', are also observed in detail.

The key element in the helping relationship is transference, which happens
when the therapist becomes a significant figure in the client's life, and the
client perceives and responds to the therapist in ways that are similar to how
they responded to significant persons in the past. Through the transference
relationship, the client is enabled to understand how the past influences the
present, becoming more autonomous and able to exert control over primi-
tive inner forces.

Humanistic counselling

This includes a variety of counselling approaches, including existential
therapy, gestalt therapy, transactional analysis, narrative therapy, and
person-centred counselling. Only the latter will be considered in detail here.

Person-centred counselling was first developed in its present form by Carl
Rogers in the 1950s and 1960s. Rogers was part of the humanistic psychology movement that began in the United States and also included Abraham
Maslow. Humanistic psychology can be described as a holistic, phenomenological theory of human nature. The individual must be considered as a unique
being in the context of family, friends, work, their past, present and hopes for
the future (holism), and as an organism that perceives and interprets events
in order to make sense of the world (phenomenology). The key concepts of
humanistic psychology are first that human beings have a natural tendency
to develop in ways that promote growth – what Rogers calls 'the self-
actualisation tendency' (Rogers, 1959, p 210), and second that this personal

growth is attained through human relationships. Humanistic counselling is based on these beliefs, and the purpose of the therapeutic relationship is to enable the client to reach his or her full potential.

Cognitive- behavioural therapy and counselling

Cognitive Behavioural Therapy (CBT) derives from behavioural therapy and cognitive therapy. Behavioural counselling is based on the assumption that all human behaviour is learned and can therefore be unlearned. Cognitive therapy maintains that thinking determines feelings and behaviour, and mal-adaptive thoughts are responsible for the problems that people experience. In combination, CBT, based on the work of Beck (1976), is increasingly popular as a treatment option for a variety of problems, including depression, anxiety, obsessive-compulsive disorder, and substance use. The therapeutic rationale for CBT is that an individual's behavioural and emotional response to a negative situation is determined by their thoughts or beliefs about the event (Palmer & Szymanska, 1996). These beliefs take the form of negative automatic thoughts, which result in an emotional consequence and CBT, therefore, looks at the relationship between cognitions, affect and behaviour (Stallard, 2002).

The goal of CBT is to increase self-awareness and improve self-control by identifying dysfunctional thoughts and beliefs that are negative and self-critical (Stallard, 2002). It is a time-limited, skills-based and collaborative approach that focuses on current problems in a practical way. It involves the use of structured exercises and homework is set so the client can practice tasks in a real-world setting. Whatever the approach, there is strong evidence to suggest that the person of the counsellor and the presence of the core conditions (see above) can positively affect the outcome of counselling (McGuiness, 2000).

The process of counselling: beginning, sustaining and closing the therapeutic relationship

Beginning the therapeutic relationship

In the mental health setting, the first encounter with the patient is often on admission, but even before this meeting, it is important to spend some time in preparation (Nelson-Jones, 2000). Ideally, counselling should take place in a quiet, private place that is free from interruptions – pulling curtains around a bed only gives an illusion of privacy! Telephones should be diverted and certainly not answered during the therapeutic time. Attention should be paid to the furniture in the room. There should be no physical barriers between the client and counsellor, chairs should be at the same level, and positioned at a slight angle to each other, not directly facing.

A clock with a clear face, positioned where it is visible to both client and counsellor, helps to keep to a time limit without any surreptitious glances at a wristwatch. This is also appropriate when working with clients in a mental health setting on a one-to-one basis. Frequently staff time is limited, and giving the patient a clear indication of how much time is available is good practice and good time management. It also enables other staff to be aware of how long the counsellor will be out of contact. A box of tissues signals that crying is permitted and acceptable (Rowan, 1996), although automatically offering a tissue to a distressed client can signal a wish to have them stop crying.

Arriving early helps the counsellor to be prepared, and seeing the client on time signals professionalism, as well as demonstrating the importance of boundaries. If this is a client who has been seen before, it's always helpful to look over previous notes and reflect on the previous session. New clients may or may not be preceded by information. In counselling settings where clients self-refer, such as drop in clinics, all the counsellor has to go on is what the client tells them. It is certainly not necessary to have comprehensive information about the client before starting. In the mental health setting, clients may have case notes or simply a referral letter. Reading these beforehand avoids unnecessary duplication of questions, which can be frustrating or distressing for an acutely ill client.

Welcoming the client is the first step in the therapeutic relationship, so it is important that the client begins to feel that he or she can trust the counsellor. Good effective use of verbal and non-verbal skills is vital. The counsellor smiles, introduces herself by name, and uses the client's name, as this is a powerful way of establishing personal contact. It can be helpful to find out what the client likes to be called – some people are more comfortable with the more informal use of first names, while others will prefer to have the counsellor use their last name and title. On entering the counselling room, the counsellor indicates where the client should sit with an open hand gesture, smiles and says: 'Please have a seat'.

Before encouraging the client to talk, the counsellor should establish the ground rules of the relationship by explaining the amount of time available and issues relating to confidentiality. The client needs to be aware from the outset that although what is discussed is confidential, there may be some instances when confidentiality has to be breached. This can be tackled by saying simple like: 'I can assure you that what we talk about in these sessions will not be shared with any one else, unless I feel that you are being harmed, or are in danger of harming yourself or someone else. If this happens, and I need to contact someone who may be better able to help you, I will tell you straight away.' Mental health clients will also need to understand the concept of team working and that they may be discussed within the team, but that confidentiality outside of the team still applies.

It can be useful to find out if the client has had any counselling before, and what they thought of it. Most counsellors will also explain what the client can expect from the sessions and what their particular way of working involves. Contracting with the client for a specific number of sessions may be left until the end, when both counsellor and client have had an opportunity to get to know each other.

It may also be appropriate to obtain some personal details and history from the client at this point if none are available. At the very least, it is vital to make sure that you have a contact address and telephone number, and to check with the client whether it's okay to contact them there: a woman in an abusive relationship may not want other family members to know she is seeking help, for instance. Counsellors differ as to whether they would formally assess a client or not. Most person-centred counsellors would not use a formal assessment, whereas a cognitive behavioural therapist would undertake a comprehensive assessment before deciding whether or not to offer counselling. In the mental health setting, the admission procedure will include a detailed assessment of mental state and risk.

Once the business details have been taken care of, the counsellor can 'give permission to talk' by using an open ended question such as 'Where would you like to start?' or 'Tell me what has led up to you coming here today'. The use of open questions encourages the client to begin to tell their story. Encouragement to continue is provided by attention giving and the demonstration of the core conditions.

Attention giving

Being accessible to the client or 'being present' for the client is attention giving. This means that all the counsellor's energy is focused on the client at that moment in time, not allowing thoughts to wander off onto what to cook for dinner! Attention can be shown towards the client by the following non-verbal behaviours:

- alert and relaxed posture;
- lean slightly towards the client;
- eye contact;
- facial expression; and
- head movements.

Observing

This is also part of attention giving, and is vitally important in the mental health setting. Observing is about being aware of one's own bodily sensations, as well as looking at the client. Observing gives important information about what the client feels about him or herself, and what frame of mind they are in. The following observational cues are adopted from Inskipp (2000).

Physical appearance

- Posture;
- Facial expressions;
- Appearance;
- Fidgeting;
- Sweating;
- Blushing; and
- Breathing.

Speech

- Slow;
- Fast;
- Able to articulate ideas clearly;
- Expressiveness;
- Tone and volume of voice; and
- Content of speech.

Thinking

- Rational or irrational thoughts; and
- Disjointed or muddled.

Emotional expression

- Anger;
- Sadness;
- Tears;
- Laughter;
- Appropriateness of emotion to speech content; and
- Incongruence between non-verbal behaviour and content of speech.

Listening

Listening is not the same as hearing – hearing is the physical process of picking up sounds; listening is an active process which requires the listener's full attention, not just to what is being said, but how it is being said. Like attention giving, 'really listening' requires that all the counsellor's energies become focused on the client. Active listening is essential in order to demonstrate empathy, and clients will feel able to talk about themselves when they feel 'listened to'. Self-awareness is important here, because a number of things can get in the way of active listening, such as physical discomfort (hunger, tiredness, a full bladder!), strong emotion, agreeing or disagreeing with the client, memories, formulating a response before the client has finished speaking, boredom, anxiety and preoccupation.

Sustaining the therapeutic relationship – using responding skills

Responding is the way that congruence, acceptance and empathy are communicated to the client, and enables the client to explore further. The word 'responsive' makes a useful mnemonic to remember what responding skills are.

R is for *Reflecting feelings* – identifying what the client is feeling, mainly from non-verbal behaviour and from what you are feeling at that moment.

Example:
'You looked quite angry just now when you talked about your mother . . .'
'I'm feeling a strong sense of sadness right now . . .'

E is for *EXPLORING* – encouraging the client to look more closely at feelings, but make sure that it is the client's agenda, and don't go off at a tangent because it sounds more interesting!

Example:
'Tell me a bit more about the situations you find frightening'
'You say you feel angry. Can you describe that angry feeling a little more?'

S is for *Summarizing* – restate briefly the main points of the session, at the end and at intervals throughout, to check understanding, to help the client to put material in perspective or to move on

Example:
'So, let me check with you – we've been talking about your relationships with people at work, and how you sometimes feel undervalued – is that right?'

P is for *Paraphrasing* – not repeating parrot-fashion, but picking up the meaning of the client's words and restating them, using your own words or the client's words, using imagery and symbolism, and checking your understanding with the client.

Example:

Client: 'I don't know how I'm going to cope, sometimes I feel as if it's all getting on top of me.'

Counsellor: 'You sometimes feel that that you can't cope, as if it's all too much to bear.'

O is for *Open questions* – closed questions can only produce the answer yes or no, and therefore don't encourage the client to go on talking. Open questions encourage the client to say more. Avoid the use of 'why?' because these can be threatening, and they also imply that the client knows why, which is often not the case.

Example:

'What made you decide to come for help at this particular point in your life?'

'In what way does your daughter's attitude affect you?'

N is for *Non-verbal* – always be aware of body language, and share your observations with the client.

Example:

'I noticed you were playing with your watch while you were talking about not having enough time'.

'That was a big sigh, I wonder what that's about?'

S is for *Silence* – don't be afraid of silence, allow yourself and the client some quiet reflection. Silences can feel much longer than they really are, so practice not responding immediately the client has finished speaking. This is often helpful for the client, as they may be thinking about what has just been said, or wondering how to continue. When clients are silent at the start of counselling, it can be helpful to offer some observations to put the client at ease.

Example:

'I can imagine it must be difficult to come and open up to a complete stranger.'

'Perhaps you're wondering where to start?'

I is for *Immediacy* – observing or discussing what is actually happening between the counsellor and the client at that moment in time, or very recently. It can help clients to voice concerns, and gives permission to talk about the relationship between client and counsellor.

Example:

'I felt quite hurt when you said there was no point in talking about your pain because I wouldn't understand. Do you think you could try telling me about it so I can at least get some idea of what it feels like for you?'

'I've noticed that you haven't been here on time for the last three sessions, and I wonder what's making it difficult for you to get here?'

V is for *Validating* – offering support and encouragement, letting the client know that their response is perfectly understandable in the circumstances.

Example:
'Of course you were upset, it had been a difficult time for you'.
'You were only a child, you couldn't be expected to protect all your family from harm'.

E is for *Empathy* – demonstrated by accurate reflection and paraphrasing, and also by expressing the deeper meaning behind what the client is saying.

Example:
Client: 'I'm 51 tomorrow, and I seem to have spent all my life doing the right thing.'
Counsellor: 'Another year older, and you still feel as if you're doing what's expected of you, not what you really want to do'.

Challenging, confronting and focusing

In order to move the client forward, it may be helpful to challenge the client a little more in order to gain a different perspective, or to encourage them to think more deeply about a particular issue by focusing on the choices available. This can also help the client to become aware of themes and inconsistencies.

Challenging and confronting can be difficult, and requires that the counsellor is aware of his or her own personal feelings. A counsellor who dislikes strong negative emotions or feels that challenging is too risky may not help the client to move on, while counsellors who enjoy challenging may be too confronting for a sensitive client. 'It is probably better on the whole to be somewhat reluctant to challenge rather than to be too eager' (Inskipp, 2000, p 87).

Examples:

Focusing:
'You say you feel as if everything you do is wrong. Can you give me an example of the last time you felt like this?'
'Can you give me an example of when that last happened?'

Challenging:
'You say you want to talk about you in the sessions, but you spend a lot of time talking about other people. I wonder if it's harder to talk about yourself?'

Confronting:
'You say you feel fine about it, but you sound a bit uncertain.'

Self-disclosure

Self-disclosure may be either the counsellor sharing some aspect of their own experience, or disclosing feelings he or she has about the client. It should only be used for the good of the client, not motivated by the counsellor's need to share. Inskipp (2000, pp 89–91) offers some useful points on the art of self-disclosure.

Advantages of self-disclosure

- The client may be encouraged to talk more openly about him or herself.
- The therapeutic relationship may be strengthened.
- It can establish an atmosphere of trust.
- It can offer a model of coping and surviving if the client sees that the counsellor has experienced similar difficulties and overcome them.

Disadvantages of self-disclosure

- Done badly, it can take the focus away from the client.
- The client may see the counsellor as a vulnerable person and worry about the counsellor's ability to contain the client's anxieties.
- Some clients may find it threatening.
- The client might feel that the therapist's personality and experiences are very different from their own, and therefore do not see self-disclosure as helpful.

Remember

- Do not disclose too early in the relationship.
- Keep it brief, and don't take the focus away from the client.
- Be aware of your motivation in wanting to share with the client.
- Don't offer the client advice based on your experiences.

Closing the therapeutic relationship

Closing the therapeutic relationship may be the closure of one counselling session, or may be the ending of the therapeutic alliance. Similar skills are needed for both. In an in-patient mental health setting, you need to help the client to be aware from admission that the therapeutic relationship will end. Mental health clients may be passed from a primary nurse in the in-patient setting to a different key worker in the community, and although the client may still be receiving support from the mental health services, it is important that each transition to a different supporting person is handled with the same sensitivity as if ending a counselling relationship. The session must be structured to allow time for endings. The client will have been told how long the session will be at the beginning, so a gentle reminder such as 'Just to let you know that we have ten more minutes' and indicating the visibly placed clock in the counselling room helps the client to realize that the session is nearing the end. Obviously it is not good practice to interrupt the client, so this needs to be flexible, but it is important that the session ends on time. Keeping to time for both beginnings and endings indicates to the client that there are clear boundaries in place, and this gives a feeling of security. In a setting where clients are seen by appointment, running over time can have disastrous consequences for the rest of the day's appointments!

The counsellor then reviews or summarizes the session or sessions for the client. This helps the client to make sense of what may have been a very disjointed session, and also provides the client with an overall impression of the progress that has been made. Summarizing at the end also provides the counsellor with the opportunity to check that they have heard the client accurately. Depending on the type of counselling being offered, there may be 'homework' tasks for the client to do and the counsellor must check understanding and the client's motivation to continue working between sessions. Where 'homework' is not an appropriate option, it is still important to ensure that the client thinks about what it will be like for them between sessions. Clients may have become upset and emotional during counselling, and the counsellor has a responsibility to ensure that the client is not leaving in too vulnerable an emotional state. Directing the client's thoughts to outside the session and offering the client some positive feedback acknowledges and reinforces evidence of the client's growth (Moursund, 1990).

Example:
'It must have taken a lot of courage to talk about this situation – I admire that. How are you feeling now?'
'That must have been difficult for you to share with someone else. How do you think you'll manage these feelings over the next week?'

Bringing the conversation down to a more mundane level, such as asking about the journey home also helps the client to prepare to face the outside world. If the sessions are continuing, then subsequent appointments need to be made, follow up arrangements after an agreed interval. When ending the therapeutic contact altogether, it is important to start discussing endings well in advance of the final appointment, and to facilitate discussion of the client's feelings about endings, how they have perceived the therapeutic encounter, and their plans for the future. Moursund (1990) points out that closure is part of the whole process of counselling, which begins with the first interview. 'By ending helping sloppily you may undo some of the good work you

have done . . . and make it more difficult for clients to return . . . in the future'
(Nelson-Jones, 2000, p 279).

Why and how to refer clients

It is important to remember that referring a client to someone else is not an
indication of failure, but evidence of your wanting the best for the client.
    What if:

- I don't have the necessary skills and/or time to help?
- I feel that someone else would be better able to help?
- The person I am trying to help is suicidal or suffering from a serious mental
  health problem?
- I find it hard to build a relationship with this person, or relate to them in
  a non-judgmental way?
  (*Source*: Adapted from Cormier & Hackney (1993))

In these instances, it may be in the client's best interests to refer them to
someone else.
    How to refer:

- Explain that there is more appropriate help available.
- Make sure the client doesn't see the referral as rejection.
- Involve the client in the referral process as much as possible.
- Continue to support the client until the referral happens, if that is what
  the client wants.
- If you are referring because you felt you couldn't work therapeutically with
  the client, reflect on what was difficult about the situation and identify ways
  in which you could manage it better next time a similar situation arises.
  (*Source*: Adapted from Cormier & Hackney (1993))

Ethical practice in counselling

Counsellors are required to adhere to a code of ethical practice. The main
bodies in the UK that register counsellors are the British Association for
Counselling and Psychotherapy (BACP), the British Psychological
Society (BPS), and the United Kingdom Council for Psychotherapy (UKCP),
and all have a published Code of Conduct to which members are expected
to adhere.
    These codes provide guidance on issues such as respecting the client,
contracting, confidentiality, competence and fitness to practice. When using
counselling skills with patients in any setting, it is important to practice in
accordance with an appropriate ethical code.

Self-awareness and supervision

Part of ethical practice involves supervision by an individual who is suitably trained to provide support and guidance. Supervision can be defined as 'a structured and formal collaborative arrangement whereby a counsellor or psychotherapist reflects regularly on their clinical work with someone who is an experienced practitioner and supervisor' (Wosket, 2000, p 201). Clinical supervision in a nursing setting is still not implemented successfully in every clinical area, although it is a recommendation for good practice. As a mental health professional working with vulnerable clients, it is absolutely essential to ensure that practice is supervised. Any one to one interventions or use of counselling skills *must* be done with the agreement of the rest of the team and a supervisory support system *must* be in place before such work is undertaken. Supervision is not just about protecting clients, but also about protecting counsellors from stress, burnout and the pitfalls of over-involvement and loss of perspective. Supervision is also a space in which the counsellor can explore their work and continue to develop their practice and self-awareness (Wosket, 2000).

References

Beck, A. T. (1976) *Cognitive Therapy and the Emotional Disorders*, New York: International Universities Press.

Brown, J. A. C. (1972) *Freud and the Post-Freudians*, Hormandsworth: Penguin Books.

Cormier, S. & Hackney, H. (1993) *The Professional Counsellor*, Boston: Allyn and Bacon.

Feltham, C. & Horton, I. (2000) Approaches to counselling and psychotherapy, in C. Feltham & I. Horton (eds), *Handbook of Counselling and Psychotherapy*, London: Sage.

Gilliland, B. E., James, R. K. & Bowman, J. T. (1994) *Theories and Strategies in Counselling and Psychotherapy*, Boston: Allyn and Bacon.

Grafanaki, S. (2001) What research has taught us about the concept of congruence, in G. Wyatt (ed.), *Rogers' Therapeutic Conditions Vol. 1 Congruence*, Ross-on-Wye: PCCS Books.

Graves, J. & Robinson J. (1976) Proxemic behaviour as a function of inconsistent verbal and non-verbal messages, *Journal of Counselling Psychology*, 23(4), 333–8.

Haase, R. & Tepper, D. (1972) Non-verbal components of empathic communication, *Journal of Counselling Psychology*, 19, 417–24.

Haugh, S. & Merry, T. (eds) (2001) *Rogers' Therapeutic Conditions. Vol. 2. Empathy*, Ross-on-Wye: PCCS Books.

Inskipp, F. (2000) Generic skills, in C. Feltham & I. Horton (eds), *Handbook of Counselling and Psychotherapy*, London: Sage.

Lambers, E. (1994a) Personality disorder, in D. Mearns (2000) *Developing Person-Centred Counselling*, London: Sage.

Lambers, E. (1994b) Psychosis, in D. Mearns (2000) *Developing Person-Centred Counselling*, London: Sage.

McGuiness, J. (2000) Therapeutic climate, in C. Feltham & I. Horton (eds), *Handbook of Counselling and Psychotherapy*, London: Sage.

Mearns, D. (2000) *Developing Person-Centred Counselling*, London: Sage.

Mearns, D. & Thorne, B. (1999) *Person-Centred Counselling in Action*, London: Sage.

Moursund, J. (1990) *The Process of Counselling and Therapy*, New Jersey: Prentice Hall.

Nelson-Jones, R. (2000) *Introduction to Counselling Skills*, London: Sage.

Palmer, S. & Szymanska, K. (1996) Cognitive therapy and counselling, in S. Palmer, S. Dainow & P. Milner (eds), *Counselling: The BAC Counselling Reader Vol. 1*, London: Sage.

Rogers, C. R. (1951) *Client-Centred Therapy*, Boston: Houghton Mifflin.

Rogers, C. R. (1957) The necessary and sufficient conditions for personality change, *Journal of Consulting Psychology*, 21, 95–103.

Rogers, C. R. (1959) A theory of therapy, personality and interpersonal relationships as developed in the client-centred framework, in S. Koch (ed.), *Psychology: Vol. 3, A Study of Science, Formulation of the Person and the Social Context*, New York: McGraw Hill.

Rogers, C. R. (1961) *On Becoming a Person*, Boston: Houghton Mifflin.

Rowan, J. (1996) The psychology of furniture, in S. Palmer, S. Dainow & P. Milner (eds), *Counselling: The BAC Counselling Reader Vol. 1*, London: Sage.

Seay, T. & Altekruse, M. (1979) Verbal and non-verbal behaviour in judgements of facilitative conditions, *Journal of Counselling Psychology*, 26, 108–19.

Stallard, P. (2002) *Think Good – Feel Good*, Chichester: John Wiley.

The Oxford Handy Dictionary (1986) (6th edn), London: Chancellor Press.

Truax, C. B. & Carkhuff, R. R. (1967) *Toward Effective Counselling and Psychotherapy: Training and Practice*, Chicago: Aldine.

Truax, C. B. & Mitchell, K. (1971) Research on certain therapist interpersonal skills in relation to process and outcome, in M. J. Lambert Bergin & Gardfield (eds), *Handbook of Psychotherapy and Behaviour Change*, Chichester: John Wiley.

Wilkins, P. (2001) Unconditional positive regard reconsidered, in J. Bozarth & P. Wilkins (eds), *Rogers' Therapeutic Conditions Vol. 3 Unconditional Positive Regard*, Ross-on-Wye: PCCS Books.

Woolfe, R. (1997) Counselling in Britain: present position and future prospects, in S. Palmer & G. McMahon (eds), *Handbook of Counselling*, (2nd edn), London and New York: Routledge.

Wosket, V. (2000) Clinical supervision, in C. Feltham & I. Horton (eds), *Handbook of Counselling and Psychotherapy*, London: Sage.

CHAPTER 15

Some Brief Psychological Therapies

JAN CONNOLLY AND SHEILA ARNOLD

Indicative Benchmark Statements

▨ The application of the helping relationship as the cornerstone of their mental health nursing practice

▨ Maintenance of therapeutic alliances with users of mental health and social care services through partnership, intimacy and reciprocity

▨ Participation in negotiation, formulation and communication of therapeutic interventions with users of mental health and social care services and their carers

▨ Application of the basic principles from the psychodynamic, behavioural social and humanistic conceptual models of mental health interventions

▨ Application of the basic principles of person-centred counselling interventions

Introduction

This chapter aims to provide the reader, (who may have little knowledge of and experience in psychotherapeutic work with clients), with a brief overview of two of the brief psychological therapies that might be used with those experiencing the more common mental health problems. Namely, Interpersonal Psychotherapy which may be used when working with clients experiencing non-psychotic depression, and Solution-Focused Therapy which, while moving away from the idea of 'problems' and towards generating 'solutions' as its name implies, may be used with clients experiencing common mental health difficulties such as depression and anxiety. The chapter begins by exploring some of the core components that are requisite to all effective therapeutic practices and progresses to providing a brief explanation of the therapies themselves.

The generation of hope

The first major component across all forms of therapy is the generation of hope. At its most simplistic, the client needs to believe that the therapy being offered will be effective in helping him/her towards problem resolution. Frank (1971) sees the generation of hope as a core mechanism across all psychotherapies. The cognitive component in the instillation of hope in the client is the setting of goals, those which should be important enough to motivate the client, and goals that motivate should, therefore, be achievable, although they might contain a degree of uncertainty. Snyder et al (1991) describe 'pathway thoughts' as being an appraisal of capabilities for finding one or more effective routes to the desired change, clients with a high degree of hope often believe that they can come up with many ways to achieve their desired goals.

Where clients are able to achieve their goals, positive emotions generally result, conversely, when goals are not achieved, the client's sense of well being is often undermined. At the onset of intervention, the establishment of working within a therapeutic alliance is extremely important. Clients have reported that one of the most important components of the therapeutic process is whether or not the client feels both liked and respected by the nurse. Whatever the specific therapy is to be, most clients need an explanatory session before its commencement. This increases the client's hopeful expectations and enhances their perceived ability to deal with their problems: perceived control is essential in maintaining improvement (Snyder et al, 1991).

Empowering the client in the course of therapy

At the beginning of interventions, many clients feel both helpless and out of control. One of the aims of *therapy*, therefore, is to help them to reclaim a sense of control over their life and problems and thus a major function of the *nurse* is to not only to provide support, but also to teach the client coping and problem-solving skills and to work in such a way with the client that he/she is empowered throughout the course of therapy. Therapy is usually perceived by the client as having been successful if or when the client feels less helpless and more in control of their own life. Snyder et al (1991) outline four areas of control that need to be assessed at the onset of therapy:

- environmental influences (how controllable are the client's circumstances);
- skills and abilities for enacting control;
- the responsibility for control; and
- the desire for control.

Clients who feel in control of their lives and problems are more likely to be motivated to continue in therapy and to persist in overcoming problems, thus clients need to have positive expectations about the outcome. Additionally, involving the client in the process of therapy strengthens a sense of control over therapeutic outcome and as therapy proceeds, it is useful for the client to see himself or herself as being responsible for the changes taking place in their lives. Initially, the nurse acts as a guide, making suggestions to the client to test out as therapy continues, the nurse's role becomes collaborative as decision-making is transferred to the client. The role of the nurse is thus to provide an environment that is both secure and allows the client freedom of choice.

In order to maximize the likelihood of a successful outcome to therapy, it is necessary for the nurse to make the following assumptions about both the client and the therapy being offered.

Assumptions about the client

Regardless of the specific therapy to be offered, most will make common assumptions about the client, the major assumption being that clients have both the strengths and resources to solve problems. As an individual, the client is responsible for his/her actions and has the capacity to change actions regardless of either background or affective state. It is also assumed that clients can change some areas of their lives. Clients who appear to be resistant and unco-operative often seem so when they feel that the nurse has not listened; has blamed or negated them in some way or is not perceived as being helpful. It is, therefore, important that the nurse believes that the client is intrinsically able to work through difficulties with the necessary support and approaches the client with a positive, non-blaming and non-judgemental attitude.

Assumptions about therapy

The major assumption about therapy is that it is both relevant to client need and that it will, therefore, be effective in helping the client to work through problems and enhance coping skills. In the two therapies out-lined in this chapter, it is also largely assumed that it is not always necessary to know the specific aetiology, history or function of a problem in order to resolve it. Therefore, the therapies referred to later may be viewed as empir-ical in nature.

Assessment considerations

Assessment is assumed to be an ongoing process: it is not necessary to have 'the right diagnosis' at the onset of therapy, however the suitability of the chosen therapy *vis-à-vis* client problems usually becomes apparent in the early stages. Risk is an important area of assessment in terms not only of risk behaviours such as suicidality or violence etc. but also in terms of the context in which therapy is being offered ie: therapy must be offered in an environment that maximizes client safety.

In the process of client assessment, key questions include 'who thinks that there is a problem?', 'what is that person complaining about?' – these questions can become the focus of therapy. Other areas of consideration include what the client wants to be the outcome of therapy and therefore ensuring that its resulting goals are both realistic and attainable. Is the client motivated towards therapy and if not, why not? It may be that a perceived lack of motivation is symptomatic of the client's affective state, in depression for example, or that the therapy offered is not appropriate to client need or equally, that the client does not perceive the nurse as being helpful in some way.

Brief psychological therapies and psychopharmacotherapy

The taking of prescribed psychotropic medication is not contra-indicated with therapy: indeed, for example, a severely depressed client might well benefit from antidepressant medication before the commencement of therapy in order to elevate mood sufficiently to improve the client's levels of interaction and to remain on it throughout the course of therapy.

Interpersonal Psychotherapy

Weissman et al (1984) first developed Interpersonal Psychotherapy (IPT) as a short-term therapy for depression. It is an empirical model of intervention, rather than aetiolgical and is based upon the belief that depression is (assumed to be) either maintained or worsened by the client's interpersonal functioning and therefore improvement in interpersonal functioning will decrease the number and intensity of depressive feelings. Klerman et al (1984) state that the improvement in depression will occur regardless of whether or not interpersonal problems are the primary cause of depression or are concomitant to it.

The main aim of IPT is the alleviation of depressive symptoms and it focuses on interpersonal functioning as the major mechanism for therapeutic change. It specifically focuses on interpersonal problems as they relate to the beginning, the maintenance and any worsening of depression and its symptoms. The focus of IPT is on the present, therapy is time-limited, usually from 12 to 16 weeks and, therefore, discussion is focused upon current difficulties and ways in which they might be improved.

IPT is conducted in three stages: the initial stage, the intermediate stage and the final sessions.

The initial stage

In the first two to three sessions, the client describes the problems for which they are seeking help. Assuming that the nurse believes the client to be depressed, the client is told that they are suffering from depression. Many clients cannot actually put a 'label' to their symptoms and in telling the client that they are depressed can help them to understand that the symptoms they are experiencing are part of a syndrome which is both common and treatable, thus giving the client hope for the future. At this point, the client is assigned 'the sick role', the client is exempted from normal social functioning and responsibilities and is told to focus upon the task of recovery. This empha- sizes the active role the client should take in therapy and the sick role is presented as inevitable but time-limited. Once they understand that these symptoms are part of depression, the client and nurse start to explore the interpersonal context of the client's depression.

The client is then asked to complete an 'interpersonal inventory' – simply, the client names; the significant people in their life; the types of relationship; ranks them in order of importance; identifies what kind of support that person gives the client – whether it is practical, emotional or motivational – and how the client reciprocates.

At this point, the client is asked to describe the changes that would improve any problematic relationships. The nurse and client then identify the specific goals of therapy and form a treatment plan for the remaining sessions.

The intermediate stage

These are sessions 4 to 12 of therapy. In the initial stage one of four target problems is defined and intermediate sessions are used to help the client work through the target problem. The target problems are grief; role disputes; role transition and interpersonal deficits.

Grief

The goals are to facilitate the client through a healthy bereavement process and to develop other relationships/interests. This should lead to a decrease in depressive symptoms through acceptance of the loss and an increase in support from others.

Role disputes

This refers to instances where both the client and at least one other signifi- cant person have differing or incompatible expectations of their relationship.

Snyder et al (2000) have noted that unresolved role disputes tend to be related to the onset and maintenance of depression. The goals of therapy are to identify the dispute; form an action plan and to modify expectations and/or communication patterns to bring about resolution.

Role transitions

A great deal of literature links depression to major life changes, retirement and unemployment being two very common examples. Generally, role transitions associated with depression are associated with feelings by the client of being unable to cope with the transition. The goal of IPT is to help the client to grieve for the loss of the old role if necessary and to acquire new sources of social support and coping mechanisms to deal with the transition.

Interpersonal deficits

Clients with interpersonal deficits have had problems throughout their lives in forming and maintaining relationships. If there is no existing relationship upon which to focus, the nurse may need to explore past relationships or even focus upon the client–nurse relationship as a starting point. In this instance communication analysis may be used to explore relationship skills, and techniques such as role-play might be used as strategies for forming new relationships.

The final sessions

In the final three or four sessions, the nurse allows the client to express any feelings about the ending of the therapy, but at the same time, encourages them to try out newly learned techniques independently. Successes throughout the course of treatment should be positively reinforced to boost the client's self-esteem and strategies for how the client will deal with future difficulties should be discussed.

Some clients, particularly those, who are chronically depressed, may require a new, longer-term therapeutic contract, however, most clients will be anxious about the ending of therapy. Klerman et al (1984) recommend that clients wait from four to eight weeks to determine whether further therapy is either appropriate and/or necessary.

Solution Focused Therapy

Solution Focused Therapy (SFT) was developed by de Shazer and Berg (de Shazer, 1985, 1988, 1991, 1994; Berg 1994) in the mid 1980s and has been used successfully in a variety of settings. This therapeutic approach is useful when working with clients in a time-limited way, for example, in acute in-patient care. It also offers the nurse a 'brief' way of working or communicating with clients which is positive and does not promote the pathologizing of the individual. It places emphasis upon the individual's personal story and recognizes that values are alternative, not normative (Anderson and Goolishian, 1992). SFT is a co-operative psychological approach that is neither 'expert' led nor diagnostic, and places emphasis upon co-constructing meaning with the client, with the nurse intervening only to the extent necessary to create movement in the client's behaviour. The past is only explored for examples of what has worked well for the client and can be used to inform possible actions the client may take in the present.

The nurse will use this short-term goal-focused therapeutic conversational (Gilligan & Price, 1993) approach to help clients talk about change by constructing solutions rather than dwelling on problems. For example, the client who dwells upon problems can be helped to talk about what they can do to make some change to their situation. This involves the nurse in making a theoretical shift away from an interpretive or directive approach to therapeutic intervention and places an emphasis upon conversations (Jones, 1999) that focus on mobilizing hope, using existing support systems and supporting the clients' strengths. In this way the client will be facilitated by the nurse in constructing their own solutions from their own experiences, building upon their past successes.

A central feature of this approach is the assumption that the problems and goals worked on are those chosen by the client and that they already have extensive resources to bring to the discussion. An important difference between solution-focused and more traditional psychotherapy, or the psychiatric tradition, is that there is very little need for a detailed history and less requirement for analysis of symptoms of illness or problems. This promotes the possibility that the conversations between nurses' and clients' would adopt a positive approach involving the view of the client and talking about their personal context assuming that they are capable of making changes and creating what they want (O'Hanlon & Weiner-Davis, 1989).

Moving away from 'problem talk' towards 'solution construction'

The nurse will find that detailed descriptions of the client's complaint may be helpful in designing interventions and care planning, but for solution-focused conversations it is not essential. The solution-focused approach involves the client in doing something different in response to their situation, and all that really needs to be known is, 'How will we know when the problem is solved or situation has been resolved?' One of the first principles is that more time is spent focusing on solutions and less time focusing on problem talk (O'Hanlon & Weiner-Davis, 1989). Elements of the desired solution are often already present in the client's life, and could become the basis for ongoing change.

The nurse does not hypothesize in advance what might be 'the client's problem' and far less 'the solution' but seeks to understand the client by listening (only) to what they say. The solution-focused style of questioning assumes that, by emphasizing the view of the person, personal meaning will emerge and establish what the client wants; what will make a difference; how they will know that things have improved and in what ways are they experiencing something of what they want now. More specifically, the nurse asks about exceptions to the problems (Molnar & de Shazer, 1987); how the client presently copes; hypothetical scaling position or movement; creating a desired scenario; a future focus and personal resources.

The nurse's discussion with the client will focus upon what they have learned from their past experiences; what they wish to leave behind and how they would have liked to have been different in the past; how that would have made a difference for them now and how they live through, or cope with, their experiences. The client's perception of the problem becomes central to the conversation and the truism 'the problem is the problem, not the person' (Walter & Peller, 1992) becomes fundamental.

The nature of the questions asked, contain assumptions within them and by asking particular questions the nurse facilitates directions toward particular answers (Walter & Peller, 1992). For example, questions relating to the cause and maintenance of problems change to an exploration of how to construct solutions. This approach involves defining what the client wants rather than what they do not want, looking for what is working and doing more of it and if what they are doing is not working then require them to do something different. A solution-focused approach encompasses a way of thinking as well as a way of conversing with clients, which then creates and enables a way of constructing solutions interactively. It is not a collection of techniques or an elaboration of a technique rather it reflects fundamental notions of change, interaction and reaching goals. The nurse's goal is to help people become more specific in their descriptions of their complaints and goals and to become more present and future oriented. This is to help clients, who present with vague complaints, to be able to present their goals more specifically, in the form of a task (de Shazer and Molnar, 1984).

Some assumptions central to the SFT approach include looking for small positive changes that would be empowering for the client. This involves the recognition and use of clients' existing strengths thereby helping them reframe problems to provide solutions by considering other interpretations of the situation and keeping concepts simple and meaningful. The focus of the talk about solutions increases the opportunities for the client to develop possible solutions. The rules proposed include 'If it isn't broken – don't fix it'; 'If it works – do more of it'; 'If it doesn't work, do something different' (de Shazer, 1994).

The assumptions underpinning this approach (de Shazer 1985, 1988, 1991, 1994) view human interaction as the context in which complaints develop and are maintained and the task of therapy is to help the client do something different. The view is taken that clients are not 'resistant' but seek change when their attempted solutions have not been working. The process of helping involves helping the client seek different meanings from their experiences that can be constructed in response to their situation. If the client explores their behaviours or interactions in another context this could lead to redefining their 'symptoms' as normal and possibly appropriate behaviours in light of the circumstances.

The idea that change is always occurring and therefore is inevitable and also that both small change and small goals are necessary are central to working with the clients' behaviour and can lead to changes in the behaviour of all involved in an interaction. SFT is a straightforward, practical, understandable, and quick-to-begin therapeutic approach that focuses on what the client wants and on ways to help clients reach their goals. A solution-focused nurse would consider talking about problems only when necessary but rather should focus more directly on helping the client construct solutions. As such it is an approach well suited to the short-term contact or brief time-limited opportunities for therapeutic interaction within in-patient stay facilities or community visits.

This approach involves defining what the client wants rather than what they do not want, looking for what is working and do more of it and if what the client is doing is not working then have them do something different. The stages of solution building typically involve the following in the first session (de Jong and Berg, 1997).

The formula first session task

By stating the goal or problem, the nurse begins the interaction and this is accomplished by asking the client what they want from the interaction. This might be with a question such as, 'What is your goal in being here?' Clients are asked to briefly describe the events that lead them to seek help.

Clients may be quite clear about what their objectives are and in this case the nurse would proceed by discussing examples of situations in which the goal or objective is already being achieved partly or occasionally. In the event that the client can't think of situations where the goal is already occurring, the nurse asks the client to think about hypothetical solutions wherein at some future time the goal is achieved. For example, looking back from the future to see how they resolved the problem. If the client has trouble conceptualizing a future situation without the difficulties then the following questioning approach is used.

The Miracle Question (MQ)

During the conversation the nurse will focus on the client's goals, exceptions, pre-treatment changes and, in general, the client's resources. The nurse does this by using their client's language, and at the same time promoting the descriptions in specific, small, positive (presence of solutions rather than absence of problems). Nurses should adopt a respectful, non-blaming and co-operative stance, working towards their client's goals from within their client's frame of reference.

The MQ is used to help the client express and shape up their desired scenario and can begin with a question such as: 'If a miracle happened tonight and you woke up with the problem solved, or you were reasonably confident you were on a track to solving it, what would you be doing differently?' Wherever possible it is helpful to obtain statements that include action, behaviour, some new way of viewing the problem, or to articulate something they will be saying to themselves or others (de Shazer, 1985, 1988; Cade and O'Hanlon, 1993; Walter and Peller, 1992). For the practical-minded who don't like miracle questions the following approach may be taken: 'If this were the last time we were to talk and parting with your the problem solved, or at least were getting on with solving it, what would you be doing differently?'

Exploring exceptions

The process of searching for exceptions to the problem can occur at any time during the interaction – after the client has had appropriate time to describe the problem (O'Hanlon, 1999). As exceptions to the problem are usually considered rare by clients, they can be surprised by anyone asking about when the problem doesn't occur. To make this transition easier for them, the nurse should use whatever opportunities and descriptions the client offers to ask 'exception finding' questions. Although the examples below use the word 'problem', once it is established what the client does when the problem doesn't occur then the questions can be phrased in those terms.

A solution-focused nurse would believe that information about problems isn't necessary; that solution construction is independent from the problem processes. After getting a statement of the problem or goal, the nurse would ask about recent changes or exceptions to the problem, rather than examining what caused or maintains the problem. The nurse would also ask questions which explore for exceptions to the problem to encourage the client to continue doing what is already working rather than trying to figure out something new which might not work.

Exception finding questions

Even when the complaint is limited to the client only or to the client's significant other, it is useful to gather information on the client's perceptions of the other person. It adds more depth and breadth to the description of the exceptions and what part others may play. These relationship questions can be expanded to include other family or personal contacts depending on the nature of the client's situation. The answers to the 'exception finding questions' provide clues (de Shazer, 1988) as to what the solution would look like to the clients and their significant others. The miracle question and the scaling questions can be used to determine which exceptions are related to the client's goals so that the steps toward a solution can be negotiated. Coping questions are used to highlight how the patient keeps going, carries on living, or isn't 'worse' given the presence of the problem. This promotes the experience or reinforces that the client is already coping in some way and empowers the person.

The nurse, moving towards a future construction, will ask the client what they will be doing when the problem is no longer troubling them. This is achieved by supporting the client as they construct solutions in the form of behavioural tasks. A presupposition within solution constructing questions is the belief that there are solutions to the client's situation; that there is more than one solution; that they are constructable: that the nurse and client can do the constructing and that solutions are *constructed* and/or *invented* rather than discovered.

Solution-focused goals

These are described in terms of what the person will be doing or thinking when their goal is reached or the problem is resolved. One way of describing goals is in verbs ending with '-ing', for example, 'I will be *listening, reminding* myself, *going* shopping, *doing* my housework, *reading* regularly, *going* to bed on time, etc' The nurse will facilitate the client in stating their goals in terms of what the client will do *now* or *soon*, rather than in the far future.

If the client is having difficulty in stating their goal according to the criteria for well-defined goals, then questions about *hypothetical solutions* can be asked. This is in order to help clients free themselves from past unsuccessful problem definitions and help them come up with a positive way to describe their goal. Hypothetical solutions are sought before exploring exceptions because hypothetical solutions encourage picturing a future where the solution has been attained. If the problem is the client's view or poor motivation and the nurse asks for 'exceptions', they could get examples of times when the client is motivated and active or the nurse could ask what the client will be doing differently (hypothetical solution) when they are motivated and active.

Formulation of well developed goals

The client is helped to generate a description of what will be different when the problem is solved through the development of specific workable goals.

Good goals meet the following six criteria:

- Goals are stated in the positive.
- Goals are stated in process (what will you be doing?) form.
- Goals are stated in the here-and-now.
- Goals are as specific as possible.
- Goals are stated in ways that are within their control.
- Goals are stated in client's own language (adapted from de Shazer, 1991)

Sometimes, a client's goals include statements about what they want others to do differently. The nurse can ask questions such as: 'What do you want different as a result of talking today?' In order to help the client return their focus to themselves and their own role in the creation of the solution, the nurse asks questions about what others will notice the client doing differently when things are better.

Other questions that help the client focus on solutions rather than problems include: 'What is working already for you and how might you do more of it?'; 'What are you doing that keeps the problem going?'; 'What would you like to try that is different from what you ordinarily do?'. These latter questions help the client move beyond the goal statement to considering exceptions to the problems, or what might comprise a hypothetical solution.

End of session feedback

At the end of the discussion, as a form of summing up, the nurse will allow time for the client and themselves to think about the conversation, by facilitating the opportunity to think about what has happened. De Shazer and Molnar (1984) suggest as a final assignment, 'Between now and the next time we meet, I would like you to observe, so that you can describe this to me next time, what happens in your life that you want to continue to have happen?' The notion is that not only will clients be more clear about what they want to continue, but also that they will be able to describe new changes that have occurred because they followed through behaviour they thought would be successful.

Evaluation of the client's progress

During subsequent contacts the nurse can focus on eliciting talk about what is better for the client, what they are doing to make that happen and what they notice themselves doing differently since the last conversation. Also, there is discussion about how the client can do more of the same. If the client reports that things are not better, then further talk should centre on how the client is coping, why things are not worse and how they can do something different to feel a sense of change and success no matter how small.

The nurse's critical awareness of the use of a solution-focused questioning and helping style of interacting with clients offers a strategy or way of talking with them that promotes and reinforces their self-esteem, facilitates experiences of success and a sense of empowerment.

Conclusion

The general aim of this chapter has been to explore aspects of the development of therapeutic nursing skills important when working with clients experiencing mental distress. For the engagement of clients the emphasis is placed upon the development of a therapeutic alliance as an essential precursor to further therapeutic endeavour. Interpersonal and solution-focused therapies are explored for the nature of nursing attitudes, knowledge and skills important when working therapeutically with clients. Importance is placed upon a positive approach and optimism, considering individual needs, the power differentials between client and nurse, the importance of non-judgemental, non-blaming and non-punitive attitudes and the consideration of difference perspectives when working with mental health and social care service users. The approaches explored examine the nature of participation in the negotiation, formulation and communication skills involved in therapeutic intervention. They also offer strategies for the enablement of users (their families and carers) in establishing their own meaningful focus or goals in the formulation of their care plans. Finally the importance of a critical awareness of the student's own understanding, attitudes and competence and needs in their present and future personal and professional development of therapeutic ways of working with clients (UKCC, 2000).

References

Anderson, H. & Goolishian, H. (1992) The client is the expert: a not-knowing approach to therapy, in S. McNamee & K. J. Gergen (eds), *Therapy as a Social Construction*, London: Sage, Ch 2. 25–39.

Berg, I. K. (1994) *Family-Based Services: A Solution-Focused Approach*, New York: WW Norton.

Cade, B. & O'Hanlon, W. H. (1993) *A Brief Guide to Brief Therapy*, London: WW Norton & Company.

de Jong, P. & Berg, I. K. (1997) *Interviewing for Solutions*, Pacific Grove CA: Brooks Cole Publishing.

de Shazer, S. (1985) *Keys to Solution: Brief Therapy*, London: WW Norton & Company.

de Shazer, S. (1988) *Clues: Investigating Solutions in Brief Therapy*, London: WW Norton & Company.

de Shazer, S. (1991) *Putting Difference to Work*, London: WW Norton & Company.

de Shazer, S. (1994) *Words Were Originally Magic*, New York: WW Norton.

de Shazer, S. & Molnar, A. (1984) Four useful interventions in brief family therapy, *Journal of Family Therapy*, 10(3), 297–304.

Frank, J. D. (1971) Therapeutic factors in psychotherapy, *American Journal of Psychotherapy*, 25, 350–61.

Gilligan, S. & Price, R. (eds) (1993) *Therapeutic Conversations*, Londn: WW Norton & Company.

Jones, A. (1999) Listen, listen, trust your own strange voice (psyhoanalytically informed conversations with a woman suffering serious illness), *Journal of Advanced Nursing*, 29(4), 826–31.

Klerman, G. L., Weissman, M. M., Rounsaville, B. J. & Chevron, E. S. (1984) *Interpersonal Psychotherapy of Depression*, New York: Basic Books.

Molnar, A. & de Shazer, S. (1987) Solution-focused therapy: toward the identification of therapeutic tasks, *Journal of Marital and Family Therapy*, 13, 349–58.

O'Hanlon, W. H. (1999) *Do One Thing Different*, New York: William Morrow & Company.

O'Hanlon, W. H. & Weiner-Davis, M. (1989) *In Search of Solutions: A New Direction in Psychotherapy*, London: WW Norton & Company, London.

Snyder, C. R. & Ingram, R. E. (eds) (2000) *Handbook of Psychological Change: Psychotherapy Processes and Practices for the 21st Century*, London: John Wiley & Sons.

Snyder, C. R., Harris, C., Anderson, J. R., Holleran, S. A., Irving, L. M., Sigmon, S. T., Yoshinobu, L., Gibb, J., Langelle, C. & Haevey, P. (1991) The will and the ways: development and validation of an individual differences measure of hope, *Journal of Personality and Social Psychology*, 60, 570–85.

UKCC (United Kingdom Central Council For Nursing, Midwifery and Health Visiting), (2000), *Requirements for Pre-registration Nursing Programmes*, London: UKCC.

Walter, J. L. & Peller, J. E. (1992) *Becoming Solution-Focused in Brief Therapy*, New York: Brunner/Mazel.

Weissman, M. M., Klerman, G. L., Rounsaville, B. J. & Chevron, E. S. (1984) *Interpersonal Psychotherapy of Depression*, New York: Basic Books.

CHAPTER 16

Person-centred Approach to the Care of Older People With Mental Health Problems

LIZ DESIRA AND GEOFF MARTIN

Indicative Benchmark Statements

■ Identification of the impact of stigma on mental health service users, their families and carers, and the motivational basis of prejudice

■ Ability to work in mental health and social care settings in a non-discriminatory way

■ A caring and empathetic attitude to users of mental health and social care services and their carers

■ Participation in the practice of psycho-social rehabilitation

■ Identification of the complexities of mental health and social care within acute settings

---

Introduction

It is thought that old age can be seen, fundamentally, as a frame of mind and perhaps older people are acting out society's expectations of how they should behave. Goffman's early work on the way we present ourselves in everyday life (Goffman, 1969) came to the conclusion that people act out the roles that are expected of them. As a result the attitude of individuals, communities and society towards older people may influence the way they behave and perhaps even feel. This chapter addresses this idea as central to an understanding of mental health problems commonly seen to occur in this group of people and will outline the range of problems as well as pointing towards ways of addressing them from a person-centred perspective.

If we agree that people act out their roles based on stereotypical ideas of how they should behave we must also conclude that there is the potential to foster prejudice toward any group of people that is stereotyped in this way. Sexism, homophobia, racism and ageism may be the result of this process and can bring about disempowerment of the individual if such prejudice exists (Croft & Beresford, 1989). Our focus is on the effect this has upon older people. We need, therefore, to consider the role that ageism can play in the lives of those subject to it and consider a person-centred approach in an effort to bring about a cultural change in the environment of care.

Person-centred care

There has been a move in recent years to adopt a person-centred approach for the care of people with dementia arising out of the work of Kitwood (1993, 1997a). This approach attempts to understand the person with dementia by a process of empathy and individualized care. The notion of 'them and us' that labels the client as damaged, different and disabled needs to be challenged. Kitwood feels that health professionals are all part of the problem. He reminds us that we are, in fact, *potentially* 'them' and should, therefore, try to care for clients as though they were our own relatives. Three key areas identified by Kitwood and Bredin (1995) to bring about change are:

- Viewing 'behaviour' as a form of communication rather than a problem to be managed. If we can understand what is being communicated we may be able to address the need and so resolve the problem.
- Physical care while important is only part of the care, it is just as important to provide age-appropriate activities and human social contact.
- The client's reality is real for them and as such should be validated rather than they be 'orientated' to our reality.

It is important that the culture changes to accommodate this different approach to care that can, according to Kitwood, maintain the person's independence and self-esteem. Alongside this approach, there needs to be ongoing audits of care, as new cultures are fragile and old ways of working can become re-established. Dementia care mapping can be used as an audit tool to monitor improvements in this area (Martin & Younger, 2000, 2001).

The role of ageism

Stereotypes can have a strong influence upon our perceptions of people, which influences and undermines our ability to interact in a person-centred way. Common notions of older people lead to images of somebody difficult, irritable and inflexible. The old man shouting abuse at the children playing outside his house confirms this view. The old lady in front of you in the super-market having a long chat at the checkout and struggling to get her purchases into the bags, underlines the standard perception of the slow, confused and perhaps lonely old lady stereotype. Old age can bring about many negative images such as useless, disabled, incapable, dependent, incontinent. As a result older people can feel worthless, devalued, unwanted, and a burden, thus affecting their self-concept and self-esteem. It is easy to link these feelings to the perceived inevitability of mental health problems such as depression, dementia and paranoia. However we need to be cautious, this jump is too great, as the majority of older people do not suffer from such problems despite having to face negative attitudes. Perhaps these attitudes arise from our reluc-tance to face our own future, our fears of loss of control, powerlessness, ulti-mately a fear of death, and anxiety about the causation and manner in which this will occur. Inexplicably we take note of the negatives, the positives do not attract the same attention.

In order to maintain the self-concept and self-esteem of older people it is necessary to acknowledge the many positive factors surrounding this age group. An understanding of the range and diversity of the lives of older people can bring us to a greater understanding of the person. Work done by The Dementia Services Development Centre in Sterling and Goldsmith's impor-tant exploration of hearing the voices of people with dementia (Goldsmith, 1996) have lead the way forward in the field of care of people with demen-tia. We can use this material to value, understand and empower older people whatever their mental health problem. The old have had many years of problem solving and had the opportunity to learn from experience and obser-vation, and through these processes have gained wisdom. The older person has much to offer and would experience better mental health if only they were afforded respect, dignity and time.

One of the most extreme consequences of ageism, prejudice and disem-powerment is elder abuse, sometimes related to the problem of 'burnout' associated with the stress of caring over a long period of time. Elder abuse is defined by Kingston and Penhale (1994) as being intentional or unintentional or the result of neglect. It causes harm to the older person, either temporary or over a period of time. It can take many forms:

- Physical abuse, which can include not providing sufficient food, negle-cting personal care needs, not requesting medical care, use of physical restraint or assault including sexual assult.
- Psychological abuse involving lack of respect, privacy and dignity, swear-ing, humiliation, harassment and verbal threats.
- Material abuse consists of misuse or theft of property or money. Abuse can take place in the person's own home, their place of residence, e.g. with family member, or in institutional settings such as nursing homes or hospitals.
- Sociological abuse involving loss of social contact and abandonment.

Any suspicion of abuse should, of course, be reported and investigated in accordance with local and professional guidelines and regulations. The Social Services Inspectorate in 1992 identified two main strategies focused around the abused elder:

- to help the person remain at home by providing appropriate services; and
- to separate the individuals involved, usually through provision of residential or nursing home care for the older person.

The latter approach was seen as a last resort and it could be argued that it is the abused elder that should remain at home with support and the abuser removed. It is clear that continuous monitoring of the situation is necessary as well as careful co-odination of services (ibid).

Common mental health problems

The most frequently seen mental illnesses in older people are dementia (organic illness) and affective disorders, depression and anxiety being the most common (functional illness). Initial presentation for these conditions can be similar so it is important that we carry out a full assessment to ensure the correct care and treatment is put into place. Signs and symptoms must be understood and accurately recorded during the assessment process to avoid confusion and misdiagnosis.

Dementia

Dementia, is more commonly seen in old age, and with an increasing elderly population it may becoming more prevalent. The various forms of dementia have features in common, although there may be variations in different types of dementia. It is important to identify which type of dementia the client has as treatment and care is different for each. For all, however, person-centred care must be a central plank of care delivery.

Alzheimer's Disease

Alzheimer's Disease is the commonest form of dementia and has the longest duration, although many theories of causation have been proposed no one conclusive factor has been identified and research continues in this area. It is difficult to give a list of typical symptoms as the disease can present differently for different people. Table 16.1 gives a comprehensive list but that is

Table 16.1 Summary of symptoms of Alzheimer's Disease

Behavioural	Cognitive	Perceptual	Mood
Tactlessness; Social withdrawal; Loss of receptive and expressive skills; Inability to plan activities; Inability to set goals; Inability to organize; Altered concentration levels; Walking; Lack of purpose; Catastrophic reactions; Poor self-care skills; Inability to maintain own safety.	Poor concentration; Pre-occupied with self; Disorientation for time; Poor ability to make choices; Impaired judgement; Impaired communication	Delusions; Hallucinations; Initially loss of recent memory; Later loss of long-term memory; Difficulty identifying visual and auditory stimulation.	Emotional lability; Frustration; Agitation; Difficulty controlling temper; Violent outbursts, verbal and/or physical.

Source: Adapted from Stokes & Goudie (1990)

not to say the people with Alzheimer's disease will show all of these and some may only show a very few, particularly in the early stages of the illness (Stokes & Goudie, 1990).

Multi infarct dementia

This consists of a step like progression of deterioration as intermittent damage occurs to parts of the brain, due to arteriosclerosis, embolus or haemorrhage. The 'stroke like' episodes result in physical and mental decline and the effected individual may experience seizures (Stokes & Goudie, 1990).

Lewy body dementia

This condition has been recognized in recent years. Lewy bodies, found in the substantia nigra, result in Parkinson's disease, however it is thought that lewy bodies found in the neocortex cause dementia. Research is still ongoing, but sufferers of Parkinson's Disease usually have lewy bodies in the neocortex and the substantia nigra, which could account for the dementia in Parkinson's disease, not a coincidental combination of Parkinsons and Alzheimer's disease as previously thought. Sufferers experience unexplained falls, loss of consciousness, hallucinations, delusions and fluctuating memory loss. Neuroleptic medication, often given for the treatment of hallucinations and delusions in other conditions, have adverse effects in Lewy body dementia and can result in death (Walton, 1999).

Less common forms of dementia

Wernicke's Encepholopathy and Korsokoff's Syndrome are associated with alcohol use and thiamine deficiency. A diagnosis of alcohol-related dementia may be difficult to establish due to difficulty in gaining an accurate drinking history. However symptoms include regular bouts of challenging behaviour, which are difficult to anticipate and understand (Stokes and Goudie, 1990).

Creutzfeldt–Jakob disease is a rare but rapidly progressive form of dementia usually occurring between the ages of 50 and 75 years. There appear to be three ways of getting this illness:

1 Sporadic Creutzfeldt–Jakob disease where there is no known cause;
2 Inherited Creutzfeldt–Jakob disease – approximately 10 to 15 per cent of cases are inherited;
3 Creutzfeldt–Jakob disease through infection through iatrogenic transmission due to contaminated surgical instruments or transplant of infected material (http://cjdfoundation.org, 2002)

The duration of the illness is usually one year, but can range from several months to two years. The early signs are insomnia, depression, confusion, personality and behavioural changes and difficulty with memory, co-ordination and vision, as the illness progresses there are involuntary, jerky movements, muscular weakness problems with language and dementia.

Depression

Assessment of the older person presenting with a low mood is extremely important in order to decide observation levels, guide interventions and assist with decisions on future care needs. It is important to distinguish sadness – temporary responses that will go away in a relatively short period of time, from depression that is more severe and enduring and requires professional help. Causation may be multi-faceted, influenced by biopsychosocial factors and vulnerability should be taken into account, a genetic predisposition to depression may be triggered by changing family and social circumstances, e.g. death of spouse, moving house, retirement, financial problems, deterioration in mobility and physical health. Medication being taken for physical conditions should also be considered as depression is a possible side effect of some drugs used to treat hypertension and inflammatory conditions such as arthritis.

Indications of depression include disturbed sleep, fatigue, loss of energy, alterations in weight and appetite, irritability, lack of self-care, loss of interest in previously enjoyed activities, low self-esteem, feelings of worthlessness and hopelessness, a change in psychomotor activity – either increased as in agitation or decreased as in retardation may be present and an inability to plan for the future.

Suicide is a risk for the depressed elderly person especially if they have been recently bereaved, are living alone, have a chronic mental illness or chronic physical illness or have a previous history of suicide attempts. Warning signs include talk about death, expressions of hopelessness and helplessness, increased use of prescription drugs and/or alcohol, not following medical advice, accumulating large amounts of medication, social withdrawal, making elaborate goodbyes to family and friends, and suddenly making or changing a will (Evans, 2000).

Some individuals may present complaining of physical problems such as constant tiredness, headaches or stomach upsets but no emotional, cognitive or behavioural symptoms. When physical illness has been excluded and possible causative factors of depression have been identified treatment for depression should be offered.

Sometimes an older person does not complain of physical complaints or present with emotional disturbance but with poor concentration and difficulty with memory and cognition, this can lead to a misdiagnosis of dementia or be put down to the normal ageing process and is known as *pseudo dementia* (Riley, 1994)

Care interventions

Consent

Before care interventions can take place, consent must be obtained. Such consent is sometimes a difficult issue with older people. Some may need longer to think about things and need more clarification and explanations, especially if they have dementia. They may canvas opinions from a variety of sources, this can be interpreted as an inability to think for themselves or make the decision, when in fact it is their way of making an informed choice. Although relatives and informal carers cannot give consent, they may try to help by stepping in too early and sometimes see things from a different perspective from the older person. Here the nurse must use careful observation of mood and verbal and non-verbal communication. Withdrawing from the conversation does not always indicate agreement, it can be giving in to what they see as pressure, or agreement because they do not want to be a nuisance or a burden. The nurse may have to act as advocate by suggesting more time for them to think, by discussing the options once more and giving support whatever the decision (Gates, 1994) Many older people see health professionals as 'all knowing', and will comply without question, care should be negotiated wherever possible and although guidance may be needed care should not be dictated. In the case of dementia, consent may have to be an ongoing process. If agreement is reached initially, because of short-term memory loss, this may later be withdrawn. The nurse must take this into account and stop care procedures until consent is reached again.

Drug therapy

Medication for the treatment of mental disorder should be used with caution as absorption and metabolism may be altered in older people (Fielo and Rizzolo, 1985). Older people frequently have a concurrent physical illness that can be affected by medication used in mental health thus preventing usage or requiring lower doses than that used for a younger person.

As there is increased risk of side effects, adverse reactions and drug inter-actions, major tranquillisers are contra-indicated for people with dementia (Stokoe, 2001). If there are incidents of challenging behaviour or agitation a person-centred approach is the best way to address it but in the interests of the patient, if there is distress or anxiety, it may be necessary to resort to some form of drug therapy. This should never be used to compensate for poor staffing levels or pressure from relatives and others to 'do something'. The drug of choice is Resperidone (Tune, 2001) but this should be given with caution and its effects monitored carefully. There are many side effects associated with the drug and so the lowest possible dose should always be prescribed.

There a number of new drugs now available for people with dementia, if in the mild to moderate phase, drugs such as Aricept (Donepezil), which can give up to two years respite (Rogers et al, 1998). It has been found to be effective in treating symptoms of memory and cognitive loss in this group of patient with Alzheimer's Disease. The patients show improvements in cognitive function as well as global function to extent of showing an improvement in activities of daily living (ibid). There is also on trial a new drug, Ebixa (Memantine), for more advanced stages of the disease which has shown encouraging results so far (Alzheimer's Society, 2002). The aim of person-centred care, however is to keep drug therapy to a minimum, particularly tranquillizing medication, which is unsuitable for this client group with no psychotic symptoms.

Medication for depression

Anti-depressant medication may be used as the only form of treatment for depression but is more frequently used in conjunction with supportive psychotherapy or cognitive behavioural therapy. Care must be taken to ensure that anti-depressant medication does not have an adverse reaction with any other medication being taken, if there are any doubts advice and guidance can be obtained for the pharmacist. Dosages used for the elderly may need to be lower than for the younger person due to altered absorption and metabolism. Discontinuation of anti-depressants should be gradual in order to avoid withdrawal symptoms such as anxiety, panic, insomnia, dizziness and gastro-intestinal disturbance. Patients living at home, especially if living alone, should be carefully monitored as compliance is often a problem due to their frail mental state rather than any deliberate intention to not take the medicine.

Tricyclic anti-depressants (TCAs) e.g.: Amitriptyline, Clomipramine, Doxeprin, are useful where agitation is present as they have sedative properties. However they have many side effects some of which can be particularly distressing to the elderly, especially blurred vision and postural hypotension which increase the risk of falling. The use of TCAs for those with cardiovascular disease poses the potential risk of sudden death.

Selective serotonin-reuptake inhibitors (SSRIs) e.g.: Fluoxetine, Paroxetine and Sertriline should be used with caution with patients who have diabetes or cardiovascular disease – conditions quite likely to be encountered in the elderly. Side effects include loss of appetite and weight loss, insomnia, agitation and anxiety, which may complicate the patient's presentation. However they are less sedating than TCAs and pose less risk to patients with heart problems.

Venlafaxine is a serotonin and noradrenaline re-uptake inhibitor (SNRI) that is proving effective in the treatment of depression in the elderly, it has less sedating effect than TCAs but should be used with caution in patients with heart disease. An advantage is that it is available as modified release that needs to be taken only once a day.

Mono Amine Oxidase Inhibitors (MAOIs) e.g. Phenilzine, Isocarboxazid, are an older group of anti-depressants which are best avoided in the elderly due to adverse interactions with certain foods and other medicines, the older person may forget they should not eat cheese, meat or yeast extract, e.g. marmite, or drink alcohol – items that may have been a regular feature in their diet. MAOIs should be discontinued at least 2 weeks before any other anti-depressants are commenced, during this time the nurse must be very alert to the risk of suicide. Extra care must also be taken in patients who have diabetes or cardiovascular disease.

Electro Convulsive Therapy (ECT) for depression

Gould (1997) states the main advantage of ECT is the speed of action, important in older people when depression is so severe suicide is a risk, or neglect of self-care poses a serious risk to health, or where medication has not been of benefit or is contraindicated. ECT remains controversial and patients and families will need clear explanations and reassurance. A doctor must do a full medical examination to ensure the patient is fit for general anaesthetic and treatment. Informed consent for treatment must be obtained.

Sensory stimulation

Multi-sensory environments are becoming increasingly popular, yet scientific evidence to support this is limited. Using sessions involving stimulation in the form of sound/music, foods, smells, massage, texture and visual stimuli may benefit sensory stimulation. It may also improve communication and trust, with reactions to stimuli being related to previous life experience and likes/dislikes. Achterberg et al (1997) observed the effects of specific pieces of sensory stimulation equipment on individuals and advised carers to use them at times of agitation for the dementia sufferer. They acknowledged the effect did not last forever but did enable the patient to be cared for in their own home for a longer period.

Reality orientation

Reality orientation (RO) though very popular at one time is now more focused on 24 hour and informal RO rather than the more focused, formal classroom RO. It is often best adapted to centre the individual in time, place and person but done so in a way so as not to cause distress. Verbal RO should remind the person who he/she is, using preferred name/title, where he/she is, what time of day it is and giving information about surroundings (Jones, 1995).

Example:
'Good morning Mr Jones, it's half past seven, are you ready to get out of bed yet, breakfast is in half an hour?'

'Good morning Mrs Brown, you're out of bed early, shall I walk to the bathroom with you, you seem to enjoy a bath first thing?'

'Hello, Miss Murray, can you smell the food, it's lunchtime? The dining room is through the red door.'

'Would you like to sit in the garden, it's a lovely Summer's day?'

'You are in hospital as you haven't been well recently.'

Sentences should be short to take account of a short attention span and in-ability to take in a lot of information, but it is important such conversations are spoken in a normal tone of voice, not condescending or as if speaking to a child.

Example:
Patient: 'That's my sister, why isn't she coming to talk to me?'
Response: 'Julie is one of the nurses working in the hospital, does she look like your sister?'

This approach helps put the individual in the current place and person. To say bluntly 'that's not your sister she died years ago' would be a harsh and cruel response.

Other ways to reinforce reality may be for staff to wear uniform, a reminder that they are in hospital or a nursing home. Calendars featuring the month pictorially in relation to the weather might give an idea of the time of the year. Large clocks should be available one with Roman numerals (these were popular in the past) and one with ordinary numerals serve as reminders of the time. Notices and signs should be large enough to be read by those with poor sight but not all in capital letters. People do not grow up reading material in capitals but in a combination of upper and lower case with the latter being the most common, people will respond better to what they are familiar. Rooms should be as homely as is practical. Signs and directional arrows should be in bright colours, red and blue being the best for visual purposes, if directional arrows to the dining room are blue the dining room door should be blue, arrows in red should lead to a red door (Holden and Woods, 1988).

Validation

Each person has their own unique experiences and memories. If someone has dementia the long-term memory can stay intact for many years. As short-term memory is lost, memories of past events become important and are valued by the individual, as a result we need to also value these memories and not undermine their validity. Feil (1992) developed validation therapy to encourage this and allow people to talk about their lives without being challenged or undermined. She identified a task following on from Erikson's 'integrity v despair' called 'resolution v vegetation'. Validation explores the emotional content behind the conversation and aims to restore dignity. Accepting that many older people may return to the past to resolve feelings about unfinished business, these feelings are validated by having someone to listen to them. As a result feelings have been acknowledged and valued. Goudie and Stokes (1989) described a further process called resolution therapy whereby there may be a hidden meaning in what is being said related to a current concern. With understanding and time such meanings can be explored and perhaps problems resolved.

The aims of validation are to:

- to restore self-esteem and self-worth;
- regain dignity;
- reduce stress;
- increase verbal and non-verbal communication;
- improve physical well being;
- reduce the need for medication;

- work towards resolving unfinished conflicts;
- prevent withdrawal; and
- relive past pleasures.

It is important that sufficient time is available for validation and communication skills are essential, the use of paraphrasing, clarification, mirroring, warmth and empathy and a non-judgemental approach are vital.

Example:

Patient   'that's my sister, why isn't she coming to talk to me?'

Response   'Julie is one of the nurses who work here, does she remind you of your sister?'

Patient   'she's over there'

Response   'did you help look after her?' or 'did you enjoy playing with her?'

These responses would allow the patient to return to past experiences with her sister.

Reminiscence

This can be used for people with dementia or depression and families caring for an older person can be advised how to use it in their home. Reminiscence is the recall of long-forgotten facts or experiences, once triggered the older person may give an account of a memorable experience. Reminiscence can be on a 'one to one' basis or as a group activity, it aims to increase interaction and socialization and reduce isolation and withdrawal, focus conversation and raise self-esteem. If it is a planned group activity, group members should have a reasonable attention span and be of a similar age. Stevens-Ratchford (1993) found gender differences in topics: men more likely to discuss work and hobbies and women families and children.

Reminiscence can serve to identify further activities e.g. using an old cookery book to chat about previous favourite foods can lead to a cookery session. Many things can be used to trigger memories: books, magazines, photographs, old films and music/songs. The latter are very popular but material from the correct era must be selected. Care must be taken that pleasant memories are evoked – what may be good for one may be bad for another – for example, the World Wars may have been exciting and challenging for some but for others the memories will be of sad or horrifying experiences (Crump, 1997).

Compiling life storybooks can give the staff an understanding of the person as a whole with a history that needs to be taken into account when viewing behaviour or planning care. All life story work of this kind can be a useful way of understanding better the person's needs and lead to a more person-centred or individualized care programme.

Coping with memory problems

Memory loss is one of the first symptoms of most types of dementia and it is useful to identify strategies that can be used to help the client function on a day-to-day basis. We are all creatures of habit and have set routines although we don't always recognize it. We wake up at approximately the same time each day even when we don't have to. Very often we take the same route to our regular destinations; we use the same supermarket because we know where to find things. Following the same pattern of behaviour makes us feel safe and secure and we are not challenged by the unknown. Although most of us can cope with something different, for older people with dementia change becomes a struggle and the more advanced the dementia the harder the struggle.

With the onset of dementia the individual may cope for many years as they have their routines and set patterns of behaviour. As the memory declines it may be necessary to advise families/carers to provide 'aide memoirs' – notes displayed in prominent places to give reminders as to what they should be doing. For example, many older people need to take medication and it is important the instructions are adhered to. The pharmacist can be asked to supply medicines in packs labelled with days, times and amounts of tablets to be taken. As dementia increases such measures may become of little use due to impaired cognitive ability. Family and carers can be advised to monitor daily activities such as shopping and meal preparation. Regular phone calls can be useful reminders as well as reassuring the person that all is well. Carers can often assist with day-to-day needs, but such help should be given in a way that does not make the older person feel undermined and disempowered.

At some point an assessment to a day unit/hospital is advantageous, as the patient will return to a familiar environment and people in the late afternoon. Continued day care may be an option for those living with a relative and give much needed respite. This will provide, not only an opportunity for continued monitoring by health professionals but also, an appropriate level of stimulation and socialization for the patient as well as giving the carer time for themselves. Admission to hospital or residential care may be required where there is disturbance of behaviour during the 24-hour cycle, or where the older person lives alone. Admission can be very stressful as it is to an unfamiliar environment with unfamiliar people. Although there is the attempt to maintain home patterns this is constrained by hospital systems and routines, e.g.: meal times dictated by delivery and safety times for keeping food warm, staffing levels may not allow for individuals to eat at different times. Sleeping patterns may be disturbed in an unfamiliar bedroom. A previously continent person may now have an 'accident' because they cannot find the toilet and do not know who to ask. As a result they can be unjustly labelled 'incontinent'.

Admission to hospital or residential care can be accompanied by anxiety that can reduce the ability to understand questions and instructions and to give appropriate responses leading to a poor assessment of the patient's abilities. It is, therefore, important to allow the patient to settle for two to three days. During this time needs for nutrition, hygiene and safety must, of course, be met and observations of abilities can be made, but these should be reviewed as they settle into the ward environment.

Personhood

To understand the meaning of 'personhood' is essential if we are to strive for a person-centred approach to care. It is important, therefore, that we move away from labelling people based on stereotypes or behaviour. Just because they may have a diagnosis of dementia or depression, it does not mean people are all the same and have the same problems and needs. The term 'personhood', coined by Kitwood (1997b), relates to the way we care for people. We must acknowledge that clients have valid experiences that should be taken into account and that these experiences are valued. The client is trying to do things, trying to communicate, not just showing 'challenging behaviour'. As individuals, clients have differing levels of awareness – we should not assume they do not understand what is happening. In their past life they were empowered individuals and should be treated as such now they are older and unwell. It is with respect, warmth and genuine interest that we should deliver person-centred care (Kitwood, 1993). The use of dementia care mapping will assist in this. Dementia care mapping (DCM) (Bradford Dementia Group, 1997) is detailed observations of behaviour and responses of people who have dementia, it provides a basis for evaluation and audit in the care of older people with dementia. An important element of DCM is the recognition of personal detractors (PDs) or malignant social psychology. These are short episodes that are thought to lead to a reduction in sense of personhood for people with dementia (Younger and Martin, 2001).

The *DCM Manual* (1997) gives examples of this:

- *Labelling* – using a pattern of behaviour (e.g. Wanderer) as the basis for describing and interacting with a person.
- *Treachery* – using some form of deception in order to distract or manipulate a person.
- *Disempowerment* – not allowing a person to use the abilities they have.
- *Accusations* – blaming a person for actions that arise from their lack of ability, or their misunderstanding of the situation.

If staff are made aware of these PDs then they can be highlighted in staff training sessions. Very often such actions are taken without thought of the consequences and by the use of training sessions these are identified and outlawed from practice. For person-centred care to become a reality staff need to learn to empathize with the client group and bring something of themselves to the care they give. It is not enough to provide physical care in a professional, impersonal way we need to see people as whole human beings with pasts that need to be taken into account. Approaches such as validation and reminiscence can be a useful way of getting staff to understand clients' feelings and meet their needs more accurately. The use of life storybooks is also a helpful tool to this end. If we want to see a fundamental change in the way we care for older people then staff must begin to listen, empathize and understand their needs rather than working on assumptions based on stereotypes and labels of older people, which are outdated and restricting in nature.

Conclusion

Older people are at risk of physical and mental illness, sometimes both, which may be inter-related or separate. They remain individuals, they and their families and carers must be listened to and empowered. They should be informed about treatment options and be encouraged to make their own choices. They have earned the right to be heard, to live out their lives in comfort, to be afforded dignity and respect, and be valued for their past experiences as well as their present life. The concept of person-centred care should not just be an ideal it should be applied to care practices as a matter of course. It is a way of maintaining a person's self-esteem and has the ability to undermine the institutionalization process that can deprive people of their identity and reconstruct them within the institutional framework (Goffman, 1969). As cognitive impairment advances the amount of interaction needs to increase not decrease.

What we are talking about is a whole change of culture that is prepared to undermine the notion of 'them and us'. Which looks on challenging behaviour as a form of communication to be understood not merely managed and to move beyond the limited parameters of providing just physical care towards the maintenance and enhancement of 'personhood'. Care of older people with mental health problems is a skilled job and unless we are prepared to adopt the new culture approach we are falling down on our duty of care.

References

Achterberg, I., Kok, W. & Salentijn, C. (1997) Snoezelan: a new way of communicating with the severely demented elderly, in M. L. Miesen & G. M. M. Jones (eds), *Care-giving in Dementia Vol. 2*, London: Taylor and Francis, 119–24.

Alzheimer's Society (2002) New hope for people with severe Alzheimer's Disease, *Alzheimer's Newsletter*, October, 1.

Bradford Dementia Group (1997) *Evaluating Dementia Care; The DCM Method*, Bradford: University of Bradford.

Creutzfeld-Jakob Disease Foundation Inc (2002) Online at: http://cjdfoundation.org

Croft, S. & Beresford, P. (1989) User-involvement, citizenship and social policy, *Critical Social Policy*, 26, 5–18.

Crump, A. (1997) Room to remember, *Elderly Care*, 9(3), 8–10.

Erikson, E. H. (1963) *Childhood and Society*, New York: Norton.

Evans, D. G. (2000) Suicide and the elderly: warning signs and helping points, online at: http://edis.ifas.ufl.edu

Feil, N. (1992) *Validation: The Feil Method How to Help the Disorientated Old-Old*, Cleveland: Edward Feil Productions.

Fielo, S. & Rizzolo, M. A. (1985) The effects of age on pharmacokinetics, *Geriatric Nursing*, 6(6), 328–31.

Gates, B. (1994) *Advocacy: A Nurses' Guide*, London: Scutari Press.

Goffman, E. (1969) *Asylums*, Harmondsworth: Penguin.

Goffman, E. (1971) *The Presentation of Self in Everyday Life*, Harmondsworth: Penguin.

Goldsmith, M. (1996) *Hearing the Voices of People with Dementia*, London: Jessica Kingsley Publications.

Goudie, F. & Stokes, G. (1989) Understanding confusion, *Nursing Times*, 85(39), 35–7.

Gould, D. (1997) Pharmacological treatments and electroconvulsive therapy, in I. J. Norman & S. J. Redfern (eds), *Mental Health Care for Older People*, London: Churchill Livingstone.

Holden, U. P. & Woods, R. T. (1988) *Reality Orientation*, London: Churchill Livingston.

Jones, A. (1995) How effective is reality orientation for elderly, confused patients? *British Journal of Nursing*, 4(9), 519–22.

Kingston, P. & Penhale, B. (1994) A major problem needing recognition: assessment and management of elder abuse and neglect, *Professional Nurse*, 9(5), 343–7.

Kitwood, T. (1993) Person and process in dementia, *International Journal of Geriatric Medicine*, 8, 541–5.

Kitwood, T. (1997a) *Dementia Reconsidered*, Buckingham: Open University.

Kitwood, T. (1997b) The concept of personhood and its relevance for a new culture of dementia care, in M. L. Miesen & G. M. M. Jones (eds), *Care-giving in Dementia Vol. 2*, London: Taylor and Francis, 2–10.

Kitwood, T. & Bredin, K. (1992) A new approach to evaluation of dementia care, *Journal of Advances in Health and Nursing Care*, 1, 41–60.

Kitwood, T. & Bredin, K. (1995) *The New Culture of Dementia Care*, Biscester: Winslow.

Martin, G. & Younger, D. (2000) Anti-oppressive practice: a route to the empowerment of people with dementia through communication and choice, *Journal of Psychiatric and Mental Health Nursing*, 7, 59–67.

Martin, G. & Younger, D. (2001) Person-centred care for people with dementia: a quality audit approach, *Journal of Psychiatric and Mental Health Nursing*, 8, 443–8.

Mitchell, G. (1997) Depression in elderly people, *Elderly Care*, 9(1), 12–15.

Riley, K. P. (1994) Depression in functional performance, in B. R. Bonder & M. B. Wagner (eds), *Older Adults*, Philadelphia: Davis, Ch16, 256–68.

Rogers, S. L., Farlow, M. R., Doody, R. S., Friedhoff, L. T. & The Donepezil Study Group (1998) A 24-week, double-blind, placebo-controlled trial of Donepezil in patients with Alzheimer's Disease, *Neurology*, 50, 136–45.

Stevens-Ratchford, R. (1993) The effects of life review reminiscence activities on depression and self esteem in older adults, *The American Journal of Occupational Therapy*, 47, 413–21.

Stokes, G. & Goudie, F. (1990) *Working with Dementia*, Bicester: Winslow.

Stokoe, R. (2001) *Keep Taking the Medicine? Antipsychotics and the Over Medication of Older People. Its Causes and Consequences*, London: Liberal Democrats.

Tune, L. E. (2001) Resperidone for the treatment of behavioral and psychological symptoms of dementia, *Journal of Clinical Psychiatry*, 62(Supp21), 29–32.

Walton, J. (1999) Young-onset dementia, in T. Adams & C. L. Clarke (eds), *Dementia Care: Developing Partnership in Practice*, London: Bailliere Tindall, 256–80.

Younger, D. & Martin, G. (2001) Dementia care mapping: an approach to quality audit of services for people with dementia in two health districts, *Journal of Advanced Nursing*, 32(5), 1206–12.

CHAPTER 17

Treating Post Traumatic Stress Disorder

GILLIAN GREEN

Indicative Benchmark Statements

▓ Participation in negotiation, formulation and communication of therapeutic interventions with users of mental health and social care services and their carers

▓ Ability to undertake comprehensive, needs-led mental health nursing assessment

▓ Application of basic principles from the psychodynamic, behavioural, social and humanistic conceptual models of mental health interventions

▓ Application of the basic principles of cognitive behavioural interventions

▓ Utilization of appropriate research and relevant evidence to support decision-making relating to the selection and individualization of mental health nursing interventions

Introduction

Growing public awareness of the impact of trauma together with the current climate of litigation and compensation issues highlights the need for all mental health professionals to gain a comprehensive understanding of the nature of reactions that may follow a traumatic experience. With a focus on Post Traumatic Stress Disorder (PTSD), this chapter will provide the student nurse with opportunity to increase awareness, knowledge and understanding of the concept of traumatic stress reactions and the complexities involved when working with traumatized individuals.

An evidence-based review of the literature addressing the concept of post traumatic stress reactions including assessment and treatment approaches will assist the student nurse in the achievement of competencies related to the care and management of such psychologically injured individuals.

Historical perspective/changing attitudes

Reactions to traumatic stressors have been documented for centuries, and historical accounts provide us with some evidence to support the notion that PTSD is not a new phenomenon, but rather a fusion of an age-old condition, resulting in redefinition and reclassification (Kudler, 2000; O'Brien, 1998).

Hudson (1990) draws attention to perhaps one of the earliest recorded cases of psychological trauma dating back to the Battle of Marathon, which is said to have taken place in 490BC. While O'Brien (1998) refers to the Welsh legends surrounding King Arthur's magician – Merlin, who in the original stories is described as a wild man, tormented by the sights and sounds of battle, took himself off to live the life of a hermit in the woods, before returning years later with magical powers. As O'Brien (1998) notes, the above presentation could suggest that Merlin experienced intrusive memories, flashbacks and avoidance, which are characteristic symptoms of PTSD.

Daly (1983) draws attention to the Diaries of Samuel Pepys, which provides his autobiographical account of subjective distress associated with the Great Fire of London – 1666. Although, it appears that the fire did not place Pepys under any direct threat, he spent a great deal of time in the immediate area, and observed a great deal of the devastation. As Daly points out, Pepys provides evidence of the development of a psychological injury associated with the fire, when he notes 'we saw the fire as one entire arch. Above a mile long – it made me weep to see it . . . so great was our fear.' Pepys also provides evidence of traumatic nightmares: 'but much terrified in the nights nowadays, with dreams of fire and of falling down houses', and suggestion that his psychological response continued for many months after the experience, when six months after the fire Pepys reports 'I cannot sleep at night without great terrors of fire, and this very night could not sleep until two in the morning through thoughts of the fire'. The diaries also provide evidence of arousal features, such as increased anxiety and an element of hyperarousal associated with an increased concern for safety when, reflecting on his coach journey home he writes 'much troubled . . . and, which is now my common practice . . . I ride with my sword drawn.'

From a clinical perspective, early interest in trauma reactions can be found in Erichsen's writing when he conceptualizes 'Railway Spine' (Erichsen, 1866), a syndrome commonly associated with events, such as collisions and other accidents producing shock, fright and physical and emotional perturbation during the early developments of the railway system (Young, 2000).

Clinical interest continued to grow, particularly in the wake of war, with emergence of terms such as 'Irritable heart' in soldiers involved in the American Civil war, World War I gave rise to the term 'shellshock' and 'war neurosis' was associated with World War II. Mental health professionals began to notice similar symptom presentations in civilians exposed to extreme stressors. However, it was the plight of the Vietnam War Veterans that appears to have had the most significant impact (Kudler, 2000; Yule et al, 1999). With the emergence of the concept of PTSD came an increased clinical interest, which has continued to grow over the years.

What constitutes a 'traumatic event'?

The experience of a traumatic event is the pinnacle to a diagnosis of PTSD, but what constitutes a traumatic event? As clinical and research interest into the concept of trauma continues to evolve, so does the identification of what constitutes a traumatic event. A number of studies have been carried out involving a variety of populations, examining the impact of numerous traumatic experiences. The next section, exploring the definition/classification of PTSD, will expand on this when examining the stressor criteria.

Definition/classification

PTSD was not formally acknowledged as a diagnostic description for psychiatric illnesses suffered by survivors of stressful events until its inclusion in the *Diagnostic and Statistical Manual of Mental Disorders* – 3rd edn (DSM-III), in 1980 (APA, 1980). This criteria were revised in 1987 (DSM-III-R APA, 1987) and underwent further revision and reformulation in 1994 (DSM-IV, APA, 1994). Current understandings are such that the individual needs to meet six criteria (A through to F) if they are to fulfil a diagnosis of PTSD (APA, 1994).

Reformulation of diagnostic criteria witnessed a broadening of the range of events that qualify as a 'stressor'; and a shift in focus from the nature of the stressor itself, to the nature of the victims 'perception' of the event. The stressor criterion (Criterion A) requires the individual to have '*experienced*' '*witnessed*' or have been '*confronted*' by an '*event or events*' that not only poses a threat to the individual themselves, but also to others. This as Resick (2001) highlights, enables a diagnosis of PTSD to be made in individuals who may not be direct victims of an incident itself, but who have had some form of involvement in the aftermath, for example rescue workers, emergency service personnel. In addition to this, incidents that do not involve direct threat to life, but which represent a threat to the physical integrity of an individual, eg: some forms of sexual assault, and as Avina and Donohue (2002) argue sexual harassment may constitute a stressor.

Criterion A appears self-explanatory, though the wording has come under criticism on the grounds that the lack of clarity leaves it open to misinterpretation and clinicians are advised to exercise caution and sound clinical judgement when making the decision about what constitutes a stressor (Avina & Donohue, 2002).

Case Study 17.1   Maria's story

Eight months ago Maria – aged 26, was violently raped at knifepoint on her way home from work, shortly after leaving the railway station. Maria was aware of footsteps behind her, but dismissed her initial concerns, telling herself that there would of course be footsteps behind her, she had after all just left a railway station, and she would not have been the only person to get off the train. Maria tearfully recounted her ordeal, recalling a sudden push from behind and a hand coming around covering her mouth. She recalled being forced into a bushy area, yards from the roadside, and then being pushed to the ground. Initially, she tried to fight off her assailant, he hit her hard on her cheek, then she felt something pressing against the side of her neck her assailant told her to stop struggling as he had a knife, and he was not afraid to use it, – He then proceeded to rape her, she felt totally overpowered and helpless as well as feeling absolutely terrified, she recalled that 'it seemed to go on for ages, I thought it was never going to end, I was just lying there wanting the ordeal to be over, but I also felt afraid of what he was going to do to next' she thought he would kill her. When he had finished he told her not to move and to stay where she was, and that if he saw her moving he would kill her, he then ran off, disappearing over a field back towards the railway station.

At assessment Maria had given up her job in the city as she felt unable to commute, she had been working from home for approximately four months, but was finding it difficult to generate business as she had lost a lot of confidence being around males who were not previously known to her. She also described feeling afraid to leave the house alone and on leaving the house would constantly feel in danger, and would keep looking over her shoulder, in addition she felt totally unable to go out alone once it was dark. She described feeling haunted by memories of what had happened to her, such memories would 'just pop in' without any warning, and they would stop her carrying on with whatever she may have been doing at the time, in addition she reported being unable to dismiss the memories which in turn was interfering with her concentration. She also reported that when she experienced the memories she sometimes could smell the perpetrator, she also experienced images associated with the event, such images included the expressions on the face of the perpetrator, she could also feel his hand over her mouth and would get split second images of what she could see as she was pushed into the bushy area. Maria reported that she regularly experienced nightmares, which were so vivid that she woke thinking the event was recurring. She described that she would feel very distressed and would often be crying on waking, she also described her heart pounding, feeling short of breath, and being afraid to return to sleep.

She described psychological and physiological reactivity at reminders of the event, and exemplified this by reporting that she felt physically sick on handling sharp knives in the kitchen, her heart would start pounding, and she would become very distressed as this reminded her of the knife being pushed against her throat, as a result she was no longer able to look at, let alone use certain knives, and she could not even contemplate cutting meat. She had previously enjoyed hosting dinner parties for friends and her husband's business acquaintances, but she felt increasingly unable to do so at assessment. Her relationship with her husband was also suffering, she felt unable to talk to her friends, family or husband about what had happened, she could not bear for her husband to touch her, and would freeze if he tried to cuddle her, she would often sit downstairs and wait for her husband to fall asleep before retiring to bed, and sexual relations were out of the question.

Maria's experience would certainly constitute a traumatic event. She was undoubtedly confronted with an event that would constitute a stressor, and from her story, she experienced feelings of intense fear and helplessness.

Features of PTSD are also divided into three main symptom clusters, which are those of re-experiencing, avoidance and arousal, each of which will now be examined and illustrated using Maria's story.

Re-experiencing (Criterion B) involves a persistent and overwhelming sense of re-living the event at one level or another through recurring distressing recollections of the event, recurring dreams of the event, acting or feeling as if the event were recurring, intense psychological distress and/or physiological reactivity to reminders of the event. Only one of the above symptoms is required to fulfil Criterion B, we can clearly see from Maria's story, that she is experiencing recurring intrusive memories of the event, nightmares, feeling as if the event were recurring, as well as psychological and physiological arousal at reminders of the event

Avoidance (Criterion C) characterized by persistent efforts to avoid thoughts, feelings, conversations, people, places and activities that remind the individual of the event. There may also be an inability to remember some aspect of the event, a diminished interest in previously enjoyed activities, feelings of detachment or estrangement from others, a restricted range of affect and a sense of a foreshortened future. Three of the above symptoms are required to meet criteria for this symptom cluster. Maria's story highlights some avoidance type behaviours, she had given up her job in the City, as she felt unable to commute, she had not been back to the railway station since the incident. In addition she avoided conversations associated with the event, in that she felt unable to talk to friends or family about what had happened to her, she was less interested in activities that she used to enjoy, being unable to prepare and host dinner parties. There is some evidence of feelings of estrangement and a definite avoidance of physical contact from her husband, and further assessment highlighted a sense of a foreshortened future, in that she did not expect to have any children and thought that her marriage would not be a success as a consequence of the rape.

Arousal (Criterion D) is characterized by difficulties in concentrating, sleep disturbance, increased levels of irritability and anger, hypervigilance and an exaggerated startle response. Individuals need to be suffering from two of these symptoms to fulfil Criterion D. From Maria's story it is quite evident that she is experiencing difficulties concentrating, sleep difficulties are also evident in that she wakes from nightmares and often feels unable to return to sleep. There is also evidence of hypervigilance, in that whenever she goes out alone she finds herself looking over her shoulder.

The fifth element of the diagnostic criteria involves the persistence of symptoms associated with re-experiencing, avoidance *and* arousal for a minimum of one month, essentially all occurring at the same time and not separately. Finally, current diagnostic criteria requires significant levels of impairment in social, occupational or other important areas of functioning as a result of the symptoms, thus a diagnosis should not be made if the symptoms are mild, or do not interfere with the individual's levels of functioning.

This chapter has focused on diagnostic criteria in accordance with DSM-IV (APA, 1994), however, it is important to remind readers that PTSD also features in the 10th edition of the *International Classification of Diseases* (ICD-10, WHO, 1992). Comparison of the DSM-IV and ICD-10 highlights subtle differences between diagnostic criteria for PTSD, though the essential diagnostic features associated with re-experiencing, avoidance and arousal symptoms are present in both DSM-IV and ICD-10.

Different reactions to trauma experiences

As O'Brien emphasizes throughout his book, exposure to traumatic experiences does not result in the development of a psychological injury in everybody, and PTSD is certainly not the only psychological injury to follow traumatic experiences. Other disorders include Acute Stress Disorder, Adjustment Disorder, Dissociative Disorder, Disorders of Extreme Stress Not Otherwise Specified, (DESNOS). (O'Brien, 1998; Resick, 2001).

Associated symptoms

Alongside the formal diagnostic criteria a number of additional symptoms, need to be taken into consideration when working with individuals presenting with post trauma reactions. One such symptom is that of guilt, originally considered as a core symptom in DSM-III (APA 1980), though it has subsequently been classified as an associated symptom.

In general feelings of guilt may be experienced at having survived a traumatic event when others did not, or such feelings may be linked to specific acts carried out by the individual in order to survive. On the other hand individuals may convey feelings of guilt associated with things that they could have done but did not, or about things that they feel could have been done differently, or that they could have done more to help others. A significant amount of work has been carried out over the years examining the concept of guilt in relation to the development and maintenance of post trauma reactions, and the role of guilt in PTSD symptom severity. (Fontana et al, 1992; Kubany, 1994; Kubany et al, 1997; Lee et al, 2001; Tangney et al, 1992).

Shame has also been associated with traumatic reactions and although shame may be considered as a concept similar to guilt, there is a growing body of evidence that highlights the importance of discriminating between them. Shame has been identified as distinctly different to the concept of guilt in that shame is an emotional response related to attempts to understand meaning and cause of the event on the part of the individual (Lee et al, 2001; Leskela et al, 2002).

Although shame has attracted less attention than guilt over the years increased interest is starting to highlight the importance of addressing shame when assessing and treating trauma reactions, which often entails the individual recounting detailed descriptions of the event as well as their responses before, during and after the event. Individuals may experience a sense of shame as a consequence of any behaviours or actions that they demonstrated or did not demonstrate at the time of the event, or about feelings and/or emotions that they experienced in relation to the event. Certainly as Lee and her colleagues (Lee et al, 2001) highlight, any therapeutic involvement that does not take into account shame may achieve little other than to exacerbate an individual's difficulties in relation to their traumatic experience.

Dissociative symptoms such as reduced awareness; derealization and depersonalization are also considered to be associated with traumatic stress reactions alongside symptoms of numbing, dissociative amnesia and flashback experiences, which are incorporated in the diagnostic criteria for PTSD (APA, 1994; Harvey & Bryant, 1999a; O'Brien, 1998; Resick, 2001). Such symptoms may be expressed in the following ways – 'the event seemed to occur in slow motion', feelings of being in a dream or a daze. Actions may be described as a sense of 'autopilot', and sensations of being outside the body, watching the event as a spectator or a sense of unreality.

As mentioned previously, PTSD is not the only diagnostic reaction to traumatic experiences. Acute Stress Disorder – which did not enter the diagnostic nomenclature until its inclusion in the DSM-IV (APA, 1994) – places significant emphasis on dissociative symptoms, requiring the presence of at least three of the symptoms identified above. In addition, there is significant evidence supporting the notion that the presence of peri-traumatic dissociation (occurring as the event is happening) is predictive of later development of PTSD (Bremner & Brett, 1997; Marmar et al, 1994). However, there is growing evidence questioning the uniqueness of the role of peri-traumatic dissociation in such a prediction (Barton et al, 1996; Brewin et al, 1999; Dancu et al, 1996; Harvey & Bryant, 1999b).

DSM-IV (APA, 1994, p 425) draws attention to other associated features of PTSD which include 'self destructive/impulsive behaviour, somatisation; feelings of ineffectiveness, feelings of despair and/or hopelessness, feeling permanently damaged, loss of previously sustained beliefs, hostility, feeling constantly threatened, impaired relationships with others or a change in previous personality characteristics'.

Co-morbidity and associated problems

PTSD does not always occur as a singular disorder, but may co-occur with other mental health disorders – often referred to as co-morbidity, and as Brady (1997) suggests, co-morbidity in individuals with PTSD may be considered as more of a norm than an exception to any rule.

An increasing number of studies have examined co-occurrence of other mental health disorders following traumatic exposure, for example Kessler et al (1995) found that approximately 80 per cent of individuals with a diagnosis of PTSD also met criteria for at least one other mental health disorder. Major depressive disorder is one of the most frequently reported co-occurring disorders with lifetime rates in the region of 50 to 90 per cent. Co-occurring substance use disorders are also among the most frequently reported with lifetime prevalence rates of between 12 and 52 per cent. (Bleich et al, 1997; Kessler et al, 1995).

Individuals may be at greater risk of developing other anxiety disorders such as generalized anxiety disorder, panic disorder, agoraphobia, obsessive compulsive disorder, social and/or specific phobias. Although a great deal of literature examining co-morbidity and PTSD exists, the true nature of the relationships from the perspective of the degree to which co-occurring disorders precede or follow the onset of PTSD continues to be the focus of significant debate (APA, 1994; Brady, 1997; Engdahl et al, 1998; Stewart, 1996; Stewart et al, 1998).

Not everybody with PTSD will meet full criteria for another mental health disorder, but they may exhibit features of them, which left un-addressed may complicate presentation, treatment and recovery processes.

Co-morbidity or the presence of features of other mental health disorders may also contribute to the development and maintenance of associated difficulties such as loss of job, financial problems, relationship/marital breakdown, criminal behaviour and social isolation to name but a few. Tom's story illustrates the contribution of co-morbidity in the development of associated difficulties.

Case Study 17.2 Tom's story

Tom retired from the Army three years ago having completed 22 years service, during which time he had spent time in Northern Ireland had been involved in the Gulf war and had also carried out peacekeeping duties in Bosnia. Although he had not sustained any physical injuries himself, he had been exposed to a significant amount of death and destruction. He was diagnosed as suffering from PTSD with co-morbid alcohol dependence.

Although Tom described himself as always having been 'a bit of a drinker', he had started to increase his alcohol intake in an effort to control his PTSD symptoms. When intoxicated Tom became physically and verbally aggressive, he had been charged on two occasions for drunk and disorderly behaviour, one occasion for disturbing the peace, one occasion for actual bodily harm, and he had been charged with driving under the influence of alcohol, which resulted in him being banned from driving.

His wife had left the marital home taking their two children with her as she had become increasingly concerned for her safety and that of the children. Tom had physically assaulted her on two occasions while drunk; he had also on one occasion 'trashed the house' and had frequently thrown inanimate objects across rooms when drunk.

His drinking increased to two bottles of spirits per day in addition to beer and cider. He had lost a number of jobs due to him either not turning up at work, or being under the influence of alcohol on arrival at work. He was spending increasing amounts of money on alcohol, and had accumulated a significant amount of debt. He had lost contact with most of his friends, the majority of which he had known from his 'Army days'. He was facing the prospect of being homeless after being threatened with eviction for nonpayment of rent, and had received a county court summons for nonpayment of a loan he had taken out two years previous to buy a car.

Prevalence rates

Examination of the literature highlights varying prevalence rates for PTSD. A small number of general population studies suggest that PTSD affects 1 in 12 adults at some point in their lifetime; and although rates of exposure to trauma are found to be lower in females than males, females reported higher rates of PTSD than males following traumatic exposure. (Breslau, 2001; Kessler et al, 1995).

As prevalence rates vary across studies, it is important when reading the literature to consider a number of possible influencing factors such as the study population, for example treatment or compensation-seeking populations. Also, definitions of traumatic exposure may vary markedly across studies, as may the definition of PTSD, particularly if the various revisions of diagnostic criteria are taken into account. It is recommended that clinician's consider the assessment instruments used in various studies, and any associated limitations.

Assessment issues/approach

Accurate diagnosis of PTSD is crucial, not only due to the complex nature of the presentation, but also due to compensation and forensic issues frequently encountered in patients with PTSD.

PTSD may be considered as a multi-dimensional disorder, and as such the use of a multi-modal assessment technique has been advocated by a number of authors as a means of establishing a diagnosis of PTSD. Such assessment, best achieved through the use of multiple reliable and valid instruments combines the relative strengths of each measure and minimizes the psychometric shortcomings of any one single measure, leading to a maximization of reaching correct diagnostic conclusions and decisions. (Keane et al, 1997; Lyons et al, 1988; Weathers et al, 1997).

Assessment measures

A number of measures have been developed that are designed to assess traumatization at one level or another. Such measures include both structured diagnostic interviews and self-report measures, the latter of which can be used as screening tools as well as employed to reach diagnosis when specific cut off scores are used.

Interested readers are referred to the work of Carlson (1997), which provides a comprehensive overview of the challenges associated with the assessment of trauma, as well as a detailed review of the various measures that may be used in a number of settings. Consideration of the *purpose* and *goals* of the assessment is important, as this may influence decisions regarding the approach selected. For example the purpose and goals of the clinician may primarily involve diagnosis and treatment planning, whereas the purpose and goals of the researcher, may primarily involve the frequency and/or intensity of levels of traumatization within a given population.

The use of structured diagnostic interviews examining all PTSD symptoms in detail is advocated, as not only are they likely to improve diagnostic accuracy, but they may well also improve treatment planning (Keane et al, 2000; Litz & Weathers, 1994). One example of such an interview is the Clinician Administered PTSD Scale (CAPS) (Blake et al, 1990), which gathers information to make a current and/or lifetime diagnosis of PTSD. This measure assesses the frequency and intensity of DSM-IV (APA, 1994) symptoms for PTSD.

Broad-based structured diagnostic interviews are also advocated. Such interviews examine a range of mental health disorders, which assists the clinician in not only assessing PTSD, but also provides the opportunity to evaluate the extent of co-morbidity (Keane & Wolfe, 1990; Weiss, 1997). The Structured Clinical Interview for DSM (SCID) (First et al, 1997) is an example of one such interview.

A number of self-report measures designed to assess PTSD symptomology have been developed (see Carlson (1997) for detailed review). Self-report measures may also be employed to provide further assessment of comorbidity. It is recommended that the evidence base for each assessment measure is examined before any decision is made regarding its employment in the assessment of PTSD, paying attention to the diagnostic criteria on which the measure was developed, the populations in which it has been used, the actual sensitivity of the measure as well as what symptoms are actually being measured, resulting in an assessment procedure that is as global as possible.

Treatment approaches

There are a wealth of data pertaining to the treatment of PTSD among different populations. Indeed whole books have been dedicated to available treatments, as such it is beyond the scope of this chapter to provide a detailed account of each approach, and interested readers are referred to the recommended reading list. A number of approaches have been used in the treatment of PTSD, to date, though as McFarlane and Yehuda (2000) suggest, there is no one single approach that has gained global acceptance. As Foa et al (2000) highlight, some treatment approaches appear effective in reducing symptoms belonging to all three symptom clusters, while others have been shown to be effective in easing symptoms associated with one symptom cluster, for example, re-experiencing, avoidance, arousal.

Treatment approaches as suggested by Resick (2001) can primarily be divided into the categories of pharmacological and psychological, though it is not unusual for patients to be offered a combination of medication and some form of psychological intervention. The International Society for Traumatic Stress Studies (ISTSS) have published practice guidelines for the effective treatments for PTSD, these guidelines provide detailed reviews of the literature and evaluation of the efficacy of each treatment modality. The guidelines also include a detailed criteria aimed at assisting the clinician in treatment selection and goal setting for individual clients (Foa et al, 2000).

A number of pharmacological treatments, capable of ameliorating PTSD symptoms, are available and include selective serotonin reuptake inhibitors (SSRI) other serotonergic agents, anti-adrenergic agents, mono-amine oxidase inhibitors (MAOI's), tricyclic anti-depressants and Benzodiazepines (see Friedman et al, 2000 for further details pertaining to the efficacy of clinical trials).

There are also a number of psychological therapies that have been utilized in the treatment of PTSD, and there is a vast literature base pertaining to the efficacy of each approach with a variety of populations. Psychological debriefing, which is an early intervention, employed with individuals soon after a traumatic experience, is one such approach (Bisson et al, 2000).

There are also a number of different forms of behavioural, cognitive and cognitive-behavioural approaches that have been employed, including exposure therapy, systematic desensitization, stress inoculation training, cognitive processing therapy, biofeedback and relaxation, many of which contain an element of exposure (see Foa et al, 2000 for further details pertaining to the efficacy of these therapeutic approaches). Cognitive behavioural therapy for PTSD is among the most studied, and as Rothbaum et al (2000) conclude, although not every patient will benefit from this approach, such interventions have been shown to be clearly effective.

Eye movement desensitization and reprocessing (EMDR) – a relatively new type of therapy utilized in the treatment of PTSD, originated from the observations of Shapiro (1995). Although some studies have demonstrated the efficacy of EMDR, several of the eight components of this approach overlap with other treatment approaches, as such, further studies are needed to identify whether or not the principles associated with the eye movements are primarily responsible for this. (Chemtob et al, 2000; Shalev et al, 2000).

Conclusion

Traumatic stress reactions have been around for centuries, but it was not until the wake of the Vietnam War that such reactions, particularly PTSD was recognized as a discrete diagnostic entity. Since its introduction in diagnostic nomenclature there has been a continued expansion in clinical and research interest into PTSD and associated disorders, which has resulted in revision and reformulation of the diagnostic criteria.

Traumatic stress reactions warrant very careful assessment due to the multidimensional nature of the presenting symptoms and associated difficulties, particularly if the assessment is to form the foundation for treatment. A number of treatment approaches have been developed, and although the evidence suggests that cognitive behavioural approaches are among the most effective to date, they are not suitable for everybody.

Due to the complex nature of traumatic stress, it has not been possible to provide an in-depth review of the concept within this chapter. Indeed many questions may have been left unanswered; if this is the case then hopefully the recommended reading list will provide you with all the information needed to answer any further questions you may have, particularly those associated with treatment approaches.

Recommended reading

Carlson, E. B. (1997) *Trauma Assessments: A Clinicians Guide*, New York: Guilford Press.

Foa, E. B., Keane, T. M. & Friedman, M. J. (eds) (2000) *Effective Treatments for PTSD*, New York: Guilford Press.

O'Brien, L. S. (1998) *Traumatic Events and Mental Health*, Cambridge: Cambridge University Press.

Resick, P. A. (2001) *Stress and Trauma*, East Sussex: Psychology Press.

Wilson, J. P. & Keane T. M. (eds) (1997) *Assessing Psychological Trauma and PTSD*, New York: Guildford Press.

Yule, W. (ed) (1999) *Post-traumatic Stress Disorders: Concepts and Therapy*, Chichester: John Wiley & Sons Ltd.

References

American Psychiatric Association (1980) *Diagnostic and Statistical Manual of Mental Disorders* (3rd edn), Washington: American Psychiatric Association.

American Psychiatric Association (1987) *Diagnostic and Statistical Manual of Mental Disorders* (3rd edn revised), Washington: American Psychiatric Association.

American Psychiatric Association (1994) *Diagnostic and Statistical Manual of Mental Disorders* (4th edn), Washington: American Psychiatric Association.

Avina, C. & Donohue, W. (2002) Sexual harassment and PTSD: is sexual harassment diagnosable trauma? *Journal of Traumatic Stress*, 15(1), 69–75.

Barton, K. A., Blanchard, E. B. & Hickling, E. J. (1996) Antecedents and consequences of acute stress disorder among motor vehicle accident victims, *Behaviour Research and Therapy*, 34, 805–13.

Bisson, J. I., McFarlane, A. C. & Rose, S. (2000) Psychological debriefing, in E. B. Foa, T. M. Keane & M. J. Friedman (eds), *Effective Treatments for PTSD: Practice Guidelines from the International Society for Traumatic Stress Studies*, New York: Guilford Press, 39–59.

Blake, D. D., Weathers, F. W., Nagy, L. M., Kaloupek, D. G., Klauminzer, G., Charney, D. S. & Keane, T. M. (1990) A clinician rating scale for assessing current and lifetime PTSD: the CAPS-1, *The Behaviour Therapist*, 13, 187–8.

Bleich, A., Koslowsky, M., Dolev, A. & Lerer, B. (1997) Post-traumatic Stress Disorder and depression: an analysis of co-morbidity, *British Journal of Psychiatry*, 170, 479–82.

Brady, K. T. (1997) Post-traumatic Stress Disorder and co-morbidity: recognising the many faces of PTSD, *Journal of Clinical Psychiatry*, 58(Supp 9), 12–15.

Bremner, J. D. & Brett, E. (1997) Trauma-related dissociative states and long-term psychopathology in Post-traumatic Stress Disorder, *Journal of Traumatic Stress*, 10(1), 37–49.

Breslau, N. (2001) The epidemiology of Post-traumatic Stress Disorder: what is the extent of the problem? *Journal of Clinical Psychiatry*, 62(Supp 17), 16–22.

Brewin, C. R., Andrews, B., Rose S. & Kirk, M. (1999) Acute Stress Disorder and Post-traumatic Stress Disorder in victims of violent crime, *American Journal of Psychiatry*, 156, 360–6.

Carlson, E. B. (1997) *Trauma Assessments: A Clinicians Guide*, New York: Guilford Press.

Chemtob, C. M., Tolin, D. F., Van Der Kolk, B. A. & Pitman, R. K. (2000) Eye movement desensitisation and reprocessing. in E. B. Foa, T. M. Keane & M. J. Friedman (eds), *Effective Treatments for PTSD: Practice Guidelines from the International Society for Traumatic Stress Studies*, New York: Guilford Press, 139–54.

Daly, R. J. (1983) Samuel Pepys and Post-traumatic Stress Disorder, *British Journal of Psychiatry*, 143, 64–8.

Dancu, C. V., Riggs, D. S., Hearst-Ikeda, D., Shoyer, B. G. & Foa, E. B. (1996) Dissociative experiences and Post-traumatic Stress Disorder among female victims of criminal assault and rape, *Journal of Traumatic Stress*, 9, 253–67.

Engdahl, B., Dikel, T. N., Eberly, R. & Blank, A. (1998) Co-morbidity and course of psychiatric disorders in a community sample of former prisoners of war, *American Journal of Psychiatry*, 155(12), 1740–5.

Erichsen, J. E. (1866) *On Railway and Other Injuries of the Railway System*, London: Walton & Maberly.

First, M. B., Spitzer, R. L., Gibbon, M. & Williams, J. B. W. (1997) *Users' Guide for the Structured Clinical Interview for DSM-IV Axis-I Disorders SCID-I Clinician Version*, Washington: American Psychiatric Press.

Foa, E. B., Keane, T. M. & Friedman, M. J. (eds) (2000) *Effective Treatments for PTSD: Practice Guidelines from the International Society for Traumatic Stress Studies*, New York: Guilford Press, 1–17.

Fontana, A., Rosenheck, R. & Brett, E. (1992) War Zone Trauma and Post-traumatic Stress Disorder symptomatology, *Journal of Nervous and Mental Disease*, 180, 748–55.

Friedman, M. J., Davidson, J. R. T., Mellman, T. A. & Southwick, S. M. (2000) Pharmacology, in E. B. Foa, T. M. Keane & M. J. Friedman (eds), *Effective Treatments for PTSD: Practice Guidelines from the International Society for Traumatic Stress Studies*, New York: Guilford Press, 84–105.

Harvey, A. G. & Bryant, R. A. (1999a) Dissociative symptoms in Acute Stress Disorder, *Journal of Traumatic Stress*, 12(4), 673–80.

Harvey, A. G. & Bryant, R. A. (1999b) The relationship between Acute Stress Disorder and Post-traumatic Stress Disorder: a 2-year prospective evaluation, *Journal of Consulting and Clinical Psychology*, 67(6), 985–8.

Hudson, C. J. (1990) The first case of battle hysteria? *British Journal of Psychiatry*, 157, 150.

Keane, T. M., Newman, E. & Orsillo, S. M. (1997) Assessment of military related Posttraumatic Stress Disorder, in J. P. Wilson & T. M. Keane (eds), *Assessing Psychological Trauma and PTSD*, New York: Guildford Press, 267–90.

Keane, T. M., Weathers, F. W. & Foa, E. B. (2000) Diagnosis and assessment, in E. B. Foa, T. M. Keane & M. J. Friedman (eds), *Effective Treatments for PTSD: Practice Guidelines from the International Society for Traumatic Stress Studies*, New York: Guilford Press, 18–36.

Keane, T. M. & Wolfe, J. (1990) Co-morbidity in Post Traumatic Stress Disorder: an analysis of community and clinical studies, *Journal of Applied Social Psychology*, 43, 32–43.

Kessler, R. C., Sonnega, A., Bromet, E., Hughes, M. & Nelson, C. B. (1995) Posttraumatic Stress Disorder in the national co-morbidity survey, *Archives of General Psychiatry*, 52, 1048–60.

Kubany, E. S. (1994) A cognitive model of guilt typology in combat related PTSD, *Journal of Traumatic Stress*, 7(1), 3–19.

Kubany, E. S., Abeug, F. R., Kilauano, W. L., Manke, F. P. & Kaplan, A. S. (1997) Development and validation of the sources of trauma related guilt survey: war-zone version, *Journal of Traumatic Stress*, 10(2), 235–58.

Kudler, H. (2000) The limiting effects of paradigms on the concept of traumatic stress, in A. Shalev, R. Yehuda & A. C. McFarlane (eds), *International Handbook of Human Responses to Trauma*, New York: Kluwer Academic/Plenum Publishers, 3–10.

Lee, D. A., Scragg, P. & Turner, S. (2001) The role of shame and guilt in traumatic events: a clinical model of shame-based and guilt-based PTSD, *British Journal of Medical Psychology*, 74(4), 451–66.

Leskela, J., Dieperink, M. & Thuras, P. (2002) Shame and Post-traumatic Stress Disorder, *Journal of Traumatic Stress*, 15(3), 223–6.

Litz, B. T. & Weathers, F. (1994) The diagnosis and assessment of Post-traumatic Stress Disorder in adults, in M. B. Williams & J. F. Somer (eds), *The Handbook of Post-traumatic Therapy*, West Port, CT: Greenwood Press, 20–37.

Lyons, J. A., Gerardi, R. J., Wolfe, J. & Keane, T. M. (1988) Multidimensional assessment of combat related PTSD: phenomenological, psychometric and psychophysiological considerations, *Journal of Traumatic Stress*, 1(3), 373–94.

Marmar, C. R., Weiss, D. S., Schlenger, W. E., Fairbank, J. A., Jordan, K., Kulka R. A. & Hough, R. L. (1994) Peri-traumatic dissociation and Post-traumatic Stress in male Vietnam theatre veterans, *American Journal of Psychiatry*, 151, 902–7.

McFarlane, A. C. & Yehuda, R. (2000) Clinical treatment of Post-traumatic Stress Disorder: conceptual challenges raised by recent research, *Australian and New Zealand Journal of Psychiatry*, 34, 940–53.

O'Brien, L. S. (1998) *Traumatic Events and Mental Health*, Cambridge: Cambridge University Press.

Resick, P. A. (2001) *Stress and Trauma*, East Sussex: Psychology Press Ltd.

Rothbaum, B. O., Meadows, E. A., Resick, P. & Foy, D. W. (2000) Cognitive-behaviour therapy, in E. B. Foa, T. M. Keane & M. J. Friedman (eds), *Effective Treatments for PTSD: Practice Guidelines from the International Society for Traumatic Stress Studies*, New York: Guilford Press, 60–83.

Shalev, A. Y., Friedman, M. J., Foa, E. B. & Keane, T. M. (2000) Integration and summary, in E. B. Foa, T. M. Keane & M. J. Friedman (eds), *Effective Treatments for PTSD: Practice Guidelines from the International Society for Traumatic Stress Studies*, New York: Guilford Press, 359–79.

Shapiro, F. (1995) *Eye Movement Desensitisation and Reprocessing: Basic Principles, Protocols and Procedures*, New York: Guilford Press.

Stewart, S. H. (1996) Alcohol abuse in individuals exposed to trauma: a critical review, *Psychological Bulletin*, 120(1), 83–112.

Stewart, S. H., Pihl, R. O., Conrod, P. J. & Dongier, M. (1998) Functional associations among trauma, PTSD and substance related disorders, *Addictive Behaviours*, 23(6), 797–812.

Tangney, J. P., Wagner, P. & Gramzow, R. (1992) Proneness to shame, proneness to guilt, and psychopathology, *Journal of Abnormal Psychology*, 101, 469–78.

Weathers, F. W., Keane, T. M., King, L. A. & King, D. W. (1997) Psychometric theory in the development of Post-traumatic Stress Disorder assessment tools, in J. P. Wilson & T. M. Keane (eds), *Assessing Psychological Trauma and PTSD*, New York: Guilford Press, 98–135.

Weiss, D. S. (1997) Structured clinical interview techniques, in J. P. Wilson & T. M. Keane (eds), *Assessing Psychological Trauma and PTSD*, New York: Guildford Press, 493–511.

World Health Organization (1992) *International Classification of Diseases*, *(10th edn)*, Geneva: WHO.

Young, A. (2000) An alternative history of traumatic stress, in A. Shalev, R. Yehuda & A. C. McFarlane (eds), *International Handbook of Human Responses to Trauma*, New York: Kluwer Academic/Plenum Publishers, 51–68.

Yule, W., Williams R. & Joseph, S. (1999) Post-traumatic Stress Disorder in adults, in W. Yule (ed), *Post-traumatic Stress Disorders: Concepts and Therapy*, Chichester: John Wiley & Sons Ltd, 1–24.

CHAPTER 18

Assessing and Engaging People with Personality Disorder

PETER MELIA AND STEPHAN D. KIRBY

Indicative Benchmark Statements

- Identification of the main characteristics and needs of the mental health and social care users and their carers

- Facilitation of therapeutic co-operation with mental health service users and their carers, taking account of those who nurses find difficult to engage

- Maintenance of therapeutic alliances with users of mental health and social care services through partnership, intimacy and reciprocity

- Awareness of the effectiveness of early interventions in mental health and social care

- Utilization of appropriate research and relevant evidence to support decision-making relating to the selection and individualization of mental health nursing interventions

---

Introduction

The very notion of a health or functional deficit related to personality is both nebulous and extravagant. While there are a number of diagnostic manuals and protocols that outline broad classifications based on behavioural symptomatology there is little consensus as to the aetiology, development, course or maintenance of such disorders. Notwithstanding this, this group of individuals continue to cause a great deal of angst and disharmony in their direct human environment, among politicians, mental health professionals, the judiciary, administrators of the criminal justice system and the general public.

Before launching into the discourse as to the classification and presentation of personality disorders we would like to remind those professionals practicing in mental health that the basis of psychiatry is statistical rather than pathological. In most areas of medicine diagnosis and treatment is guided by determinable and measurable pathology (X-rays, blood tests, CAT or PET scans etc.). Few areas of psychiatry have, however, any such identifiable pathology and diagnosis and therefore treatment is consequently based on the presence or absence of significant clusters of behaviour. This is as true for personality disorders as it is for other psychiatric disorders, but in some cases is confused by the observation that some individuals may legally be diagnosed as 'antisocial' or 'psychopathic' while actually being quite content with their lot and happy to blame others for the consequences of their behaviour.

It was once glibly muted by a legal counsel at a Mental Health Review Tribunal (MHRT) that the client was illegally detained as the MHA (1983) (HO & DoH, 1983) clearly states detention for treatment is only permissible when the individual concerned 'suffers' from a psychopathic disorder. In this case counsel argued the client 'does not suffer from a psychopathic disorder but actually enjoys it'. The MHRT Chair thanked counsel for an interesting legal debate but sent the client back for further treatment. This does to some extent further enforce the debate that the treatment of individuals diagnosed as having a personality disorder must be self-directed and where this is not present then treatment is useless if not impossible. Notwithstanding this there is growing evidence that there is tangible benefit to the provision of psychological and pharmacological treatments to this group of individuals (Bateman & Tyrer, 2003, Craissati et al, 2003).

Partly as a result of this there has been a great deal of debate over many years as to whether this issue is best dealt with by the criminal justice or mental health system but in the new (draft at time of writing) Mental Health Bill (HO & DoH, 2000) there is a clear message that from henceforth the issue of personality disorder and Dangerous & Severe Personality Disorder (DSPD – this term is used to differentiate between personality disorders and psychopathy) is the legitimate responsibility of psychiatry. Similarly there has been a political lobby for the provision of legislation enabling preventative detention for this group of individuals but this is unlikely to happen as will be outlined later in this chapter.

The recent work carried out jointly by the Department of Health and Home Office regarding the review of legislation and services to provide care for individuals suffering from personality disorders and those classed as 'dangerous and severely personality disordered', highlights the difficulty presented by this group. In the case of those diagnosed or classified as DSPD there is also a clear mandate that the protection of the public is a priority.

This very process has to some extent forced the debate as to whether the issue of personality disorder exists as a health, psychological or social phenomenon (or, of course, a mixture of all three). This is not helped by the 1983 Mental Health Act's rather nebulous definition of Psychopathic Disorder as a: 'persistent disorder or disability of mind (Whether or not including significant impairment of intelligence) which results in abnormally aggressive or seriously irresponsible conduct on the part of the person concerned' (HO & DoH, 1983).

While this legally facilitates the detention of any individual considered to pose a risk of violent or other behaviours deleterious to the well being of the general public, it offers no indication as to what a 'psychopathic disorder' might or might not be. In the absence of any tangible consensus as to the aetiology, development, maintenance or pathology of personality disorders, classification has been based on statistically significant clusters of behaviour and associated psychopathology.

Dilemmas in defining psychopathy and personality disorder

The debate as to the existence (or otherwise) of personality disorder and its usefulness as a concept of aberrance in psychological health or functioning continues. The nebulousness of this very concept is compounded further by the (as yet) poorly defined distinction between psychopathy and personality disorders. Using the categorical scales of assessment outlined initially by Cleckley (1976) and more comprehensively by Hare (1984, 1991) the distinction is relatively clear, as the scoring system offers an indication of the extent of psychopathic disorder according to the absence or presence of common personality traits and interpersonal styles associated with psychopathy. This model offers a view of psychopathy that is quite distinct from other personality disorders with no automatic link to the current range of diagnoses available in the medical manuals.

Other theorists challenge the very notion of disorders of personality being a continuum of personality functioning from health to disorder and adopt a dimensional rather than categorical model of assessment. Blackburn (1992) asserts that a more comprehensive measure of personality can be gleaned by using a measure of assessment where the starting point is the extent to which an individual creates interactions as a combination of power (dominance v submissiveness) and affinity (hostility v friendliness). In this model the distinction between psychopathy and personality disorder is not as easy to make but generally the characteristics associated with psychopathy would be most apparent in those who maintain high dominance and high hostility scores.

Similarly the postmodern and deconstructionist view considers personality disorder to be a social construct used to describe behaviours that fall outside dominant social norms and expectations. Included within this are behaviours appearing contradictory, self-defeating, bizarre and apparently motiveless, in effect, behaviours with little epidemiological or aetiological basis. This explanation of psychopathy is based upon a model in which the meaning of deviant lifestyle is construed as a clinical pathology (Levenson, 1992). As Levenson (1992) points out, however, apparently motiveless actions are frequently evident in the behaviours of individuals who do not attract any psychiatric diagnosis and, he asserts, these are not indicative of disorder. Rather they imply an unwillingness on the part of the observer, sentencer or health professional to examine or accept atypical or expressed motive.

Other social science writers, for example, Illich (1977) enhance this argument through an analysis of the ideology, background and value systems of the professions and systems that seek to define personality disorder. They encompass the notion that the construction of personality disorder and particularly psychopathy, serves society's needs to define and reinforce what is 'normal' via the abjection of what is 'abnormal'. Following this argument would imply an inherent tautology that personality disorder is anything that powerful sections of society define as abnormal. This would lead to some questioning of the motives of those groups involved in classifying individuals as personality disordered and/or psychopathic.

Social historians are quick to point out the previous status of homosexuality as a perversion often encompassed in mental health and criminal legislation in western societies. In Britain, homosexuality was 'treated' (up until the 1960s) as a mental and criminal disorder founded similarly on the (then) prevalent perspective of moral turpitude. The change in the dominant ideology demonstrates an acknowledgement of the rights of those who do not fall completely into a society's notion of the norm. It also highlighted the limitations of 'treating' those alleged disorders that are morally formulated rather than scientifically devised.

There is also some evidence that the traits described as characteristic of personality disorder and psychopathy are, in fact, more evenly distributed throughout our society than frequently thought. From both an individual and anthropological point of view, some of these traits may be both useful and adaptive in certain circumstances (e.g., armed services, ruthless business management, animal experimentation, abattoir/butcher workers etc.). Levenson (1992) argues that a new and more accurate definition of psychopathy would be that of a life philosophy founded upon the trivialization of others and which he sees as becoming increasingly widely distributed throughout (Western) societies. This is a recurrent theme in many psychodynamic approaches.

Classification and description – medical

The ICD-10 (World Health Organization, 1992) notes that individuals suffering personality disorders usually come to the attention of social care, criminal justice or mental health care staff because of a gross disparity between (their) behaviours and the prevailing social norms. Such disorders are characterized by:

- a callous unconcern for the feelings of others;
- gross and persistent attitude of irresponsibility and disregard for social norms, rules and obligations;

- incapacity to maintain enduring relationships though having no difficulty in establishing them;
- very low tolerance to frustration and a low threshold for the discharge of aggression including violence;
- incapacity to experience guilt or to profit from experience, particularly punishment; and
- marked proneness to blame others or to offer plausible rationalizations for the behaviour that has brought the individual into conflict with society (World Health Organization, 1992).

Similarly the DSM-IV (American Psychiatric Association, 1994) describes personality as a composite of personality traits, which are:

> enduring patterns of perceiving, relating to and thinking about the environment and oneself and are exhibited in a wide range of important social and personal contexts. It is only when personality traits are inflexible and maladaptive and cause either significant functional impairment or subjective distress that they constitute personality disorder.

In addition it goes on to describe the general diagnostic criteria for personality disorder as being:

- An enduring pattern of inner experience and behaviour that deviates markedly from the expectations of the individual's culture, the pattern being manifested in two or more of the following areas:
  - cognition – ways of perceiving and interpreting the self, other people and events;
  - affectivity – the range, intensity, lability and appropriateness of emotional response;
  - interpersonal functioning; and
  - impulse control.
- The enduring pattern is inflexible and pervasive across a broad range of personal and social situations.
- The enduring pattern leads to clinically significant distress or impairment in social, occupational or other important areas of functioning.
- The pattern is stable and of long duration its onset being traced back to adolescence or early adulthood.
- The enduring pattern is not better accounted for as a manifestation or consequence of another mental disorder.
- The enduring pattern is not due to the direct physiological effects of substance (e.g., a drug of abuse, a medication or a general medical condition such as head trauma or brain injury) (American Psychiatric Association, 1994).

Important to note here is that the classification of 'psychopathic disorder', as described by the Mental Health Act (HO & DoH, 1983) incorporates all diagnostic categories of personality disorder within the medical manuals (ICD-10 & DSM-IV). There is, however, no automatic correlation with the pattern of interpersonal functioning outlined by the psychological manuals the PCL-R (Hare, 1985) and CIRCLE (Blackburn, 1993).

This particular client group maintain this taut relationship with the environment in which therapy takes place. The skills required by staff to maintain the therapeutic endeavour under these circumstances are complex and in order to develop more adequately the necessary specialist skills we need first to examine more exactly the challenge of the client group. To some extent the characteristics can be demonstrated by examining the diagnostic categories particular to the client group coming to the secure psychiatric services. The most neatly outlined is that of the DSM-IV (American Psychiatric Association, 1994) which identifies ten diagnostic categories in three clusters based on how the individual's disorder presents itself in the human environment.

In this, as can be seen in Table 18.1, Cluster A disorders are characterized by individuals who neither seek nor want human contact and will avoid it to as great a degree as possible. Cluster B disorders are characterized by individuals maintaining a commitment that the world hates them and they're going to hate it right back. While Cluster C disorders are characterized by individuals who feel they have little or no control over their own lives and will seek either to over-compensate by rigidly controlling their environment and activity or to get others to take over that responsibility.

Classification and description – psychological

A persuasive notion of psychopathy is that described initially by Cleckley (1976) and later developed by Hare (1985) into the most widely used and validated measure for the assessment of psychopathy (the PCL-R). This measurement tool discards the broader and more tentative descriptions of personality disorders and recognizes those features normally associated with psychopathic personality disorder into a distinct clinical entity including criteria such as egocentricity and callousness. While this is enormously helpful in assessment and identification of the impact of a disorder on the presentation of the patient, it requires sophisticated translation into treatment programmes. Moreover it does lend itself to the lay notion that there is an inherent and automatic relationship between personality disorders and serious offending behaviours creating the notion that serious offenders and psychopaths are one and the same and that they are in fact a homogenous group.

Using this categorical scale of assessment the distinction is relatively clear as the scoring system offers a system for measuring the extent of psychopathic

Table 18.1   DSM-IV Axis II diagnoses

Cluster	Personality disorder	Characteristic traits
Cluster A	Paranoid	Distrusts others' motives; expects to be harmed, abused, let down or rejected; preoccupied with issues of loyalty and trustworthiness; bears grudges; misreads events as directly hostile towards him/her self.
	Schizoid	Social detachment; Emotionally controlled in interpersonal settings (often appearing cold or flat in affect); solitary and aloof; little interest in sexual contact with others; indifferent to social feedback.
	Schizotypal	Interpersonal deficits with cognitive or perceptual distortions and associated eccentric behaviour; acute sensitivity to self (perceives events as directly relating to self); odd beliefs or magical thinking reflected in speech and behaviour; excessive social anxiety.
Cluster B	Antisocial	Disregards and violates rights of others with impunity; fails to observe social and legal proprieties; deceitful; impulsive; irritable and aggressive; reckless with regard to safety of self and others; irresponsible; lacking in remorse.
	Borderline	Poor self-image (abjection) and identity disturbance; impulsive; intense fear of rejection or abandonment; severe mood swings and poor mood control; intense emotional attachments (love/hate); recurrent self-injury or suicidal behaviours; self defeating/sabotaging.
	Histrionic	Excessively emotional; needs to be centre of attention; shifting and shallow expression of emotion; overly concerned with physical appearance; melodramatic/theatric; over-estimates degree of intimacy in relationships; sexually seductive/provocative in appearance.
	Narcissistic	Intense grandiosity and need for admiration; superiority without commensurate achievements; exploitative; lacks empathy or feels justified mistreating others; arrogant and haughty; sense of entitlement (rules are there for others); fantasist (power, brilliance, ideal love etc.)
Cluster C	Avoidant	Socially inhibited; feels inadequate; hypersensitive to negative social feedback; sense of being socially inept, unappealing or inferior; excessive rumination about failure and embarrassment.
	Dependent	Intense need to be cared for; submissive and clinging in relationships; looks for others to make their decisions; excessively seeks nurturance and support; feels helpless when alone.
	Obsessive-Compulsive	Inflexible perfectionism that interferes with task completion; preoccupation with rules, lists and order to the point that the purpose of the task is lost; inability to balance competing priorities causing indecisiveness and protractedness; rigidity in personal beliefs, values, ethics and morality discounting those of others.

Source: Adapted from American Psychiatric Association (1994)

Table 18.2 Categorical evaluation of psychopathy

Psychopathic Personality – Cleckley (1976)	Psychopathy Checklist – Hare (1984)
Superficial charm and good intelligence	Glibness/superficial charm
Absence of delusions or irrational thinking	Grandiose sense of self-worth
Absence of neurotic manifestations	Need for stimulation/proneness to boredom
Unreliable	Pathological lying
Untruthful and insincere	Cunning/manipulative
Lacks remorse	Lack of remorse or guilt
Social behaviour inadequately motivated	Shallow affect
Fails to learn by experience	Callous/lack of empathy
Egocentric and incapable of love	Parasitic lifestyle
Emotionally slow	Poor behavioural controls
Lacks insight	Promiscuous sexual behaviour
Socially unresponsive	Early behaviour problems
Objectionable behaviour after drinking	Lack of realistic long-term plans
Suicide threats and gestures without serious attempts	Impulsivity
	Irresponsibility
	Failure to accept responsibility for own actions
Impersonal sex life	Many short term marital relationships
No consistent goals	Juvenile delinquency
	Revocation of conditional release
	Criminal versatility

Source: Adapted from Cleckley (1976) and Hare (1984)

disorder according to the absence or presence of common personality traits and interpersonal styles associated with psychopathy (see Table 18.2). Briefly, though, Hare's (1985) PCL-R is a twenty factor assessment, each with a potential score of 0, 1 or 2, where:

0 = not present;
1 = intermittent (outline under what circumstances it becomes present);
2 = a regular and common feature of the individual's presentation.

The end score is therefore in the range of 0–40 and broadly, the interpretation by experienced clinicians, is that the higher the score the more profound the extent of the disorder. At its extreme end (25+) the view is generally that the extent of the individual's psychopathic disorder is so profound they are unlikely to benefit from the range of treatments currently available. Consequently many individuals diagnosed as suffering a psychopathic disorder and detained in secure psychiatric establishments under the provisions of the Mental Health Act (HO & DoH, 1983) would not meet the criteria for psychopathy as measured by the PCL-R. Conversely many individuals detained in prison under the provisions of the Criminal Justice Act (Home Office, 1994) would meet the criteria for psychopathy as measured by the PCL-R but do not access mental health services either due to an unwillingness to cooperate with the assessment process or because they are currently deemed 'untreatable'.

Blackburn's typology cluster (CIRCLE)

This dimensional model of interpersonal functioning (Blackburn, 1993) (Figure 18.1) challenges the more categorical scale of measurement suggesting a continuum of personality development from normal to abnormal as used by Hare et al and the associated suggestion that personality disorder is a standard diagnosis. In fact it has been demonstrated by Blackburn and Maybury (1985) that the very notion of a personality disorder leads to the enormously misleading notion of homogeneity.

Assessment of personality in the normal range would score within the inner

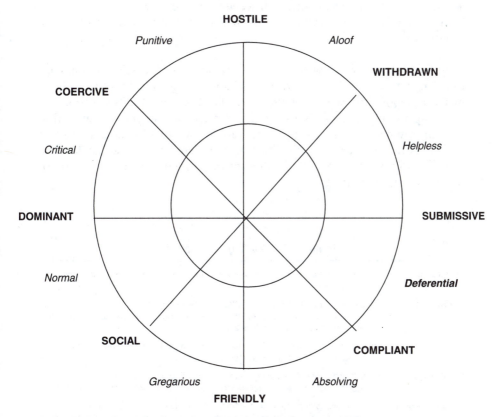

Figure 18.1 Chart of interpersonal relationships in a closed living environment
Source: Adapted from Blackburn (1993)

circle and demonstrates fluidity in the range and repertoire of interpersonal skills available to the individual. Where there is deviance the score on the particular axis exceeds the boundary of the inner circle and indicates not only an exaggerated (e.g. hostility) or deficit (e.g. submissiveness) component of interpersonal functioning but also an associated over-reliance on this aspect of interpersonalness. That particular characteristic of the individual's behaviour tends to be more rigid and he or she will have an impaired reper-toire of skills available in other areas of interpersonal functioning. Blackburn and Maybury (1985) demonstrated that within the classification of antisocial personality disorder alone there are four distinct clusters of personality, namely:

- Primary (impulsive, aggressive, hostile, extroverted and self-confident with low to average anxiety);
- Secondary (hostile, impulsive, aggressive, socially anxious, withdrawn, moody and low in self-esteem);
- Controlled (defensive, controlled, sociable and very low anxiety);
- Inhibited (shy, withdrawn, controlled, moderately anxious and low-self esteem).

They further noted that not only were this group of individuals heterogenous but that the nature of the disorder was largely responsive to their environ-ment, as opposed to being a purely internalized process. This notion of psy-chopathy and personality disorder being dimensional rather than categorical has similarly been considered by other leading psychologists in this area and of note is the so called 'big five' factors considered by Costa and McCrae (1991) (as shown in Table 18.3) to be the major components or domains of interpersonal functioning.

Table 18.3　The 'big five' factors

Neuroticism	Stable *v* unstable image of self in relation to the environment (esp. the human environment)
Extroversion	Sociability *v* socially isolative and the processes by which this is achieved (i.e. the process is as important as the factor – an individual may seek social inclusion but does so by bullying or intimidation)
Openness	Openness to new situations and experiences which are life enhancing and developmental *v* closetedness and insularity
Agreeableness	Affinity *v* hostility – this can be likened to the principal dimensions of hostility/friendliness and dominance/submissiveness used by Blackburn et al.
Conscientiousness	Do activities take place to define the individual's belonging to a tradition (community, culture or such) or are they simply the quickest way of getting an outcome?

Source: Adapted from Costa & McCrae (1991)

A word on the judiciary and DSPD

Detention for treatment under mental health legislation is somewhat fraught with this client group as it is facilitated on the basis of prophesy rather than history. The Mental Health Act (1983) (HO & DoH, 1983) enables an individual to be held for long periods of time, against their will, on the basis of risk, which of course means what they might do in the future. This is in contrast to detention under the criminal justice system (e.g. prison), where individuals are detained for a fixed period of time 'under pain of punishment' for some past act of which they have been found guilty (*history*). Mental health law accepts responsibility as being diminished by mental disorder but facilitates continued detention while we, the clinicians, consider the individual may offend again in the future (*prophesy*).

Furthermore, though it is not the purpose of this chapter to consider the role of the judiciary, but in relation to the issue of DSPD (Dangerous and Severe Personality Disorders) it has been suggested that the use of legislation to enable 'preventative detention' is not likely to gain support but that 'anticipatory detention' is perfectly possible. This is in relation to the postulation that individuals such as Michael Stone (who was at liberty to kill a mother and child on a London Common despite being well known to the psychiatric and criminal justice agencies) should be detained under mental health legislation before they commit any serious offence.

The distinction here is that *prevention* is an enclosure from which there is no egress while *anticipation* is a fluid state requiring continual assessment and re-assessment enabling discharge (should the individual's anticipated risk become lessened). In effect, preventative detention is permanent and gives regard only to an individual's history of offending. Anticipatory detention, however, is less rigid and allows detention to continue only when it can be demonstrated that there are reasonable grounds to anticipate the individual would present a risk to others if at liberty. This would, however, be largely reliant upon the development of a medical/psychological process for assessing risk and formulating a competent and comprehensive prediction measure.

This has caused considerable confusion with regard to the strength of evidence confirming the existence of personality disorders or otherwise and has been further amplified by the language of 'dangerous and severe' in relation to this category. In particular the use of the term 'dangerous' implies a permanent state. Clearly this is highly misleading as offending of any type is closely related to the environment and circumstance. We know of no individual who presents a continuous risk to his/her environment 24 hours per day, seven days per week – and so on. The issue then is to determine the individual's propensity to harm others and under what conditions that propensity is likely to be realized. In effect this is better referred to as 'risk' rather than dangerousness.

Similarly the concept of severity is difficult to apply to this category of disorder. Too often the term is actually applied to the *offending* behaviour rather than the *extent* of the individual's disorder. Various proposals for categorizing severity or justifying the use of the term have been asserted. These include utilizing both psychological and medical diagnostic procedures to focus on developmental components of personality. The psychological tools gauge dynamic and interpersonal factors such as superficiality, lying, impulsivity and lacking empathy. The suggested criteria for imposing the label of 'dangerous and severe' includes having three or more Axis II diagnoses from the ICD-10 or DSM-IV; a score of 30+ on the Hare Psychopathy Checklist-Revised (PCL-R), or a combination of the two (PCL-R score of 30+ with two axis II diagnoses or PCL-R score of 25+ with three or more axis II diagnoses).

It is currently the case that the continued use of the 'D' and 'S' part of the DSPD label is quite likely to be dropped. The 'PD' component is also not looking altogether likely to remain. Irrespective of the language adopted, however, it remains the commitment of both the health and criminal justice services, driven by Government, that some development of services for this client group must take place. These services will aim to tackle the issue of mental health care and to protect the public.

Working with personality disordered clients

In the human environment this translates into relationships being highly charged and often emotionally intense to the point where social interactions occur in a corrupted and exploitative manner. Such individuals demonstrate emotional extremes far beyond any continuum imagined in common social interactions and often punctuated with a language constructed in superlatives and hyperbole. Levels of anger and hostility are particularly high and are most commonly focused towards those on whom individuals are most reliant, in effect the family and those health care professionals involved in the care and support of the client.

In relating to others, such individuals maintain a deeply ingrained expectation that they will be harmed, exploited, let down, rejected and otherwise abused and they will enter into relationships with this expectation (subconsciously) in mind. Consequently such individuals will continually test issues of loyalty and fidelity within relationships, demonstrating an intense concern for, and preoccupation with, the protection of self but showing little evidence of concern for others within their sphere of social interaction. They will often demonstrate seriously irresponsible and thrill seeking behaviours with short-term immediate gratifications, but with little or no concern for the possible consequences. They will often demonstrate an exaggerated moral outrage if they feel their own personal rights or wants have been violated, but will disregard the rights of others, demonstrating no remorse for having wronged another and showing no capacity to experience guilt or to profit from experience, often to the point where they will actually feel justified in having hurt or mistreated others.

Such individuals are apt to be self-centred and egocentric, whose own sense of entitlement precludes the capacity to recognize or experience how their actions may affect others within the environment. It is important to realize that some, or even many of these characteristics, may appear in any or all of us at given times within our lives. A formal diagnosis of Personality Disorder, however, would only be considered where such traits were present as a constant and pervasive feature of the individual's life and interactional styles.

Similarly in the living environment such individuals demonstrate no constancy in any value base or moral regulatory system but may feign a range of differing commitments depending on the circumstance at any given time. Such individuals are noted to develop a remarkable ability to rationalize their own actions to an exceptional degree, often shifting responsibility for their own actions and avoiding introspection through a process of blame, complaint and protest. They will constantly invite collusion from others via a range of linguistic and interpersonal techniques developed over very long periods of time.

Such processes are deeply ingrained within the mindset of clients suffering from such chronic and damaging disorders and these can relatively easily be explored through the life history of individuals suffering these disorders. They can most commonly be seen as having come from home circumstances which may be severely abusive and neglectful; will have had problems in schooling and local environment due to conduct disorders in childhood; will have demonstrated excessively indulgent behaviours of an almost epicurean intensity in relation to drugs, alcohol and early sexual experience through adolescence; there will be a pattern of seriously irresponsible or 'thrill seeking' behaviours, shifting into criminal offences (usually of increasing severity) through adolescence and into early adult life; such individuals will often have come to the attention of the criminal justice system at a relatively early age. Indeed many will have resided in care homes, Special Schools and Young Offender Institutions before reaching the age of 18. Most will have experienced some period of incarceration within a penal institution.

Dynamic issues and relationship as a therapeutic tool

Working with this client group then the issue of boundaries in interpersonal relationships is fundamental to the therapeutic process, both for the protection of the carer and to aid the progress of the client. The research is clearly emerging that the benefit of treatments afforded to the patient are heavily influenced by the quality of the relationship between patient and therapist (Bowers, 2000; 2003). Most important here is that while it seems an absolute imperative that the practitioner maintains a stolid professional detachment it is equally imperative that he or she promotes a positive and motivational perspective as to the potential outcomes and benefits of treatment approaches.

Similarly the need for the practitioner to avoid exhibiting negative attitudes is vital as there are clear links between the inculcation of negative attitudes; the concomitant dynamic of nurses becoming alienated from disliked patients and a resulting increase in untimely discharge and resultant suicide of PD patients (Adler, 1973, Gunderson, 1984).

Clearly at the outset, the relationship between the client and care staff is relatively neutral with clear boundaries dictated by professional etiquette and cultural expectation. The process of assessment and treatment, however, can challenge the social construction of a neutral relationship, as the discussion will often relate to the most intimate and intrusive components of the client's life, experience and feelings. This can be particularly difficult for the carer who will spend long periods of time with the client exploring a range of private and public experiences. By consequence this process predicates the sharing of the kind of sensitive and often intimate information that is most commonly confined to close and intimate relationships. Without careful and ongoing supervision carers can lose sight of the boundaries that define their professional roles in relation to the personality disordered client and professional impropriety and boundary disintegration is not uncommon. In a review of major security breeches involving staff collusion in the high secure hospitals it was noted that in all such cases the client inviting such collusion and professional misconduct was personality disordered (Fallon, et al 1999). To the knowledge of the authors no in-depth research has been carried out on this matter but it is apparent that health care professionals rarely compromise professional boundaries with severely mentally ill or learning disabled clients but all too frequently do so with personality disordered clients.

It is apparent then that there are unusual, and at times, exceptionally convoluted and complex inter-personal dynamics at play in the formulation of the relationship between the personality disordered client and his or her carer and this can leave even the most experienced and professional care staff vulnerable to boundary violations. Gutheil and Gabbard (1993) note three degrees or levels of challenge to relationship boundaries, namely boundary crossing; boundary violation and sexual misconduct. They further note that the care environment can predict the violation of boundaries as 'various group therapeutic approaches or therapeutic communities may involve inherent boundary violations' Gutheil and Gabbard (1993, p 189).

In Forensic Mental Health settings this can be even more complex given the nature of offending behaviours that bring individuals into contact with the secure mental health care services. While the patient may well be unhappy with components of his or her life, the construct of the disorder predicates that the client will generally tend towards a denial or minimization of responsibility for offending behaviours and often offer complex rationalizations as to how the root of his or her problems is with someone else. The client will essentially seek validation to the point of collusion from care staff. As in all relationships they will be most strongly drawn towards those individuals who are less challenging and more accepting of their view of the world and inter-pretation or rationalization of events.

This whole process is founded on a tension that while the relationship is focused on attempting to challenge therapeutically the way the client perceives their (human) environment and relates to others, there is a constant need to validate their individuality and self-determination and this can have the effect of actually reinforcing the way they perceive their position. Inherent in this process then is an acknowledgement that the carer is, in this regard, acting as a change agent and that the therapeutic relationship must therefore, be constructed accordingly. In practice this means there must be a clear under-standing from the outset that the carer will be challenging aspects of the indi-vidual's inter-relatedness but that this must be done with the active involvement of the client and with a properly assessed and agreed formula-tion of which area(s) of the client's interpersonal functioning are to be addressed. Only by having a clear formulation of target areas to be addressed, a clear plan of how the therapist or carer is going to isolate those areas of interpersonal functioning and a clear idea of expected or desired outcomes can such a therapeutic relationship be possible.

Splitting and secrets

The process of splitting in groups is well identified and recorded in the aca-demic literatures related to this field and put simply it is a process of making an individual or group feel different (normally better or worse) to their peers or those around them. In practice the negative splitting behaviours are often quickly picked up, for example a client may claim he or she is being victim-ized by a specific member of staff (or staff group) by not facilitating a request that they claim others do (even if this is contrary to policy). In this, the patient is both exerting a pressure on staff (who are attempting to maintain consis-tent practice), to alter or 'bend' the rules and creating conflict between care team members. While such dynamics do create tensions they are normally easily diffused where good communication is maintained as care staff clarify policy and practice by discussing the client's claims of what is and isn't allowed between themselves and re-asserting or reviewing agreed protocols (Gorney, 1994; Singer, 1965).

More destructive than this, however are the seductive components of split-ting, which are far more easily missed and can actually have a greater impact. For example when the client invests an apparent trust and confidence in a par-ticular member of the care team and tells them 'you're the only one I can talk to, they (other clinical team members) are not interested'. This is further com-plicated and distorted when the patients invite the therapist to maintain 'secrets' often in the name of confidentiality 'Can I tell you something that I've never told anyone before' or 'I really need to talk about something that's really private but you have to promise it won't go outside this room.' This is often used to compound the notion that the therapist is different to his or her peers as it is explained 'they (other clinical team members) will use it against me or to wind me up, they wouldn't understand anyway!' This can be particularly divisive when more than one discipline is involved and can lead to major conflicts among the clinical care team.

The level of conflict generated by such dynamics can be powerful and the ultimate effect is usually an avoidance or loss of sight of core matters in relation to the care of the patient and an over investment in day-to-day management issues and the 'power plays' that occur within groups. Moreover such splitting among clinical team members frequently results in factions within the clinical team and these dynamics are quickly recognized and further exploited by the client. The effect is in any case deleterious both to the care of the client and the functioning of the clinical team.

With this in mind it is essential that all care staff, irrespective of their individual professions, are able to discuss aspects of relationship with personality disordered clients and particularly explore linguistic reflections of how the client views the relationship. In inpatient services it is frequent that carers will discuss, with each other, claims by a client that other carers have facilitated some action contrary to a particular policy but it is rare indeed that carers will report that a particular client has told them they are 'better' or 'more caring' than other care staff, yet these are powerful indicators that the relationship with the client is shifting from a therapeutic to a personal dimension. As innocent and unimportant as it may seem such dynamics are in fact hugely damaging as they work at various levels to confirm the clients view that their problems emanate from others and are therefore beyond their scope of responsibility or influence. Such selective use of confidentiality is tantamount to collusion.

Rejection

Like many components of interpersonal relationships, identifiable aspects or processes can be complex and multi-faceted. Certainly the process of rejection by a client can be a powerful yet highly complex relationship issue in that much as the nature of those disorders here discussed are such that clients often expect to be exploited, harmed, abused and let down and approach relationships with that expectation in mind. As a result they can be possessive and defensive in relationships, continually testing loyalties and ardently searching for signs that a 'let down' is imminent.

At its most basic level then a rejection from the client is merely a defence mechanism from one who fears being rejected by someone close (in this case the carer) and will negate the possibility by rejecting them first. Literally the patient will reject you before you get the chance to reject him or her. The effect of this as a contributory factor in the deconstruction of professional boundaries or therapeutic relationships and the shift towards personal friendships or more intimate relationships is profound. It is a human trait that in a social circumstance where rejection occurs we assume some level of personal responsibility and a desire to rectify any wrongs done, or perceived to have been done. In this, the staff will often attempt to rectify the relationship with the client by seeking the cause of the rejection rather than exploring the psychopathology of his or her feelings, thoughts and behaviours. Carers are, by necessity, constantly vigilant to the demeanour of all clients and when the client becomes hostile towards someone with whom they have previously had a good relationship it is common for that staff to attempt discourse to establish why the relationship has altered. In this, questions like 'are you annoyed with me?' or 'have I done something to upset you?' can unintentionally change the nature of the relationship shifting it to a personal, rather than professional or therapeutic level as such utterances focus on the carer's actions rather than those of the client.

Melia et al (1999) observe that following such a rejection experience these attempts to rectify the situation can be met with a highly intense level of anger and hostility as a result of the perceived wrongdoing, mitigated by phrases like 'I can't believe you of all people would do that to me' or 'I thought you were different, I thought I could trust you!' The discomfort phase following such an incident can last for days before a gradual 'softening' occurs and the relationship resumes its previous status but, by consequence, is less professional and more personal.

Over prolonged periods of time such rejection experiences can have extremely undesirable and cumulative effects on even the most qualified and experienced of staff. Unchecked this can lead to prolonged duress stress disorders in some members of staff but more importantly can lead to staff losing sight of their own value base and conduct boundaries to the point where they may avoid challenging an issue or enforcing a policy, for fear of provoking the discomfort of a rejection experience and its inevitable aftermath. At worst such processes can also lead to a fragmenting of boundaries to the point where the carer may agree to 'bend the rules', thus establishing a level of intimacy based on 'shared secrets' but masquerading as trust.

This will frequently demonstrate itself in terms of challenges to the normal social proprieties of interpersonal and professional boundaries. The client will often invite the therapist to collude in their perspective of conflict, seek validation for offending behaviours and take their side against any perceived enmity or aggression. This will often be asserted in the name of 'trust'. It is the experience of the authors that trust, when forced or invited, can be a false and misleading mentor and should be avoided. If the therapist maintains an entirely impartial demeanour and acts at all times with absolute professional integrity trust will follow as a natural process in the development of the truly therapeutic relationship.

Conclusion

While the very concept of a health or functional deficit related to personality remains somewhat nebulous with some health care professionals believing this is little more than an attempt to medicalize a social issue, the impact for individuals who 'suffer' personality disorders (and especially the so called 'dangerous and severely personality disordered' client) on their human environment is considerable. At the launch of the *Managing Dangerous People With Severe Personality Disorder* (HO & DoH, 1999) document the former Secretary of State (Frank Dobson) addressed a professional audience indicating the view that the traditional model of psychiatric care has both failed to provide effective care and treatment for Dangerous and Severely Personality Disordered clients and to protect the public from them. The planned changes in legislation will dramatically alter the framework of care and intervention for such individuals, placing far greater responsibility on the range of professionals, including psychologists, involved in their assessment, treatment and detention.

From this it is clear that the current psychiatric services are not adequately equipped to provide the comprehensive and intensive treatment programmes necessary to facilitate good and safe care to this client group and there needs to be radical changes and the development of new services. This will almost certainly involve an entirely new model of staffing as there is little or no evidence that the traditional model of having a doctor, nurse, social worker, psychologist, occupational therapist and so forth is in any way appropriate to the needs of this client group. We would assert that a grass-routes reformulation of what services are required and who is best equipped to provide that service needs to be undertaken.

References

Adler, G. (1973) Hospital treatment of borderline patients, *American Journal of Psychiatry*, 130, 32–5.

American Psychiatric Association (1994) *Diagnostic and Statistical Manual of Mental Disorders*, 4th Edn, Washington DC: APA.

Bateman, A. & Tyrer, P. (2003) Effective Management of Personality Disorder, in *Personality Disorder No Longer a Diagnosis of Exclusion*, London: HMSO, online at: http://www.doh.gov.uk/mentalhealth/personalitydisorder.htm

Blackburn, R. (1992) Criminal behaviour, personality disorder and mental illness: the origins of confusion, *Criminal Behaviour and Mental Health*, 2, 66–77.

Blackburn, R. (1993) *The Psychology of Criminal Conduct: Theory, Research and Practice*, Chichester: John Wiley & Sons.

Blackburn, R. & Maybury, C. (1985) Identifying the psychopath: the relation of Cleckley's criteria to the interpersonal domain, *Personality and Individual Differences*, 6, 375–86.

Bowers, L. (2000) *Practitioner Client Relationships: Maintaining Positive Regard For Vulnerable Clients*, London: UKCC.

Bowers, L. (2003) *Dangerous and Severe Personality Disorder*, London: Routledge.

Cleckley, M. (1976) *The Mask of Sanity*, St Louis: Mosby.

Costa, P. T. & McCrae, R. R. (1991) *Neo Five Factor Inventory*, Odessa FA: Psychological Assessment Resources.

Craissati, J., Horne, L. & Taylor, R. (2003) Effective treatment models for personality disordered offenders, in *Personality Disorder No Longer a Diagnosis of Exclusion*, London: HMSO, online at: http://www.doh.gov.uk/mentalhealth/personalitydisorder.htm

Fallon, P., Bluglass, R., Edwards, B. & Daniels, G. (1999) *Report of the Committee of Inquiry into the Personality Disorder Unit, Ashworth Special Hospital*, London: HMSO.

Gorney, J. E. (1994) On limits and limit setting, *Psychoanalytic Review*, 81(2), 259–78.

Gunderson, J. (1984) *Borderline Personality Disorder*, Washington: American Psychiatric Press.

Gutheil, T. G. & Gabbard, G. O. (1993) The concept of boundaries in clinical practice: theoretical and risk management dimensions, *American Journal of Psychiatry*, 150, 188–96.

Hare, R. D. (1984) A research scale for the assessment of psychopathy in criminal populations, *Personality and Individual Differences*, 1, 111–17.

Hare, R. D. (1985) A comparison of procedures for the assessment of psychopathy, *Journal of Consulting and Clinical Psychology*, 53, 7–16.

Hare, R. D. (1991) *Manual for the Revised Psychopathy Checklist*, Vancouver, Canada: University of British Columbia.

Home Office (1994) *Criminal Justice and Public Order Act (1994)*, London: HMSO.

Home Office & Department of Health (1983) *The Mental Health Act 1983*, London: HMSO.

Home Office & Department of Health (1999) *Managing Dangerous People with Severe Personality Disorder, Proposals for Policy Development*, London: HMSO.

Home Office & Department of Health (2000) *Reforming the Mental Health Act, Part I: The New Legal Framework, Part II: High Risk Patients*, London: HMSO.

Illich, I. (1977) *Limits to Medicine: The Medical Nemesis and the Expropriation of Health*, Harmondsworth: Penguin.

Levenson, M. (1992) Rethinking psychopathy, *Theory and Psychology*, 2(1), 51–71.

Melia, P., Moran, A. & Mason, T. (1999) Triumvirate nursing for personality disordered patients: crossing the boundaries safely, *Journal of Psychiatric and Mental Health Nursing*, 6, 15–20.

Singer, E. (1965) *Key Concepts in Psychotherapy*, New York: Random House.

World Health Organization (1992) *ICD-10 Classification of Mental and Behavioural Disorders: Clinical Descriptions and Diagnostic Guidelines*, Geneva: WHO.

CHAPTER 19

The Influence of Dual Diagnoses

DOMINIC WAKE

Indicative Benchmark Statements

▪ Participation in the assessment and management of factors of co-morbidity and precursors to mental illness

▪ Recognition of relapse signatures in users of mental health and social care services

▪ Application of the fundamental knowledge of psychopharmacology

▪ Participation in techniques useful in increasing adherence to appropriately pre-scribed mental health medication and other treatments

▪ Assertiveness, conflict management and problem-solving skills within the multi-disciplinary mental health and social care team

Introduction

When considering the problem of dual diagnosis, the student first needs to be aware that the term 'dual diagnosis' means different things to different people. In the context of this chapter we are referring to clients with mental health problems who also have problems resulting from their alcohol and/or substance use. However, most authors, including Rassool (2002); Frischer and Akram (2001) and Copello et al (2001) agree that the term 'dual diagnosis' is more usually applied to clients with serious mental illness, such as schizophrenia or bi-polar affective disorder. Usually, there are two terms that are applied to the combination of mental illness and substance use: dual diagnosis and co-morbidity. Weaver et al (1999) prefer the second term for the above reasons and also because it avoids speculation as to whether substances are used or misused. Rassool (2002) states that there has been a recent move away from thinking in terms of 'dual diagnosis' towards a more accurate description of clients with 'complex needs'.

In 1976, the World Health Organization (WHO) published a paper that described the alcohol-dependence syndrome (Edwards & Gross, 1976). The WHO then went on to outline the related psychological, social and physical problems related to alcohol dependence (Edwards et al, 1977). This relationship between alcohol/substance use and psychiatric disorders is complex and has many manifestations. According to Crome (1999, p 154):

- Substance use (even one dose) may lead to psychiatric syndromes.
- Harmful use may produce psychiatric syndromes.
- Dependence may produce psychological symptoms.
- Intoxication from substances may produce psychological symptoms.
- Withdrawal from substances may produce psychological symptoms.
- Withdrawal from substances may lead to psychiatric syndromes.
- Substance use may exacerbate pre-existing psychiatric disorder.
- Psychological morbidity not amounting to a 'disorder' may precipitate substance use.
- Primary psychiatric disorder may lead to substance use disorder.
- Primary psychiatric disorder may precipitate substance use disorder which may, in turn, lead to psychiatric syndromes.

From the above list, it becomes clear that there are many reasons why a client may be informed that they have a dual-diagnosis. This makes the treatment options difficult to work out for the clinician and even harder for the client to follow and comply with. We must also consider the fact that as both substance use and mental health problems are very common, the two are likely to occur together by mere coincidence. However, one of the major problems faced by clients and clinicians alike is that because the symptoms of substance use and substance withdrawal can resemble psychiatric symptoms, a psychiatric diagnosis can only be confidently established when the client is not currently abusing alcohol or drugs (Mueser et al, 1995). For this reason, many clients with histories of extensive substance use, are advised that if they want help and treatment for their mental health problems, they must first abstain for a period of time which may, in some cases, be *at least* six months.

This is a tall order for some and an impossibility for most. Many clients feel that they are not taken or treated seriously and are left in a 'Catch 22' situation with their drug of choice seen by themselves as their only reliable form of medication for relief of their symptoms and their psychiatrist seeing the drug as the cause of the symptoms. Indeed, many clients are so incensed at what they see as 'psychiatry's misunderstanding of their situation' that they set out to prove their doctor wrong. They sometimes embark on a period of abstinence (with or without support from services) often to be told later that six months of abstinence is not long enough and they should continue to abstain and suffer psychiatric symptoms for longer.

The National Service Framework for Mental Health (DOH, 1999) report that:

Around half of those reporting any substance misuse disorder have experienced other mental health problems. Of individuals seeking help for substance misuse, more than half have had a mental disorder in the previous six months. It is not unusual for around 30% of those seeking help for mental health problems to have current substance misuse problems. Assessments of individuals with mental health problems, whether in primary or specialist care, should consider the potential role of substance misuse and know how to access appropriate specialist input. The likelihood that substance misuse will increase suicide risk must also be considered.

Maslin et al (2001) sum up the relationship thus: 'All studies point to the considerable likelihood that staff working within mental health and substance misuse services will be coming into frequent contact with clients who have severe mental health problems and use substances problematically.'

Prevalence

Frischer and Akram (2001) report that relatively little is known about the extent of co-morbidity and most prevalence estimates relate to the USA. However, in the UK, the Office for Population Censuses and Surveys survey of psychiatric morbidity (Farrell et al, 1998) show that men were three times more likely than women to be alcohol dependent and twice as likely to be drug dependent (Meltzer et al, 1995). Glass & Jackson (1988) carried out the first study of its kind in the UK and found that 10 per cent of the patients with mental health problems they studied were found to have an alcohol problem. Of the patients with drink problems, 40 per cent had a dual diagnosis and associations were noted between alcoholism and neurosis, personality disorder, drug addiction, affective psychosis and schizophrenia (Crome, 1999). Crome (1999) goes on to suggest that European and American studies indicate that up to one-half of substance users have a psychiatric disorder, while approximately one-third of psychiatric patients have a substance use disorder. People with schizophrenia outnumber all other psychiatric diagnostic groups in the percentage of co-morbid substance abuse/dependence diagnoses. Substance use is endemic among the disadvantaged people within our society who are variously described as 'living on the margins' or 'socially excluded'. Most worryingly, there is an increased risk of relapse as the rate of non-compliance with treatment increases greatly in mental health patients who use illicit drugs and alcohol (Gournay et al, 1997; NHS Advisory Service, 1996).

Violence and offending

Johns (1997) warns that the epidemiological data available consistently shows that substance use is a major risk factor for violence. Certain substances and alcohol are linked to an increased propensity towards violence. Most worryingly in recent years is the short-term or chronic use of crack cocaine. The effects of using crack cocaine are reported as intense feelings of an increase in libido, increased self-confidence and raised energy levels.

Could this have a direct link with sexual offending behaviour? Parker and Bottomley (1997) estimated that on average, crack cocaine users spent approximately £20,000 each year on feeding their crack habit. Hodge (1993) believes that violence cannot be psychopharmacologically attributed to substance use, however, he also reports that intoxication with alcohol is often accompanied by temporary cognitive deficits, autonomic arousal and irritability. Intoxication with either drug, or often both can of course lead to aggressive feelings and hostile behaviour.

One of the biggest problems faced by crack cocaine users is that there is no access to substitute prescribing, as there is for heroin users. This is because unlike heroin, there is no recognized physical withdrawal syndrome associated with stimulants such as amphetamines, cocaine or crack. The relationship between violence and the withdrawal syndrome depends on the substance, the individual, history and setting. However, most features of withdrawal are familiar to the clinician and are widely accepted to be unpleasant experiences. However, most crack users report psychological withdrawal symptoms, including aggression and acute dysphoria, that manifest shortly after the drug has worn off due to its very short-lived effect (approximately 20 mins).

Goddard (1991) reports that heavy drinkers have been found to be 4.6 times more likely to experience aggressive feelings and 10 times more likely to have been involved in violence in the past week. In the *Report of the Confidential Inquiry into Homicides and Suicides by Mentally Ill People* (Boyd, 1996), it was found that in 18 per cent of homicides in England, the use of alcohol or other substances was present in the immediate period leading up to the killing. Boyd (1996) also found that of the suicides reported, 33 per cent of the cases had been involved with the use of alcohol, drugs or solvents in the period prior to the act of suicide. This study also reports that up to 90 per cent of people who take their own lives are mentally ill and that there is a more particular risk for mentally ill people who use substances or drink heavily.

The Task Force to Review Services for Drug Misusers (DoH, 1996) was established in 1994 by the Department of Health to review the effectiveness of drug services delivered in England and to devise and deliver recommendations to the Government. This Government task force commissioned the National Treatment Outcome Research Study (NTORS), (Healey et al, 1998) which went on to fund several major research studies of both mainstream and specialist drug services. One study followed over 1000 users over a period of 18 months, including those users who dropped out of treatment. The NTORS study (Healey et al, 1998) showed that many substance users who were in treatment for their substance use showed significant levels of psychiatric morbidity. Suicidal thoughts, feelings of hopelessness, anxiety and depressed mood were widely reported but the NTORS study (Healey et al, 1998) also showed that after only four weeks in treatment, all types of psychological symptoms were significantly reduced. Further to this, *Purchasing Effective Treatment and Care for Drug Misusers* (DoH, 1997) recommended that in seriously mentally ill persons, because the misuse of drugs and/or alcohol is a significant risk factor in the prediction of future violent behaviour, liaison between the services is vital in order to minimize the risk to the client and society. Unfortunately, according to Phillips (2000), communication and collaboration between substance misuse and forensic mental health services often remain fractured and limited both at a clinical and organizational level.

Motivation

Why do people who are mentally ill use drugs? Apart from the same reasons as the rest of society, there are some specific motivations for people with mental illness to use drugs. Lamb (1982) suggests that substance misuse in this group represents an opportunity to move away from the 'mental' label and to forge an alternative identity for themselves that may at least be more socially acceptable. Bergman and Harris (1985) report that substance misuse among people with schizophrenia is about their opportunities for increasing social interactions, or at least to move within 'none mental illness circles and with people who are not mentally ill'. More recent studies report that people with schizophrenia who use substances are attempting to self-medicate for the relief of their symptoms. On the subject of symptoms, Miller et al (1989) suggest that the relief of extra-pyramidal side effects, encountered as a result of taking prescribed anti-psychotics, is a strong motivation to experiment with illicit drugs.

Therapeutic strategies

On 1 March 1999, the London Evening Standard printed an article with the headline, 'Drug Dealing Rife in Mental Wards' (Revill, 1999). The story reported the death, after a suspected overdose of heroin, of a young female patient who was an in-patient, receiving treatment for depression in one of London's mental hospitals. On one level, there are frequent reports of conflict between staff, patients and substance use. Then, at the other end of the scale, there are serious concerns regarding the physical safety of mental health staff and patients due not only to the effects of intoxication but this in combination with psychiatric symptoms and the frequently reported violence associated with certain areas of the drug scene invading the mental health setting. This is compounded further by the reported risks regarding the influx of clients who use substances to psychiatric wards and the resulting management, treatment and integration problems. Barker (1998) reports that there is a shortage of partnerships between acute psychiatric admission wards and community drug services for the purposes of treatment and discharge planning. There may be even less access to specialist substance misuse services for people who have a mental illness and are in the care of mental health services. After ten years of working in the field of substance use, it is certainly the author's experience that treatment in one setting by one part of a mental health service can hinder rather than help the prospect of the client gaining access to other service options. This may be due to several factors including the pressure to attend to one's own patients and not accept even joint responsibility for patients seen to be under the care of another service.

Illicit drug use often raises legal, moral and attitudinal problems for society as a whole and this is reflected in the reactions from staff and clients alike. For many years, the social environment of psychiatric wards has been a concern. This led Maxwell Jones (1952, 1968) to identify the need not only to recognize the power of psychiatric units as social milieu and the need to manage that as well as the care of patients individually, but just as importantly, the considered use of that milieu in a positive, therapeutic way. Cohen et al (1999) report that in many mental health wards and departments the staff regularly need not only access for their clients but also specialist advice and consultation from substance use services, whether statutory or voluntary. At the very least, argue Cohen et al (1999) the situation appears to require an extended consultative role for substance use services. Unfortunately, following the publication of the Government's strategy on drugs, *Tackling Drugs to Build a Better Britain* (The UK Anti-Drugs Coordination Unit, 1998), it became clear to substance use service providers that extending their role was not what the government had in mind. In the aforementioned white paper, the government set a target for all statutory substance use services to double their treatment caseloads by the year 2008. The government clearly believes that what is important is getting more substance users into the existing treatment systems rather than extending the scope and setting for treatment.

Maslin et al (2001) completed a study to assess the training and support needs of staff working within mental health and substance use services, working with dual diagnosis clients in central Birmingham. The study involved 136 staff, working in community-based services, who completed a questionnaire. The central question posed by this study was, 'Are front-line clinicians appropriately equipped to work with clients who have combined severe mental health and substance use problems in terms of knowledge, skills and confidence?' Maslin et al (2001) found that mental health staff had been working significantly longer in mental health services than substance misuse staff had been working in substance misuse services. Results showed that the majority of staff had experience of working with this client group and saw the work as a significant part of their role. Their study found that there was a need to integrate care through improving links between services and providing information and training for staff. Some mental health staff identified a need for a greater understanding of basic issues such as 'what drugs actually look like' and 'what presenting symptoms relate to different drug types'. The study by Maslin et al (2001) was based on self-report data. It has been suggested that outcomes will be substantially improved if these training needs are addressed (Derricott & McKeown, 1997; Drake and Osher, 1997). O'Neill (1993) reports that feelings of anger, frustration, incompetence and powerlessness are common among mental health professionals who encounter and/or work with people with dual diagnosis.

A number of writers have presented increasing evidence for the effectiveness of treatment for substance use (Gossop et al, 1998; Johns, 1994). These studies can show that outcomes improve in approximately 30 per cent of clients treated. Crome (1999) suggests this is important for several reasons:

- Treatment of substance problems often ameliorates psychiatric problems.
- Psychopathology is associated with poorer prognosis and treatment of psychopathology improves prognosis.
- Increasing severity of dependence is related to increasing psychological and psychiatric problems and that treatment of these additional psychiatric problems, improves prognosis.
- Psychopathology is also associated with higher HIV prevalence and risk-taking behaviour.

Emerging themes for dual diagnosis treatment

- People can get better without the help of treatment services.
- Individuals with substance problems demonstrate the capacity for change despite severe problems.
- The particular components of treatment that yield beneficial results are not presently identifiable.
- Engaging patients in a long-term relationship is important in improving outcome.
- The health care costs of untreated cases is more than treated.
- Minimal interventions e.g., GP advice, may produce significant health gain.
- Intensive treatment for severe problems should be an option as it can be associated with improvement.
- Combined treatments, e.g., psychological and pharmacological, may prove to be very effective. (Crome, 1999)

In the drugs field, the overriding theme of treatment has been one of harm reduction and substitute prescribing (DoH, 1996). The results of these linked strategies have been to attract people into drug treatment services and to hinder, for the time being at least, the progress of HIV infection. However, keeping people in treatment has been more problematic, despite obvious improvements in their functioning, due to widespread short-term prescribing policies. It must also be said that while the threat of HIV is still present, HIV is now becoming much more of an issue to harm-minimization strategists.

Pharmacological Interventions

- *Detoxification*: In-patient or community based; mainly for alcohol and/or opioids. Seen by many clinicians and service users as the main purpose of treatment. By no means always appropriate and often unsuccessful. Clients may be offered detoxification even several times a year over the course of their sometimes long-term problem. The treatment may last from a week for 'alcohol clients' to over a year for heroin/opioid users. The process is one of starting the client on an agreed dose that treats the withdrawal syndrome, so that they are physically well enough to function without their drug of choice. The next step is 'weaning' the client off the prescribed drug over an agreed period of time. As one can imagine, reaching agreement on dose and rate of dose-reduction is often the stumbling block.
- *Maintenance or substitution*: Mainly for opioid users, sometimes benzodiazepine and amphetamine users may be offered substitution, depending on circumstances (and in the past, depending on local use patterns). With the purpose of minimizing the harm caused by prolonged drug use, this treatment is often seen by clinicians and service users as the 'soft option' as there is usually little pressure on the client to 'come off' the prescribed drug. Service users and providers make a clear treatment decision that their aim is for the client to become 'illicit drug free' as opposed to drug-free. Usually offered to older and longer-term service users; the treatment may last many years.
- *Anti-craving medication*: For clients with alcohol problems who have problems with craving for alcohol once detoxified, a drug called Acamprosate can be prescribed. The medication can be backed up by teaching and supportive material, which some clients appreciate.
- *Relapse prevention medication*: Naltrexone has been used for years in the treatment of opioid overdose (often referred to by service users as the heroin antidote). It blocks the receptor sites in the brain thus preventing the effects of heroin/opioids. Taken on a daily basis, the client is unlikely to use heroin/opioids because they will feel no effects from their drug of choice. However, if a client continues to use heroin/opioids, the Naltrexone will induce severe withdrawal symptoms. Disulfiram (Antabuse) has also been used for many years to treat abstinent clients with alcohol problems who feel unsafe about maintaining their abstinence. Disulfiram

interferes with the breakdown and absorption of alcohol in the body and taken daily, can be a powerful disincentive to drink alcohol. The effects from drinking alcohol after taking Disulfiram are extremely unpleasant and have proved fatal.

● *Treatment of co-existent mental health problems and/or medical problems.* Often, in cases of dual diagnosis, there is inadequate communication between prescribers resulting in medication regimes for mental health problems that may be at odds with regimes for substance use (and vice versa). Close liaison and effective communication between all service providers must be achieved to fully understand the clients and their problems. A good background understanding of the commonly used substances and their effects/side effects is vital in understanding the nature of problems encountered and likely treatment options.

Accurate assessment

One of the main problems faced by both mental health and substance misuse staff alike is the need for an accurate assessment of a client's substance use pattern to determine the extent of their use, the problems caused and the potential for withdrawal syndromes. The ICD 10 (WHO, 1987) lists the range of psychoactive substances as alcohol, opioids, cannabinoids, sedatives/hypnotics, cocaine, stimulants including caffeine, hallucinogens, tobacco, volatile solvents, poly drug use and other substances. Crome (1999) states that, in general, chronic use and intoxication with depressant drugs and withdrawal from stimulants may produce symptoms akin to a depressive disorder. Chronic use of stimulants may mimic psychotic illness, e.g., amphetamine psychosis. On the other hand, withdrawal from depressant drugs may result in symptoms of anxiety/panic/phobic disorders. The clinician has the choice from a variety of instruments for the assessment of substance related problems, including dependence. For clients with alcohol problems there is the Severity of Alcohol Dependence Questionnaire or SADQ (Stockwell et al, 1979). For clients with drug problems there is the Severity of Opiate Dependence Questionnaire or SODQ (Burgess et al, 1989). However, many clients who use drugs do not stick to their main drug of choice and will use other drugs regularly or opportunistically. These first two assessment tools deal specifically with physical dependence but there are associated problems for client who use drugs with no recognized physical withdrawal syndrome, eg: cocaine and cannabis. An absence of physical dependence does not preclude a client from serious drug-related problems.

There are other assessment tools that cover both dependence and other drug related problems. The Drug Abuse Screening Test or DAST (Skinner, 1982), for example, includes both dependence and related problems. Each of these assessment tools take a fair amount of time on the part of client and clinician to complete and this in itself can cause problems. For the sake of promoting client engagement with your service, the clinician should be prepared to allow for several sessions in which to complete a full assessment of a client who may have more to occupy their mind (e.g., their chaotic lifestyle), rather than helping the clinician to complete their task. The importance of a fair and accurate assessment cannot be overstated.

Over the past few decades, many instruments have been devised for the assessment of mental health problems. There are instruments for assessing specific mental health problems. For depression, for example, there is the Beck Depression Inventory (BDI) (Beck et al, 1988) and there is the Zung Self-Rating scale (Zung, 1986) as well as the Profile of Mood States (McNair et al, 1992). One assessment tool in particular, the Structured Clinical Interview for DSM (SCID) (Spitzer et al, 1987), for example, actually questions clients as to whether they believe their mental health symptoms could be as a result of substance use. According to Crome (1999), most clinicians would agree that a detailed psychiatric history with corroborative information (usually in the form of toxicology) is the cornerstone in the management of dual diagnosis clients.

Once the clinician has assessed the problems faced by a client with dual diagnosis, treatment options need to be negotiated with the client. There is no point in aiming to address problems that the client fails to recognize or of expecting the client to cease from doing something that they perceive to gain benefits from. Ley et al (2001) report that although there is at this point a lack of evidence to support particular treatment interventions, there is agreement that the management of clients' problems must be integrated into mainstream services such as the Assertive Outreach services. Copello et al (2001) believe there are many good reasons for this, which include the need for developing and maintaining engagement with the client and also the sheer prevalence of the problem. They advocate an integrated shared care approach in which the clients' drug and mental health problems are addressed by the same clinician. This clinician could be from the mental health setting but care could also be shared between mental health and substance misuse services. Copello et al (2001) advocate what they call Cognitive Behavioural Integrated Treatment or CBIT.

Families and significant others

In the summer of 2001, the author interviewed 20 parents of heroin users in a localized (but unpublished) research study. The area where the parents live offers probably the cheapest heroin (in the UK) to users as young as 12. More than anywhere else in the UK, a significant number of these young initiates inject from the outset of their heroin using career. The findings of this small piece of research were that the parents felt rejected by substance use services but more important were their feelings towards their children. The majority of those parents stated categorically that they would prefer their sons and daughters to die rather than go through more of the suffering they had experienced as a heroin user.

Conclusion

For many years, drug users were thought of as loners living apart from society and close family involvement. However, this is the exception rather than the norm. Most people who use drugs, even in an addictive cycle, are dependent also on support from their partners and their families. It is the responsibility of service providers to offer more than just advice to the families and partners of people with drink and drug problems as the effects on family life and relationships can be devastating.

Reference

Barker, I. (1998) Mental illness and substance misuse, *The Mental Health Review*, 3, 6–13.

Beck, A. T., Steer, R. A. & Garbin, M. G. (1988) Psychometric properties of the Beck Depression Inventory: twenty five years of evaluation, *Clinical Psychology Review*, 8, 77–100.

Bergman, H. C. & Harris, M. (1985) Substance abuse among young adult chronic patients, *Psychosocial Rehabilitation Journal*, 9, 49–54.

Boyd, R. (1996) *Report of the Confidential Inquiry into Homicides and Suicides by Mentally Ill People*, London: Royal College of Psychiatrists.

Burgess, P. M., Stripp, A., Pead, J. & Holman, P. (1989) The severity of opiate dependence in an Australian sample: further validation of the SODQ, *British Journal of Addiction*, 84, 1451–60.

Cohen, J., Runciman, R. & Williams, R. (1999) Substance use and misuse in psychiatric wards, *Drugs: Education, Prevention and Policy*, 6(2), 181–94.

Copello, A., Graham, H. & Birchwood, M. (2001) Evaluating substance misuse interventions in psychosis: the limitations of the RCT with 'patient' as the unit of analysis, *Journal of Mental Health*, 10(6), 585–7.

Crome, I. B. (1999) Substance misuse and psychiatric comorbidity: towards improved service provision, *Drugs: Education, Prevention and Policy*, 6(2), 151–74.

Department of Health (1996) *The Task Force to Review Services for Drug Misusers: Report of an Independent Review of Drug Treatment Services in England*, London: HMSO.

Department of Health (1997) *Purchasing Effective Treatment and Care for Drug Users*, London: HMSO.

Department of Health (1999) *The National Service Framework for Mental Health Modern Standards and Service Models*, London: HMSO.

Derricott, J. & McKeown, M. (1997) Dual diagnosis: future directions in training, *Psychiatric Care*, 3, 34–7.

Drake, R. E. & Osher, F. C. (1997) Treating substance abuse in patients with severe mental illness, in: S. W. Henggeler & A. B. Santos (eds), *Innovative Approaches for Difficult to Treat Populations*, Washington DC: American Psychiatric Association.

Edwards, G. & Gross, M. M. (1976) Alcohol dependence: a provisional description of a clinical syndrome, *British Medical Journal*, 1, 1058–61.

Edwards, G., Gross, M. M., Keller, M., Moser, J. & Room, R. (1977) *Alcohol-Related Disabilities*, (WHO Offset Publication No. 32), Geneva: WHO.

Farrell, M., Howes, S. & Taylor, C. (1998) Substance misuse and psychiatric comorbidity: an overview of the OPCS National Psychiatric Morbidity Survey, *Addictive Behaviours*, 23(6), 909–18.

Frischer, M. & Akram, G. (2001) Prevalence of comorbid mental illness and drug use recorded in general practice: preliminary findings from the General Practice Research Database, *Drugs: Education, Prevention and Policy*, 8(3), 275–80.

Glass, I. B. & Jackson, P. (1988) Maudsley Hospital survey: prevalence of alcohol problems and other psychiatric disorders in a hospital population, *British Journal of Addiction*, 83, 1105–11.

Goddard, E. (1991) *Drinking in England and Wales in the Late 1980s*, London: HMSO.

Gossop, M., Marsden, J. & Stewart, D. (1998) *National Treatment Outcome Research Study: NTORS at One-Year*, London: Department of Health.

Gournay, K., Sandford, T., Johnson, S. & Thornicroft, G. (1997) Dual diagnosis of severe mental health problems and substance abuse/dependence: a major priority for mental health nursing, *Journal of Psychiatric and Mental Health Nursing*, 4, 89–95.

Healey, A., Knapp, M., Astin, J., Gossop, M., Marsden, J., Stewart, D., Lehmann, P. & Godfrey, C. (1998) Economic burden of drug dependency, *British Journal of Psychiatry*, 173, 160–5.

Hodge, J. E. (1993) Alcohol and violence. in P. J. Taylor (ed.), *Violence in Society*, London: Royal College of Physicians, 127–37.

Johns, A. (1994) Opiate treatments, *Addiction*, 89, 1551–8.

Johns, A. (1997) Substance misuse: a primary risk and a major problem of Comorbidity, *International Review of Psychiatry*, 9, 233–41.

Jones, M. (1952) *Social Psychiatry: A Study of Therapeutic Communities*, London: Tavistock.

Jones, M. (1968) *Beyond the Therapeutic Community: Social Learning and Social Psychiatry*, London: Yale University Press.

Lamb, H. R. (1982) Young adult chronic patients: the new drifters, *Hospital and Community Psychiatry*, 33, 465–8.

Ley, A., Jeffrey, D., McLaren, S. & Siegfried, N. (2001) *Treatment Programmes for People with Both Severe Mental Illness and Substance Misuse*, The Cochrane Library (4). Oxford: Update Software.

Maslin, J., Graham, H. L., Cawley, M., Copello, A., Birchwood, M., Georgiou, G., McGovern, D., Meuser, K. & Orford, J. (2001) Combined severe mental health and substance use problems: what are the training and support needs of staff working with this client group? *Journal of Mental Health*, 10(2), 131–40.

McNair, D. M., Lorr, M. & Dropplemann, L. F. (1992) *EdITS Manual for the Profile of Mood States (POMS)*, San Diego, CA: Educational and Industrial Testing Service (EdITS).

Meltzer, H., Baljit, G., Petticrew, M. & Hinds, K. (1995) *OPCS Surveys of Psychiatric Morbidity in Great Britain. Report 2. Physical Complaints, Service Use and Treatment of Adults with Psychiatric Disorders*, London: HMSO.

Miller, F. T., Busch, F. & Tanenbaum, J. H. (1989) Drug abuse in schizophrenic and bipolar disorders, *American Journal of Drug and Alcohol Abuse*, 15, 291–5.

Mueser, K. T., Nishith, P., Tracy, J. I., DeGirolamo, J. & Molinaro, M. (1995) Expectations and motives for substance use in schizophrenia, *Psychiatric Clinics of North America*, 13(4), 613–32.

NHS Health Advisory Service (1996) *The Substance of Young Needs. Children and Young People: Substance Misuse Service*, London: HMSO.

O'Neill, M. M. (1993) Countertransference and attitudes in the context of clinical work with dually diagnosed patients, in J. Solomon, S. Zimberg & E. Shollar (eds), *Dual Diagnosis: Evaluation, Treatment, Training and Program Development*, New York: Plenum.

Parker, H. & Bottomley, T. (1997) The rock repertoire: crack cocaine, polydrug use and criminal careers, *Probation Journal*, 44, 26–31.

Phillips, P. (2000) Substance misuse, offending and mental illness: a review, *Journal of Psychiatric and Mental Health Nursing*, 7, 483–9.

Rassool, G. H. (2002) *Dual Diagnosis: Substance Misuse and Psychiatric Disorder*, Oxford: Blackwell Science.

Revill, J. (1999) *Evening Standard*, 1 March.

Skinner, H. A. (1982) The Drug Abuse Screening Test (DAST), *Addictive Behaviours*, 7, 363–71.

Spitzer, R. L., Williams, J. B. W. & Gibbon, M. (1987) *Structured Clinical Interview for DSM-III-R*, New York: New York State Psychiatric Institute.

Stockwell, T., Hodgson, R., Edwards, G., Taylor, C. & Rankin, H. (1979) The development of a questionnaire to measure severity of alcohol dependence, *British Journal of Addiction*, 74, 79–87.

The UK Anti-Drugs Co-Ordination Unit (1998) *Tackling Drugs to Build a Better Britain: the Government's 10-year Strategy for Tackling Drug Misuse*, London: The Stationery Office.

Weaver, T., Renton, A., Stimson, G. & Tryer, P. (1999) Severe mental illness and substance misuse, *British Medical Journal*, 318, 137–8.

Williams, B., Durant, M. A. & Drummond, D. C. (1995) A questionnaire to measure drug related problems in opiate users, Personal communication.

World Health Organization (1987) *Tenth Revision of the International Classification of Diseases*, Geneva: World Health Organization.

Zung, W. W. K. (1986) Zung self-rating depression scale and depression status inventory, in N. Sartorius & T. A. Ban (eds), *Assessment of Depression*, Heidelberg: Springer Verlag.

CHAPTER 20

Psychosocial Interventions for People with Serious Mental Illness

MIKE FLEET

Indicative Benchmark Statements

▨ Identification of the needs and main characteristics of mental health users and carers

▨ Contribution to the care and treatment of service users with severe mental illness which is underpinned by the stress/vulnerability model and a biopsychosocial approach

▨ Participation in the provision of evidence-based family intervention programmes for service users with severe mental illness

▨ Utilization of appropriate research and relevant evidence to support decision-making relating to the selection and individualization of mental health nursing interventions

▨ Recognition of the prodromal signs of mental illness

Introduction

There has been acceptance that the experience of those suffering mental illness is 'fundamentally non-understandable' (Jaspers, 1959). This is not quite so – *it is* normal to hallucinate or have 'odd' ideas, sometimes (Haddock & Slade, 1996; Kingdon & Turkington, 1994).

For many years there has been an emphasis in mental health services to maintain service users in the 'community'. However, maintenance is a service-led aim rather than a client-led aim. Service users want to recover their lives and their roles in society (Bentall, 1990; Romme & Escher, 1989; Warner, 1994).

The National Service Framework For Mental Health (DoH, 1999) has demanded the utilization of evidence-informed practices and social inclusion of service users, thus providing a challenge for society in general and mental health nursing in particular. Since the 1950s neuroleptic medication has enjoyed a hegemony in the treatment of this client group but a significant minority of clients continue to experience hallucinations and delusions (Curson et al, 1988).

Psychosocial Interventions (PSI) are a comprehensive range of evidence-informed approaches to the care and treatment of people with serious mental illness (Birchwood & Tarrier, 1996, Gamble & Brennan, 2000). Interventions can be divided into the two broad categories; working with families and individual approaches.

This chapter is aimed at enabling the reader to develop an awareness of the knowledge base(s) necessary to offer service users, and their families, collaborative interventions. This will be through the exploration of each of the categories of psychosocial interventions and the evidence base for their inclusion in treatment strategies with people with serious mental illness. It is intended and hoped that this will enhance the reader's awareness of collaborative working with service users and their families.

The role of engagement

Before undertaking any discussion of psychosocial interventions it is essential to consider the role of engagement with the client or family. The goal of engagement is to form a trusting relationship or working alliance that will enable the worker to support the client through treatment. Voluntary engagement may take place only if the client sees that a relationship with the worker can be of benefit. Sometimes clients do not engage with services. There can be several factors involved in this decision including: poor past history of service contact; personality issues, racism, substance use/misuse and/or lack of trust.

Sometimes services do not engage with clients. Again there are several factors including: substance use/misuse, personality issues; past history; and services not being available. There are a number of avenues that may aid the process of engagement: practical assistance; empathic interviewing; crisis intervention; forming an alliance with the family or other social network members; and ensuring that legal constraints are sensible (Sainsbury Centre for Mental Health, 1998).

Psychoeducation

Underpinning psychosocial interventions is the stress/vulnerability model (Zubin & Spring, 1977) describing the multifactorial nature of serious mental illness. The model explores the predisposing, precipitating and perpetuating (biological, emotional, intellectual and sociological) factors in the development and progress of serious mental illness (Gottesman, 1991). The model emphasizes the fact that 'psychotic' experiences are *not* abnormal (Haddock & Slade, 1996; Kingdon & Turkington, 1994). In general, people develop their own subjective models of illness in order to make sense of ill health, and this model will influence the assimilation of any new information offered to them.

These models help the client and the family to attempt to cope with and control the distressing consequences of the illness. Information given by professionals will be accepted (or possibly rejected) on the basis of the model held. To change the client's model requires us to give detailed help as to how a new way of looking at the illness translates into more effective management strategies. One way of doing this is to consider a stress/vulnerability explanation for symptoms.

Stress is defined as a force that acts upon the system in such a way as to place the system under strain. Stress can be either from life events or ambient. Ambient stress is that owing to generally living in the twenty-first century. How one reacts to this stress is dependent on several factors including mood and emotional state as well as timing. Life event stress results from episodes of case specific and high levels of stress.

Vulnerability is the person's disposition to manifesting symptoms and involves several factors. These factors are either inborn or acquired. Inborn factors include genetic predisposition and potentially physical health. Acquired factors include early experiences, coping strategies, the social context, life events and personality (possibly).

The Stress Vulnerability Model examines the interplay of stress and vulnerability in the manifestation of mental illness symptoms. An example being how people experiencing a high level of stress can manifest psychiatric symptoms, when there is no other obvious predisposing factor. This occurs in such situations with prisoners of war or hostages. Whereas people with lower levels of stress can develop symptoms when there is a higher degree of vulnerability.

Working with families

As Kane & McGlashan (1995, p 825) state: 'The original notion of the family as agent of disorder is no longer tenable.' There have been several studies of the effect of the family on the prognosis of clients experiencing schizophrenia. Seminal work was undertaken in the 1960s (Brown & Rutter, 1966) developing the concept of Expressed Emotion (EE) suggesting that stressful factors in the person's home environment and particularly in the family were associated with higher levels of relapse. Clients living in high EE environments have a significantly higher relapse rate than clients living in low EE environments (Brown et al, 1972; Kavanagh, 1992). The level of contact with high EE relatives is also important. Vaughan and Leff (1976) found that over a 9 month period clients living in a high EE environment and not taking medication had a relapse rate of 92 per cent; compared with 15 per cent for those clients not taking medication but living in low EE environments. Even when fully adherent to medication relapse rates were 53 per cent and 12 per cent respectively. The rate for those clients taking medication and with low contact time with high EE families was 15 per cent. This suggests rather dramatically that medication is helpful but expressed emotion in the client's immediate environment has a significant effect.

In cognitive–behavioural family intervention, schizophrenia is seen as having a genetic predisposing influence that can occur in families functioning perfectly well. The family does not exert a causal influence but can influence the course of the illness. The family is seen as an ally in the treatment package for the client with schizophrenia. The aim of the work is to help families cope better with the sick family member. The worker makes no interpretations for the family but sets out to give information, advice and guidance. The worker encourages the family to be active in discussing the information and to work together with the worker to find solutions to their problems. The worker is active in engaging the family with various agencies, such as the National Schizophrenia Fellowship.

Common elements of cognitive–behavioural family intervention include a positive approach and empathetic working relationship; a 'here and now' focus; a problem-solving approach; psychoeducation and enhancing communication and coping skills. Several systematic reviews have found the efficacy of cognitive–behavioural family intervention, the most recent (Pharoah et al, 2002) found that family intervention may decrease relapse rates and hospitalization. These interventions may also increase adherence to medication and improve social impairment.

Several studies have shown that psychoeducation and psychosocial interventions are effective in delaying relapse in clients (Fadden 1998, Hogarty et al, 1986, 1991, Kottgen et al, 1984; Tarrier et al, 1988, 1989, 1991). Psychoeducation also aids engagement (Birchwood et al, 1992). Family interventions take several forms including cognitive–behavioural family intervention (Barrowclough & Tarrier, 1992) for individual families or even multifamily groups (Atkinson & Coia, 1995; Leff et al, 1989, 1990).

Individual approaches to psychotic phenomena

Assessment

Before employing any interventions it is essential that a thorough assessment of the client's problems and goals are undertaken. The purpose of assessment is to develop a hypothesis upon which it is possible to base care and deliver this care: enabling retesting of the hypothesis. A care plan is only as good as the information it is based on (Richards & McDonald, 1990). Owing to the complex nature of the problems people experience, assessment takes multiple forms looking at symptoms, social functioning and needs assessment. Many assessment formats use 'objective' rating scales, such as the Brief Psychiatric Rating Scale (BPRS) (Overall & Gorham, 1962) or the Manchester Symptom Severity Scale (KGV) (Krawiecka et al, 1977). These can point to the direction of further assessment, such as The Psychotic Symptom Rating Scales (PSYRATS) (Haddock et al, 1999).

Further from these 'objective' scales other formats make use of semi-structured interviews (Fox & Conroy, 2000). One such assessment is functional analysis. Employing listening skills such as summarizing, paraphrasing, expressing empathy, functional analysis looks at the main features of any problem; the *what*, the *when*, the *where*, the *why* and the *with whom* of the problem. The assessment then considers the frequency; the intensity, the duration and the onset of the problem. Following on from this a behavioural analysis is undertaken. The behavioural analysis seeks to examine what happens before the problem occurs, the antecedent (A); what happens when the problem occurs, the behaviour (B); and what are the consequences of the problem (C).

According to Richards and McDonald (1990), for each element of the A B C it is essential to know:

- physical environment the client is in at the time;
- physical sensations the client experiences;
- cognitive processes the client experiences;
- emotions the client experiences at the time;
- social environment the client is experiencing; and
- behaviour the client engages in at the time of the trigger, the problem or the consequences.

From this it is then possible to hypothesize, to develop a 'problem statement' which can be owned by the client. A statement that is in the client's own language, not in jargon, that clearly describes the problem and its impact on their life, as well as the subsequent consequences. The natural follow-on from this would then be a 'desired outcome': a goal statement. What would the client want to do in relation to the problem? Focusing on positive changes rather than simply making the 'problem' stop. The goal should be realistic, attainable and reflect the client's wishes. These then lead on to individualized interventions.

Social skills training

The negative symptoms of schizophrenia and poor social skills are the most difficult to cope with for users and families (Leff & Vaughan, 1985). The lack of social skills decreases the ability to deal with stressors leading to increased social dysfunction and social isolation. Skills training increases the clients' comfort in social settings through improving social skills in the training setting (Halford & Haynes, 1991, 1995). There is strong evidence that skills training improves skills acquisition and moderate evidence for generalization of skills and social adjustment. However, the same evidence shows that skills training is poor at the reduction of symptoms (Smith et al, 1996).

Skills training is an educational, skills building exercise, not psychotherapy; a tennis coach does not get a group of students together to *talk* about hitting the ball or how they *feel* about it. Talking and self-exploration are for other groups and sessions. An important aspect is never to underestimate the cognitive deficits of the client. There may be problems with memory, attention and higher-level problem solving. Sometimes asymptomatic clients can appear to maintain lucid conversations, seem to learn and respond affirmatively to questions about whether they understand or not. While some clients can be easily distracted, don't remember or are so concrete that they are unable to transpose skills from situation A to situation B.

Coping strategy enhancement

Every one has a different perception of the illness they experience and how they attempt to cope with the demands imposed by it. In dealing with the illness and its effects the majority of people make efforts to 'cope'. Coping can be considered to be any action carried out with the intention of producing a positive outcome (Barrowclough & Tarrier, 1992).

The coping strategies that people use look at either problem-focused or emotion-focused coping. Problem-focused (direct) coping attempts to deal directly with the situation to make it more manageable; this involves activities such as information seeking, support seeking, learning new skills and active participation in treatment. Emotion-focused (palliative) coping attempts to either manage the emotions generated by the illness or people may choose to distance themselves from potentially overwhelming emotions.

Some coping strategies have beneficial effects for the individual with little or no harmful consequences. These are known as adaptive coping strategies. Sometimes strategies appear to have beneficial effects in the short term but are actually harmful in the medium to long term, leading to more emotional distress, detriment to physical health, causing people to react badly and/or lower self-esteem.

In general, various researchers (Carr, 1988; Falloon & Talbot, 1981; Tarrier, 1987) have found three groups of strategies, behaviour control, lowering physiological arousal and cognitive coping methods. The aims of coping strategy enhancement are to increase the effectiveness of current coping strategies: to decrease the use of harmful coping strategies and to introduce novel methods of coping. The first phase in coping strategy enhancement is to assess the type and nature of the symptoms: looking at a comprehensive overview of the antecedents and precipitating conditions for each symptom. The second stage is to elicit the client's emotional response to each symptom finally looking at the consequences of the emotional response usually in terms of the client's behaviour. The next stage is to examine current methods of coping (Tarrier et al, 1990, 1993). This enables the worker to help the client to strengthen current positive coping strategies, by selecting only one symptom upon which to work, and working with that symptom until there is a noticeable improvement, the chances of success are improved. By breaking each component of the strategy down they can be taught separately and practised intensively until they become automatic.

Tarrier (1987) gives many examples of techniques for use in coping strategies. Some of these are shown in the following subsections.

Behaviour control

- Distraction involving passive diversion – such as listening to a Walkman (Collins et al, 1989);
- distraction involving active diversion – playing a musical instrument or writing a diary;
- physical change involving body movement – rest, relaxation or sleep; or activity such as walking, running or swimming; and
- indulgence – such as eating, drinking or smoking.

Cognitive control

- Suppression of unwanted thoughts or perceptions;
- redirection of attention towards neutral, comforting or less distracting ideas; and
- problem-solving – focusing on resolving some difficulty or planning a future task.

Medical care

- Using or changing medication.

Distraction

- Listening to music, reading aloud, watching TV;
- counting backwards from 100; and
- describing an object in detail.

Interacting

- Telling the voices to go away;
- talking to the voices while pretending to use a mobile phone; and
- agreeing to listen to the voices at particular times.

Activity

- Walking;
- tidying the house;
- having a relaxing bath;
- playing an instrument, singing; and
- going to the gym.

Social

- Talking to a trusted friend or member of the family;
- phoning a helpline;
- avoiding people;
- going to a drop-in centre; and
- visiting a favourite place.

Physical

- Using earplugs; and
- breathing exercises and relaxation methods.
  (Source: Adapted from Tarrier 1987)

The choice of coping strategy to be taught or strengthened is a collaboration between the worker and the client. It is pointless trying to get a client to play the piano as a coping strategy if they are tone-deaf and have no interest in it!

Cognitive–behavioural approaches to psychotic phenomena

The majority of early studies into the efficacy of cognitive–behavioural approaches to serious mental illness took the form of individual case studies (Haddock et al, 1993) Controlled studies of larger groups have taken place (Garety et al, 1994; Tarrier et al, 1993). One important factor in the effective delivery of cognitive–behavioural interventions is the training, or otherwise, of the providers of the interventions. In many areas a little knowledge is more detrimental than no knowledge at all (Elkin et al, 1989; Kingdon et al, 1996). Positive outcomes from the use of cognitive–behavioural approaches have been well-documented (Garety et al, 1997; Tarrier et al, 1998). The aim of CBT with psychotic symptoms is to help clients gain knowledge about schizophrenia and its symptoms, to overcome helplessness, reduce distress from symptoms, reduce dysfunctional emotions and behaviour and to help them analyse and modify beliefs and assumptions (Haddock & Slade, 1996).

Effective treatment depends on the clients' motivation and the distress associated with the positive symptoms (Sellwood et al, 1994). One approach to helping clients cope with hallucinations or delusions looks at initially destigmatizing and normalizing the symptoms. Under the 'right' circumstances such as increased stress or physical illness for example it is commonplace to hallucinate. Therefore it would be perfectly in order for the worker to share any experiences of odd ideas or 'voices' they have had. Coupling this with education about automatic thoughts may enable the client to view their experience in a less 'dreadful' light. One concept to consider before examining delusions and hallucinations is that of automatic thoughts.

Automatic thoughts occur spontaneously and without effort from the person concerned. They cannot be switched off or consciously controlled. Automatic thoughts are often verbal, they can occur as images or in a vague way – often occurring as fragments or partial thoughts flashing through the brain. Automatic thoughts may be sensible but they can also be unreasonable, impossible or bizarre. If they do not come to conscious awareness they cannot be recognized but they can still evoke a strong emotional response. Automatic thoughts can be about anything we have experienced or learnt or read or been told. It is perfectly normal to have automatic thoughts. The emotions, cognitions and behaviours triggered by these automatic thoughts depend to a great extent on the belief systems that individuals hold. This could lead on to discussion of how and why voices might have occurred. There have been several theories explaining the cause of auditory hallucinations.

One theory is that of misheard inner speech. When we think, we can be aware of using words and talking in our thoughts, inner speech. Whether through the random generation of inner speech (Hoffman, 1986) or through a faulty monitoring of inner speech (Frith, 1992) this speech is unexpected and alien, and the experiencer attributes the speech to external sources. It may be relatively easy for the brain to misattribute these inner words as coming from some external source. Once the words have been misattributed it would be then natural to 'hear' them as a real sound.

A second theory is that of hallucinations being vivid automatic thoughts. The thoughts are so vivid and strong as to appear to come from the outside world. It is important to convey that experience is not the same as 'fact'. For example it is very easy to misinterpret everyday events, such as hearing your neighbour beating up his wife, when in fact it was the television you heard next door. Sometimes it is appropriate to discuss beliefs held in the past but no longer held, such as Father Christmas or the tooth fairy, beliefs that were held with great conviction but are no longer.

At their very core, delusions are beliefs. We develop beliefs to help us make sense of our experiences and perceptions. We all have a unique set of beliefs that represent our particular way of generalizing about the world and our part in it. Beliefs enable us to attempt to understand what is going on and how to respond appropriately. In a normal healthy state we have a self-serving bias in that we tend to believe things that go in our favour and ignore or reject things that go against us. Many people are also prone to thinking errors, these are errors in the way we think about and, therefore, perceive events:

Errors in thinking

- *Arbitrary inference* – conclusion drawn without weighing up the evidence or considering alternatives.
- *Selective abstraction* – pay attention to the wrong cues.
- *Overgeneralization* – an example is a friend lets us down therefore 'he hates me'.
- *Magnification* – making a mountain out of a molehill.
- *Dichotomous thinking* – things are either black or white, good or evil.
- *Catastrophization* – if things go at all wrong, a disaster will follow.
  (*Source*: Adapted from Beck et al, 1979)

One theory in delusional beliefs is that deluded clients exhibit greater biases in their reasoning processes (Bentall et al, 1994).

Our beliefs develop from our experience of the world; internally generated experiences (thoughts, feelings, imagination) as well as direct experiences of the world. We also develop beliefs from other people's experience of the world and the culture. Beliefs are powerful self-reinforcers as we interpret situations according to our beliefs and these interpretations then serve to reinforce our existing beliefs. This is a distorted interpretation. If a belief is strongly held then even contradictory evidence can be used to reinforce the belief.

Another important aspect is that of selective attention. Evidence that supports a belief is noticed whereas evidence that contradicts a belief is trivialized or ignored. In order to look at delusional beliefs and hallucinations, it is necessary to help the client to look at, and perhaps challenge the non-psychotic beliefs that influence the delusions or hallucinations. These non-psychotic beliefs may be beliefs relating to self-esteem or body image, or even basic general knowledge issues. It is then necessary to modify the delusions, or delusional beliefs about voices. This can be begun by assisting the client to make general anxieties or beliefs specific, this allows for more targeted intervention such as logical reasoning and finding evidence for and against the beliefs, offering alternative explanations and employing reality testing or experimentation.

The purpose of CBT with delusions is to strengthen the rational/reasoning part of the person to argue against and influence the intuitional part. It encourages the split between 'feeling' and 'knowing'. Encouraging the patient to act on knowledge rather than the 'feeling'. Being able to argue rationally against a delusional belief will diminish the impact that the delusional thoughts would have on emotions and behaviour (Nelson, 1997). With specific reference to auditory hallucinations, interventions can look at disempowering the voices: gathering evidence to disprove what the voices say: showing that voices cannot inflict physical harm and that the voices are liars or are ignorant. This enables the client and the worker to directly question and challenge the voices, emphasizing that the voices cannot compel action.

Facilitating early intervention in relapse

Each relapse in illness increases the risk of residual symptoms (Shepherd et al, 1989) and social disability (Hogarty et al, 1991). Despite the best combination of medication and psychological interventions the risk of relapse cannot be eliminated (Linszen et al, 1998). Before relapsing many clients perceive a reduced well-being. The majority of clients then initiate some change in behaviour to enable them to cope with the early signs (McCandless-Glincher et al, 1986). The perceived lack of control over the relapse of psychotic symptoms can lead to depression (Birchwood et al, 1993). Many studies have found consistently that subtle changes in behaviour, thought and affect occur before the emergence of frank psychosis (Birchwood et al, 1989; Herz & Melville, 1980).

There are four general categories of early signs of relapse. First, *anxiety* or *agitation* such as irritability, sleep problems, tensions, fear, anxiety. Second, *depression* or *withdrawal*, the client can become quiet, withdrawn, depressed or low with poor appetite. The third category is *disinhibition* resulting generally in aggression, restlessness or stubbornness. Finally, *incipient psychosis* in which the client behaves as if hallucinated, feels they are being laughed at or talked about or exhibiting odd behaviour. In fact the early warning signs of relapse generally occur in the predictable order of non-psychotic phenomena, such as depressed mood, sleep and appetite disturbances and withdrawal. These dysphoric symptoms are then followed by increasing emotional disturbance which are ultimately followed by the development of frank psychotic phenomena (Docherty et al, 1978).

While clients express a strong interest in learning about the early warning signs of the illness and relapse (Mueser et al, 1992), there are problems in helping clients to develop an understanding of their individualized relapse signatures. These problems can be owing to either client or service factors. The identification of early signs by a clinician requires monitoring every two weeks, so there could be a heavy service commitment. Clients may hide symptoms as relapse approaches, while persisting symptoms may mask early signs of impending relapse. Regular monitoring of mental health, although a traditional task of the mental health professional, has increased value when considering relapse management. It is important to develop a baseline against which changes can be discerned and measured, allowing the reinforcement of discrimination of the changed perceptual, cognitive and affective processes through use of appropriate labels. The whole process allows the worker to educate individuals, carers and other professionals about the precise nature of a relapse signature. This helps to promote the clients' engagement with services, sharing responsibility for warning sign detection between individuals, carers and professionals.

Assuming that early warning signs are detected there are three main categories of intervention. Collaborative early intervention; cognitive approaches and targeted medication:

- *Collaborative early intervention* looks at engagement and education, education needs to be continuous as it is easy to lose a skill if it is not used or practised. This is a feature of a trusting relationship and places some responsibility on clients and relatives.
- *Cognitive approaches* look at identifying the attributions the client makes with respect to the symptoms whether it is external attribution or social attribution and also considering how the client is catastrophizing the situation. They may believe that as they relapsed last time after experiencing these signs they will do so again. It is then time to reframe the client's situation, reattribution that emphasizes control, such as verbally challenging the 'voices' or the 'odd' ideas; offering hypothetical contradiction while searching for alternatives, and helping with stress management and the rehearsal of coping skills.
- *Targeted medication* can be helpful. Several studies (Carpenter et al, 1990; Gaebel et al, 1993; Jolley et al, 1989, 1990) have shown the efficacy of targeted medication in relapse management, after one year the relapse rate in people regularly taking medication but increasing or changing when signs appear could be a quarter that in a targeted medication only group (Jolley et al, 1990). After two years the relapse rate is half that for the targeted medication only group (Carpenter et al, 1990; Jolley et al, 1990). Therefore, while targeted medication could be of value, continuous maintenance medication may be more valuable to the client.

Enhancing adherence to medication regimes

As we have seen above maintenance medication may be more beneficial to the client than targeted medication. However, people with long-term illnesses frequently do not adhere fully to their treatment regime. There are as many reasons for non-adherence, including negative effects of medication, lack of trust in the therapeutic relationship, interference with life-style, family issues, seeing no need to take prescribed medication.

Although it has been subject to criticism (Perkins & Repper, 1998), compliance therapy (Kemp et al, 1997) has been found to have positive effects on client outcomes. Compliance therapy is a cognitive psychoeducational approach to enhancing the client's motivation to adhere to a prescribed regime. The basis of compliance therapy is a modification of motivational interviewing (Miller & Rollnick, 1991) emphasizing personal choice and responsibility in a non-blaming atmosphere.

Conclusion

The challenges faced by people with serious and enduring mental illness are similar to those faced by anyone else in the twenty-first century, many and varied. Thankfully the interventions that can now be offered for these problems are many and varied. The supremacy of neuroleptic medication continues to hold but the limitations of cure-based approaches are becoming more apparent. Limitations such as experiencing cure-based strategies but disabilities remain; continuing attempts to effect a cure causing demoralization for clients and workers often leading to hopelessness. The focus on a 'cure' as the only way that life can be meaningful, implys that life with a disability is not worthwhile, while devaluing support and care.

As we have seen in this chapter there are many interventions beyond medication that can help people to live their lives to their optimum capacity, not simply maintaining the status quo.

Psychosocial interventions are not merely a comprehensive collection of interventions for people with serious mental illness, they are a different way of working with people. A collaboration based on mutual respect, dignity and an attempt at understanding something that many people would prefer to believe was 'fundamentally non-understandable'.

References

Atkinson, J. M. & Coia, D. A. (1995) *Families Coping with Schizophrenia: a Practitioner's Guide to Family Groups*, London: Wiley.

Barrowclough, C. & Tarrier, N. (1992) *Families of Schizophrenic Patients: Cognitive Behavioural Intervention*, London: Chapman & Hall.

Beck, A. T., Rush, A. J., Shaw, B. F. & Emery, G. (1979) *Cognitive Therapy of Depression*, New York: Guilford.

Bentall, R. P. (ed.) (1990) *Reconstructing Schizophrenia*, Routledge: London.

Bentall, R. P., Kinderman, P. & Kaney, S. (1994) The self, attributional processes and abnormal beliefs: towards a model of persecutory delusions, *Behaviour Research and Therapy*, 32, 331–41.

Birchwood, N. & Tarrier, N. (eds) (1996) *Innovations in the Psychological Management of Schizophrenia: Assessment, Treatment and Services*, Chichester: John Wiley.

Birchwood, M., Smith, J. & MacMillan, F. (1989) Predicting relapse in schizophrenia: the development and implementation of an early signs monitoring system using patients and families as observers, *Psychological Medicine*, 19, 649–56.

Birchwood, M., Smith, J. & Cochrane, R. (1992) Specific and non-specific effects of educational intervention for families living with schizophrenia: a comparison of three methods, *British Journal of Psychiatry*, 160, 806–14.

Birchwood, M., Mason, R., MacMillan, J. F. & Healy, J. (1993) Depression, demoralisation and control over illness; a comparison of depressed and non-depressed patients with a chronic psychosis, *Psychological Medicine*, 23, 387–95.

Brown, G. W. & Rutter, M. (1966) The measurement of family activities and relationships: a methodological study, *Human Relations*, 19, 241–63.

Brown, G. W., Birley, J. L. T. & Wing, J. K. (1972) Influence of family life on the course of schizophrenic disorder, *British Journal of Psychiatry*, 121, 241–58.

Carpenter, W. T., Hanlon, T. E., Summerfelt, A. T., Kirkpatrick, B. M., Levine, J. & Buchanan, R. W. (1990) Continuous versus targeted medication in schizophrenic outpatients, *American Journal of Psychiatry*, 147, 1138–48.

Carr, V. (1988) Patients' techniques for coping with schizophrenia: an exploratory study, *British Journal of Medical Psychology*, 61, 339–52.

Collins, M. N., Cull, C. A. & Sireling, L. (1989) Pilot study of persistent auditory hallucinations by modified auditory input, *British Medical Journal*, 299, 431–2.

Curson, D. A., Patel, M. & Liddle, P. F. (1988) Psychiatric morbidity of a long-stay hospital population with chronic schizophrenia and implications for future community care, *British Medical Journal*, 297, 819–22.

Department of Health (1999) *National Service Framework for Mental Health: Modern Standards and Service Models*, London: HMSO.

Docherty, J. P., van Kammen, D. P. & Siris, S. G. (1978) Stages of onset of schizophrenic psychosis, *American Journal of Psychiatry*, 135, 420–6.

Elkin, I., Shea, M. & Watkins, J. (1989) National Institute of Mental Health treatment of depression collaborative treatment programme, *Archives of General Psychiatry*, 46, 971–82.

Fadden, G. (1998) Family intervention, in C. Brooker & J. Repper (eds), *Serious Mental Health Problems in the Community: Policy, Practice and Research*, London: Bailliere Tindall, 159–83.

Falloon, I. R. H. & Talbot, R. E. (1981) Persistent auditory hallucinations: coping mechanisms and implications for management, *Psychological Medicine*, 1, 329–39.

Fox, J. & Conroy, P. (2000) Assessing clients' needs: the semi-structured interview, in C. Gamble & G. Brennan (eds), *Working With Serious Mental Illness: A Manual for Clinical Practice*, London: Bailliere Tindall, 85–96.

Frith, C. D. (1992) *The Cognitive Neuropsychology of Schizophrenia*, Hove: Erlbaum.

Gaebel, V., Frick, W. & Kopcke, M. (1993) Early neuroleptic intervention in schizophrenia, *British Journal of Psychiatry*, 163, 8–12.

Gamble, C. & Brennan, G. (eds) (2000) *Working with Serious Mental Illness: A Manual for Clinical Practice*, London: Balliere Tindall/RCN.

Garety, P. A., Kuipers, L., Fowler, D., Chamber, I. F. & Dunn, G. (1994) Cognitive–behaviour therapy for drug-resistant psychosis, *British Journal of Medical Psychology*, 67, 259–71.

Garety, P. A., Fowler, D., Kuipers, E., Freeman, D., Dunn, G., Bebbington, P., Hadley, C. & Jones, S. (1997) London-East Anglia randomised controlled trial of cognitive–behavioural therapy for psychosis: II predictors of outcome, *British Journal of Psychiatry*, 171, 319–27.

Gottesman, I. (1991) *Schizophrenia Genesis; the Origin of Madness*, Oxford: Freeman.

Haddock, G. & Slade, P. D. (1996) *Cognitive-Behavioural Interventions with Psychotic Disorders*, London: Routledge.

Haddock, G., Bentall, R. P. & Slade, P. D. (1993) Psychological treatment for auditory hallucinations: two case studies, *Behavioural and Cognitive Psychotherapy*, 21, 335–46.

Haddock, G., McCarron, J., Tarrier, N. & Faragher, E. B. (1999) Scales to measure dimensions of hallucinations and delusions: the Psychotic Symptoms Rating Scales (PSYRATS), *Psychological Medicine*, 29, 879–89.

Halford, W. & Hayes, R. (1991) Psychological rehabilitation of chronic schizophrenic patients: recent findings on social skills training and family psychoeducation, *Clinical Psychology Review*, 23, 23–44.

Halford, W. & Hayes, R. (1995) Social skills in schizophrenia: assessing the relationship between social skills, psychopathology and community functioning, *Social Psychiatry and Psychiatric Epidemiology*, 30, 14–19.

Hertz, M. & Melville, C. (1980) Relapse in schizophrenia, *American Journal of Psychiatry*, 137, 801–12.

Hoffman, R. E. (1986) Verbal hallucinations and language production processes in schizophrenia, *The Behavioural and Brain Sciences*, 9, 503–48.

Hogarty, G. E., Anderson, C. M., Reiss, D. J., Kornblith, S. J., Greenwald, D. P., Javan, C. D. & Madonia, M. (1986) Family psychoeducational, social skills training and maintenance chemotherapy in the aftercare of schizophrenia: I: one year effects of a controlled study on relapse and expressed emotion, *Archives of General Psychiatry*, 43, 633–42.

Hogarty, G. E., Anderson, C. M., Reiss, D. J., Kornblith, S. J., Greenwald, D. P., Ulrich, R. F. & Carter, M. (1991) Family psychoeducational, social skills training and maintenance chemotherapy in the aftercare of schizophrenia: II: two year effects of a controlled study on relapse and adjustment, *Archives of General Psychiatry*, 48, 340–7.

Jaspers, K. (1959) *General Psychopathology*, Manchester: Manchester University Press.

Jolley, A. G., Hirsch, S. T., McRink, A. & Machanda, R. (1989) Trial of brief intermittent neuroleptic prophylaxis for selected schizophrenia outpatients: clinical outcome at one year, *British Medical Journal*, 298, 985–90.

Jolley, A. G., Hirsch, S. T., McRink, A. & Wilson, L. (1990) Trial of brief intermittent neuroleptic prophylaxis for selected schizophrenia outpatients: clinical and social outcome at two years, *British Medical Journal*, 301, 837–42.

Kane, J. M. & McGlashan, T. H. (1995) Treatment of schizophrenia, *Lancet*, 346, 820–5.

Kavanagh, D. (1992) Recent developments in expressed emotion and schizophrenia, *British Journal of Psychiatry*, 160, 601–20.

Kemp, R., Hayward, P. & David, A. (1997) *Compliance Therapy Manual*, London: Maudsley Hospital.

Kingdon, D. G. & Turkington, D. (1994) *Cognitive Behavioural Therapy of Schizophrenia*, New York: Guilford Press.

Kingdon, D. G., Tyrer, P. & Murphy, S. (1996) The Nottingham Study of neurotic disorder: influence of cognitive therapists on outcome, *British Journal of Psychiatry*, 169, 93–7.

Kottgen, C., Sonnichsen, I., Mollenhauer, K. & Jurth, R. (1984) Group therapy with families of schizophrenic patients: results of the Hamburg Camberwell Family Interview study III, *International Journal of Family Psychiatry*, 5, 83–94.

Krawiecka, M., Goldberg, D. & Vaughan, M. (1977) A standardised psychiatric assessment scale for rating chronic psychotic patients, *Acta Psychiatrica Scandinavia*, 55, 299–308.

Leff, J. & Vaughan, C. (1985) *Expressed Emotion in Families: its Significance for Mental Illness*, New York: Guilford.

Leff, J., Berkowitz, R., Shavit, N., Strachan, A., Glass, I. & Vaughan, C. (1989) A trial of family therapy versus a relatives' group for schizophrenia, *British Journal of Psychiatry*, 154, 58–66.

Leff, J., Berkowitz, R., Shavit, N., Strachan, A., Glass, I. & Vaughan, C. (1990) A trial of family therapy versus a relatives' group for schizophrenia: two year follow-up, *British Journal of Psychiatry*, 157, 571–7.

Linszen, D., Lenior, M., de Haan, L., Dingmans, P. & Gersons, B. (1998) Early intervention, untreated psychosis and the course of early schizophrenia, *British Journal of Psychiatry*, 172(suppl33), 84–9.

McCandless-Glincher, L., McKnight, S., Hamera, E., Smith, B. L., Peterson, K. & Plumlee, A. A. (1986) Use of symptoms by schizophrenics to monitor and regulate their illness, *Hospital and Community Psychiatry*, 37, 929–33.

Miller, W. & Rollnick, S. (1991) *Motivational Interviewing: Preparing People to Change Addictive Behaviour*, New York: Guilford Press.

Mueser, K. T., Bellack, A. & Blanchard, J. (1992) Comorbidity of schizophrenia and substance abuse: implications for treatment, *Journal of Consulting and Clinical Psychology*, 60, 845–55.

Nelson, H. (1997) *Cognitive Behavioural Therapy with Schizophrenia*, Cheltenham: Stanley Thornes.

Overall, J. E. & Gorham, D. R. (1962) The Brief Psychiatric Rating Scale, *Psychological Reports*, 10, 799–812.

Perkins, R. & Repper, J. (1998) Softly, Softly, *Mental Health Care*, 2(2), 70.

Pharoah, F. M., Mari, J. J. & Streiner, D. (2002) Family intervention, *Cochrane Database Systematic Review (4)*.

Richards, D. & McDonald, B. (1990) *Behavioural Psychotherapy: A Pocket Book for Nurses*, Oxford: Heinemann.

Romme, M. A. J. & Escher, A. D. M. A. C. (1989) Hearing voices, *Schizophrenia Bulletin*, 15, 209–16.

Sainsbury Centre for Mental Health (1998) *Keys to Engagement*, London: Sainsbury Centre for Mental Health.

Sellwood, W., Haddock, G., Tarrier, N. & Yusupoff, L. (1994) Advances in the psychological management of positive symptoms of schizophrenia, *International Review of Psychiatry*, 6, 201–15.

Shepherd, M., Watt, D., Falloon, I. & Smeeton, N. (1989) The natural history of schizophrenia: a five-year follow-up in a representative sample of schizophrenics, *Psychological Medicine*, Monograph Supplement 15.

Smith, T. E., Bellack, A. S. & Liberman, R. P. (1996) Social skills training for schizophrenia: review and future directions, *Clinical Psychology Review*, 16(7), 599–617.

Tarrier, N. (1987) An investigation of residual psychotic symptoms in discharged schizophrenic patients, *British Journal of Clinical Psychology*, 26, 141–3.

Tarrier, N., Barrowclough, C. & Vaughan, K. (1988) The community management of schizophrenia: a controlled trial of behavioural intervention with families to reduce relapse, *British Journal of Psychiatry*, 153, 532–42.

Tarrier, N., Barrowclough, C. & Vaughan, K. (1989) Community management of schizophrenia: a two year follow-up of a behavioural intervention with families, *British Journal of Psychiatry*, 154, 625–8.

Tarrier, N., Harwood, S., Yusopoff, L., Beckett, R. & Baker, A. (1990) Coping Strategy Enhancement (CSE): a method of treating residual schizophrenic symptoms, *Behavioural Psychotherapy*, 18, 283–93.

Tarrier, N., Lowson, K. & Barrowclough, C. (1991) Some aspects of family interventions in schizophrenia. II: financial considerations, *British Journal of Psychiatry*, 159, 481–4.

Tarrier, N., Beckett, R., Harwood, S., Baker, A. & Yusopoff, L. (1993) A trial of two cognitive-behavioural methods of treating drug-resistant residual psychotic symptoms in schizophrenic patients I: outcome, *British Journal of Psychiatry*, 162, 524–32.

Tarrier, N., Yusupoff, L., Kinney, C., McCarthey, E., Gledhill, A., Haddock, G. & Morris, J. (1998) Randomised controlled trial of intensive cognitive behaviour therapy for patients with chronic schizophrenia, *British Medical Journal*, 317, 303–7.

Vaughan, C. & Leff, J. P. (1976) The influence of family and social factors on the course of psychiatric illness, *British Journal of Psychiatry*, 129, 125–37.

Warner, R. (1994) *Recovery from Schizophrenia: Psychiatry and Political Economy*, (2nd edn), London: Routledge.

Zubin, J. & Spring, B. (1977) Vulnerability: a new view of schizophrenia, *Journal of Abnormal Psychology*, 89, 260–6.

CHAPTER 21

Mental Health Nursing within Secure Conditions

STEPHAN D. KIRBY AND DENIS A. HART

Indicative Benchmark Statements

- Consider the power differential between users of services, carers and mental health and social care workers

- Ability to undertake comprehensive, needs-led mental health nursing assessment

- Identification of the needs, characteristics and key principles of care for a range of subgroups of people with severe mental illness across the age and setting continua

- Identification of the need for lifelong learning within the modernized functions and organizations of the mental health and social care sector

- Critical awareness of own competence and needs for future mental health nursing professional development

Introduction

This chapter seeks to explain the:

- current part played by mental health nurses in secure or forensic settings;
- ethical dilemmas mental health nurses face when balancing care, control and custody; and
- implications for training and professional development.

For many years forensic mental health nursing has been shrouded by a veil of secrecy, ignorance and misinformation and mental health nurses regarded as providing the smiling and caring face of patient containment. However, recently forensic nursing has come to be recognized as: 'a specialist branch of psychiatric nursing' and forensic nurses have began to see themselves first and foremost as mental health nurses because of the way they seek to practice as well as because they are wholly and solely registered as such. Forensic nurses have thus begun to adopt a holistic and health focused approach to practice rather than a pathogenic or single systems approach to care (Tarbuck et al, 1999).

Nurses have been employed in prisons for generations but regarded as 'ancillary' to those with real expertise in dealing with aggressive and difficult prisoners, the prison officers, rather than as having a well-defined role of their own giving them a remit to practice and treat.

Slowly, as a result of conscious raising by authors such as Goffman (1961), there has begun to develop a new consensus, or common understanding, as to the *specific* role of forensic mental health nurses irrespective of whether they practice in:

- High, medium or low levels of security;
- Prison or health care setting; or
- Patient- or community-based setting (supervision of discharged patients or prisoners.

The forensic nursing role and the law

To understand the forensic mental health nursing role and the duties placed on those who take up the role, we need to begin by discussing the legal context of practice. The law maintains that we may be culpable if we make: errors of commission; or errors of omission. An error of commission means, essentially, knowingly doing something we should not have done. Most ordinary people who run into trouble with the law fit this category whether for example, through trespass, dropping litter, fraud, theft or violent conduct. Errors of omission have particular implications for professionals and usually arise out of the Common Law 'general duty of care'. They essentially entail a person failing to do something that they should have done which usually results in actual harm to someone else.

The General Duty of Care as applied to secure facilities

The General Duty of Care forms the basis of liability from which both civil claims and sometimes criminal charges can be brought. The first step taken to establish whether negligence has occurred is to identify who had the duty of care for the individual at the time of the injury or incident. Normally this would be the staff on duty if the injury occurred in a hospital, care home or nursing home.

The second step is to establish whether the 'standard of care' was adequate and appropriate. The person bringing an action for negligence must be able to show: 'that the professional failed to reach the standard of practice required by the law, essentially to act in a manner acceptable to their professional peers' (Montgomery, 1997, p 166). This principle is known as the *Bolam Test*. Essentially a claim of negligence will not be upheld if peers testify that the actions of the accused were 'proper'.

The third step to be taken is to establish that harm or injury has actually occurred. The rationale for this is that civil law compensates victims for injuries and hence it would be illogical to award damages to a person who may have been neglected but has sustained no harm or injury as a consequence. Case study 21.1 is provided to help you to think through the issues just presented.

Case study 21.1

A visitor to your (secure) ward is given a personal (safety) alarm (as per the Unit policy) upon arrival. After 10 minutes of discussion in a quiet room the patient he is visiting tells him that if he really believed he was becoming stable and responsible then he'd give him the alarm as a sign of trust. The visitor does so. Ten minutes later the patient becomes agitated and seriously assaults the visitor leaving him unconscious. The patient rejoins the rest of the ward and staff only find the visitor 15 minutes later.

If this incident were actually to happen then you may have thought that there was some liability as actual harm has occurred. However, neither you (as a nurse) nor the Hospital could really be held to blame. The alarm was given to the visitor to acknowledge that personal safety is an important issue on the ward/Unit and that each person has a responsibility for their own safety including *whether or not to seek help*.

The patient's behaviour was classic manipulation and the visitor was foolhardy enough to hand over the alarm. The hospital will investigate the incident and take the opportunity to 'review its procedures', but the only hint of possible negligence would arise from the question why it took staff 15 minutes (after the patient left the room) for staff to discover the injured visitor. In undertaking such a procedural review, the hospital is effectively ensuring that it has met all of its obligations and potential liabilities under Health and Safety at Work legislation.

In cases where staff have behaved negligently, Dimond (1998) has identified four key courses of action that could be taken against health professionals to make them accountable:

- civil law;
- criminal law;

- employment law; and
- professional registration.

As employers have a liability under law, it is obvious that they will seek to clarify the roles of staff as much as possible as this deflects some liability away from them and onto others, such as forensic mental health nurses.

The General Duty of Care and forensic mental health nursing

Nurses tend to see themselves primarily as fulfilling a caring role – perhaps best summed up as 'put the patient at the centre of care' (Macleod Clark & Maben, 1998) and, in so doing, are, to some measure, protecting themselves from claims of negligence. The world of forensic mental health nursing is less simple because it is carried out with people who have committed criminal offences and are invariably housed in secure facilities for very specific reasons. At all times we must remember that, contrary to popular belief, we are, nurses first and agents of social control second. Forensic nurses clearly operate within a dichotomy which is created by their conflicting custodial role and their role as agents of therapeutic change. Irrespective of the environment, we have a responsibility for maintaining patient safety and adapting the physical care environment to enhance the promotion of the patients' (mental and physical) health.

By now the reader should be coming to the conclusion that there are some things different about working within a forensic or other secure environment. But what exactly? You may have thought about the context of practice with locked wards, security checks and overt and covert personal and environmental safety measures. You may then have gone on to think about the *nature* of the offences committed by the patients and at the need to provide positive robust treatment to effect rehabilitation so as to minimize the risk of repeat offending when released. You may also have thought about how to effectively 'contain' these prisoner patients/mentally disordered offenders and provide controls on the ward that ensure the safety of all on a day-to-day basis, while attempting, in parallel therapeutic interventions.

A number of key articles have been written on this important topic, notably: Niskala (1987), Ogle (1990), Burrow (1993a, b, c), Byrt (1993), Benson and Ducanis (1995). The general premise throughout these articles is that the forensic nurse working with people who have offended or are in secure environments will experience a role conflict between pursuing the General Duty of Care, treating and helping people and feeling uncomfortable *either* as to the acts committed by the patient, e.g., sexual abuse of children *or* working in an environment which prioritizes the restriction of liberty.

Forensic mental health nursing raises many dilemmas with which the nurse must wrestle on a daily basis, none more problematic than the formation of effective and therapeutic personal relationships with difficult, manipulative, psychotic and/or dangerous patients and having respect for patients, who *could* be deemed not to deserve it, by virtue of their offending and offensive behaviour.

Ogle (1990, p 12) provides us with a helpful personal statement:

> the population of people to which I provide health care are persons that have com-
> mitted crimes, some of the those crimes horrendous. Personally, I do not want to
> know the crimes committed, I want to be able to provide quality health care to
> inmates of the institution. It is not my job to judge them. Society and the judicial
> system make those decisions.

Forensic nursing and ethics

As Ogle (1990) has explained, the ethical principle of respect for patients is fundamental to the forensic nursing task, in that it requires that nurses retain respect for mentally disordered offenders, without prejudice or favour, irre- spective of their capacities, capabilities, social status, offences, behaviour or values. This, therefore, places all patients as equals as human beings and assigns them equivalent rights and responsibilities based on the assumption that as 'persons' they have worth.

Forensic mental health nurses have all the responsibilities afforded to them by the General Duty of Care but they must also ensure patients reside in both a safe and secure environment. Empowerment is one of the core values expected of mental health nurses in the promotion and development of safe yet secure environments We have a unique capacity to influence patients' day- to-day experiences of living through and living with their mental distress. The extent to which nurses are prepared to share power with them is critical in both a practical and a moral sense. It is clear that in contemporary mental health practice, patients and nurses are talking and listening together more. What is open to question, however, is both the quality of their discussions and the boundaries of the debates. We need to ask ourselves whether we are functioning at a therapeutic and meaningful level or simply providing an outlet for social discourse when claiming to have 'consulted' and 'listened'.

The emerging role of the forensic mental health nurse

Forensic mental health nurse's activities concern: 'The employment of those skills necessary to address the needs of the ill individual who has offended, or is likely to offend, or who remains the subject of detention within the terms of legislation' (ENB, 1989). To help forensic mental health nurses resolve moral dilemmas and find their identity Burrow (1993c) attempted to analyse the role of the forensic nurse by identifying a number of key features:

- an increasing focus on a distinctive, predominantly 'offender' client group;
- acute assessment skills of mental disorder and dangerousness;
- the safe control of the therapeutic environment; and
- intervention strategies aimed at targeting a client's health promotion and offending propensities.

This agenda, however, emphasizes a tension already contained within the UKCC *Code of Professional Conduct* (UKCC, 1998) whereby nurses are asked to safeguard and promote the interests of individual patients and clients and serve the interests of society.

A model of nursing care whereby the nurse adopts at least a moral point of view of caring shows a: non-indifference about what happens to persons. This provides a *context* for forensic practice whereby the mental health nursing competences, provide a content of greater relevance being: (as included in the Relevant Benchmark Statements at the head of this chapter)

- Provide a caring and empathic attitude to users of mental health and social care services and their carers;
- The application of helping relationships as the cornerstone of mental health nursing practice;
- Contribute to the development of culturally sensitive packages of mental health and social care;
- Consider the power differential between users of services, carers and mental health and social care workers; and
- Contribute to the audit process used to monitor the quality of mental health nursing in all settings.

The forensic nurse should be aware how people behave when they are mentally disordered, and how this behaviour may be linked to various types of offending, aggression and violence. A key aspect is the ability to address the needs of a mentally disordered individual while also developing a trusting therapeutic nurse–patient relationship. One of the key beliefs of all mental health nursing must be that 'people are not the problem – the problem is the problem' (Barker, 1995).

Burrow (1993c) further argues that a range of phenomena apply, which specifically define the nurse's role:

- The client category consists overwhelmingly of offenders with psychiatric pathology.
- Nurses contribute towards the therapeutic targeting of any mental disorder or offending behaviour related to psychiatric morbidity.
- These care strategies are largely incorporated within institutional control and custody of patients.

- The configuration of patient pathology, criminal activity, therapeutic inter-ventions and competencies, court/legal issues and custodial care creates the need for a formidable and accelerating knowledge base.
- The advocacy role is different from that in other nursing specialities, embracing both the de-stigmatization and the decriminalization of the patient group.
- Clients' potential for future dangerousness requires the formulation of risk assessment strategies.

The capability framework for modern mental health practice *The Capable Practitioner* (Sainsbury Centre for Mental Health, 2000) combines the notions of the reflective practitioner with that of the effective practitioner, dividing capabilities into five areas:

- *ethical practice* – this makes assumptions about the values and attitudes needed to practice;
- *knowledge* – lays the foundations of effective practice;
- *process of care* – describes the capabilities required to work effectively in partnership;
- *interventions* – capabilities specific to evidence-based, biopsychosocial approaches to mental health care; and
- *application* – capabilities as they apply to specific service settings or func-tions, e.g. assertive outreach, crisis resolution.

The public perception

Whereas forensic nurses are expected to show 'non indifference' and act from a perspective of empathy and care, public attitudes to mental illness are rad-ically different. Murphy (1993) found that the general public regarded men-tally ill people as 'unworthy' and attitudes towards them consisted mainly of, fear and a lack of sympathy resulting in personal and community rejection. At best, society's attitudes towards mentally ill people has always been patroniz-ing benevolence (*we* know what's best for *you*) but when the mentally ill patient is also an offender, and held in a secure environment or both, then the public concern is not just doubled, but multiplied a hundred fold.

Recently the Government has sought to: *establish A National Service Framework for Mental Health* (DoH, 1999); *develop A Competence-based Exit Profile for Pre Registration Mental Health Nursing* (Northern Centre for Mental Health, 2000); *reform* The Mental Health Act (1983) and *reorganize services Modernising Mental Health Services* (DoH, 1998). This proposed how future services should be clustered:

- Supportive Services – working with patients and serviced users, their families and carers to build healthier communities;

- Sound Services – to ensure that patients and service users have access to the full range of services that they need;

and perhaps more important for our present purpose:

- Safe Services – to protect the public and provide effective care for those with mental illness at the time they need it.

MIND as part of its own contribution to the review process has pointed out that the term 'mentally disordered' offender is both an unhelpful and oppressive one, resulting in mentally disordered offenders being held in hospital for longer periods than people who are held in prison having committed similar offences. Consequently MIND proposes that much of the role conflict experienced by forensic nurses could be removed by regarding those mentally ill people (who have offended and are being detained in secure hospitals) as 'patients' first and foremost and by establishing an independent advocacy service. The latter would particularly help resolve the dilemma, whereby: 'Nurses act as power brokers in pseudo roles of advocacy for the mentally disordered offender, balancing their rights with those of psychiatry and the State' (Tendler, 1995).

Mentally disordered offenders still require care, therapy and treatment and control and containment but by *prioritizing* mental health problems and thereby locating offending behaviour within the illness itself, forensic nurses should gain a clearer sense of purpose and direction. By separating out advocacy, as MIND proposes, and locating it within an independent body, further conflicts of role are removed.

Relationships

The collaborative nature of present-day forensic health and social care expects and demands a care arena where relationships and alliances between the patients, their families and carers and the range of professionals are seen to be the cornerstones of the treatment process. This is not only to promote a culture of patient empowerment, where patients take more responsibility for their lives and their actions, but also to support and facilitate greater client engagement with their condition. One of the core functions is to enable patients to form, maintain and end satisfying personal relationships, in a manner that is meaningful to the individuals and ensure the safety and security of all parties while being relevant and appropriate to the context of both the care setting as well as the interests of wider society. Whatever mental health nurses do under the guise of effective care, it *must* involve a complex system of interpersonal relations (Barker, 1995) and Barker expands this by saying that the essence of care is human meeting human and the content of those meetings involves interaction, exchange and influences,

– we couldn't discuss caring without invoking interpersonal relations and vice versa.

It is and has been proposed that effective nurse–patient relationships are distinguished by a dynamic mutual learning process (Kirby, 2001; Kirby & Cross, 2002). This is a relationship that is utilized by both parties – the patient who helps the nurse to understand (in their own use of words) how they conceptualize, rationalize, explain and cope with their individual and specific mental health problems, and the nurse who learns from the patients' experiences as a result of their mental health problems – both positive and negative. This will allow treatment strategies to be more meaningful and contextual.

However, Safran et al (1990) pose a series of questions to be asked by the nurse before entering into a therapeutic alliance:

- Can I permit myself to enter into the private world(s) of this patient, explore their feelings without judging them (which is especially relevant in the case of serious and heinous offences), and in some significant and honest way, respond in a manner that lets them know that I have listened and I want to provide whatever assistance or comfort that I can?
- Can I see this person as being unique in his/her reaction to illness?
- Can I see what is different, and the same, about this person so that any insight or assistance I may give is the most useful to this patient?'.

At all times the nurse must have an awareness of their first duty not to harm the patient – directly or indirectly, by omission or neglect. Nothing should override the patient's best interest or the nurses' common sense. Numerous texts (Dickes, 1975; Fulton, 1997; Kirby & Cross, 2002; Repper et al, 1994; Speedy, 1999; Sullivan 1998) have been written describing the necessary conditions and practitioner behaviours that promote a therapeutic alliance.

Williams and Dale (2001) identified six specific professional values that are inherent in all mental health work but which they stress have particular relevance to the challenges in working with mentally disordered offenders:

- Value 1 – Respect for the patient as a human being, regardless of behaviour, offending history or diagnosis;
- Value 2 – Acceptance and application of current concepts of ill health and needs for care and treatment operated by the medical and psychiatric professions;
- Value 3 – Not judging patients;
- Value 4 – Applying an equally high quality of care to every patient;
- Value 5 – Treating all patients with equality and fairness; and
- Value 6 – Maintaining confidentiality.

Interpersonal boundaries and especially the fear of boundary violations are fundamental issues within any therapeutic process, both for the protection of the staff member and to aid the progress of the patient. Boundaries within professional practice are used to define acceptable conduct and limits of practice. Most of the literature, particularly within psychotherapy, has focused upon the area of sexual misconduct, this being an extreme example but helps to identify the relationship complexities in mental health care (Dale, 2001). Given that the therapeutic relationship can be quite intense, this is an area that all professionals need to be acutely alert for any potential or actual violations. Compromise would appear to be the key concept associated with this therapeutic dilemma, the compromise that such an inappropriate relationship can bring to patient care and to the multi-disciplinary team functioning as well as both personal and professional standards (Humphreys & McClelland, 2001; UKCC, 1998).

Ensuring care needs are met in secure facilities

The only real difference between the care of the mentally disordered offender and the care of any other patient is that these people have lost their liberty through dangerous or offending behaviour. We *need* to contain them and be aware of their potential possibilities for criminal or dangerous behaviour while providing care. Ogle (1990, p 12), contextualizes the issue well, 'Of the utmost importance is a respect for the environment in which I work. I can never forget where I am and the risks involved', adding, 'but I also have a job to do and that job is to deliver quality health care to the inmate population'. On the other hand, Burrow (1993a, p 21) reminds us that: 'the already proven dangerous propensities of the mentally disordered client group demand a considerable caution while they are being managed within treatment facilities'. It is thus imperative that the building which accommodates mentally disordered offenders is completely secure and has no design faults; has been tested by others with expertise in escaping; and that staff have been fully trained in security procedures including those to be adopted in the event of an emergency. Once these measures have been taken role conflict should be dramatically reduced leaving the forensic nurse confident in the environment so as to be able to care and treat with greatly reduced constraint.

Hart (2000) has previously argued that the most effective way of managing dangerous people is to:

- ensure a physically secure environment;
- train staff in intervention techniques and use these consistently;
- provide a low key atmosphere on the ward encouraging tranquillity;
- respect patients rights and attempts to provide care based upon *individual* need.

Through such empathy the need to react in a violent or abreactive manner is greatly reduced.

Assessment of risk

Assessment of risk of the individual should already have been undertaken *prior* to their admission, as part of the pre-admission process. Essentially, someone, somewhere has attempted to match the potential risk posed by an individual to the level of security offered in the clinical setting. Our key purpose in assessing risk is to develop an individual's risk management programme thereby reducing the risk of harm or injury to the patient and to other people. In so doing, we are responding to the principle of 'think safe then think intervention'.

Risk to others

Regardless of the characteristics of the individual, we know that there are two major circumstances where the risk of aggressive behaviour may be increased, namely:

- whenever the level of inhibition is reduced; and
- whenever the level of frustration is increased.

On their own they increase the risk of violent outbursts but added together they can form, for some people, a lethal cocktail.

The risk from the person or the risk from the situation?

As stated earlier, a lot of risk management tends to focus on the patient rather than on situations and contexts. We offer the argument that this in an unhelpful approach and can contribute to the creation of a tense and fractious environment. An alternative would be to ensure that routines and procedures are designed through negotiation, are patient sensitive and as unobtrusive as possible, so that daily life can be more relaxed and environmental triggers to anger and violence thereby minimized.

Then incorporate in each individual patient's care and treatment plan an analysis of the aggressive behaviours they pose to themselves or to others as part of their mental conditions and thereby develop an agreed strategy as to how they should be managed if their aggressive behaviour is triggered.

Moore (1996, p 9) makes the point effectively:

because a sound assessment of risk will be based on the formulation of the mechanisms underlying the behaviour, it will automatically identify those processes which appear to be key elements in increasing or reducing such risk. These may involve only the assessed individual (for example, where a crucial skill deficit, or deviant drive is highlighted) or may extend to others (where marital stressors or difficulty in relating to residential staff may be identified triggers).

Audit of risk on the ward is the starting point for producing a safe environment for all and sets the context for assessing the needs of the individual patient including the aetiology of any aggressive behaviours and effective techniques for de-escalation.

Assessing patients' needs

Barker (1997, p 17) explains that: assessment tries to gain an *overall picture*: one that describes positive characteristics as well as problems. A full assessment describes the skills, assets and other positive features of a person. On the flip side of the coin can be seen his list of handicaps, disabilities or other dysfunctions and in doing so, we should abide by, 'the spirit of a more objective approach: becoming more aware of our biases and prejudices'.

What we are doing in assessment is looking at the *strengths*, *needs* and *problems* of the *individual* patient and how these can be best met. You may not like what someone has done, but nevertheless our job is to treat the person with dignity and respect separating out the person from their presenting behaviour for: 'if psychiatric and mental health nursing assessment leads anywhere, it may lead to the nurse and the person-in-care considering further the story of the person's life and to re-authoring that story, through the therapeutic process of nurses' relationship with the person' (Barker, 1997, pp 13–14). Barker goes on to illustrate how the assessment process has six component questions, which the assessor must ask of themselves:

- Why am I doing this assessment?
- What is the aim of the assessment?
- When should I assess?
- How will I get the information I need?
- How will I judge what this information means?
- How might the person function under different conditions?

Forensic mental health nurse competencies and education

Kirby & Maguire (1997) identified six key skills that are inherent in the day to day working of the forensic mental health nurse.

- the assessment and management of dangerousness;
- risk assessment and management;
- psychodynamic psychotherapies;

- assessment of offending behaviour;
- management of personality disorders with associated offending behaviour; and
- understanding associated ethical issues in the management of the mentally disordered offender.

These key skill areas have been expanded through ongoing continuing professional development and lifelong learning. A clinically focused framework comprising of eight competency statements within three overarching domains has been developed. Each competency statement comes with its own series of benchmarks, which offers the student a range of (suggested) activities to demonstrate achievement of the particular competency. These are the product of a consensus workshop (undertaken by the by the National Board for Nursing, Midwifery and Health Visiting for Scotland (NBS, 2000) resulting in the identification of broad areas of competence specific to forensic mental health nurses in a range of clinical settings.

The identification of core competencies is viewed as an integral element in both continued lifelong learning and determining the specific roles of forensic mental health nurses. This competency framework relates to fitness for purpose and is supportive of statutory, national and professional criteria. In addition the competencies inform the educational and developmental needs of staff, though it is accepted and acknowledged that many will be appropriate for other members of the multi-disciplinary team (NBS, 2000).

Watson and Kirby (2000) have argued that it is difficult to develop evidence-based practice when forensic nurses themselves have been unsure of the competencies they need to develop and acquire. They recommend that pre-registration nurse training must equip nurses to work with mentally ill people in environments that are intrinsically not safe; and that some basic principles of secure care and core competencies to develop and maintain safe care environments must be included and legitimized in the curriculum. This new found commonality has now been recognized and given new impetus with the development of National Occupational Standards as outlined in *The Capable Practitioner* (Sainsbury Centre for Mental Health, 2000), see Table 21.1.

Conclusion

Mental health nurses care for the vulnerable, the sad and the lonely but forensic mental health nurses' clients are more vulnerable and more prone to episodes of enduring and debilitating mental health problems and behaviours (offending or otherwise) that require specialized environments and skills. In essence, 'forensic nurses do it behind locked doors'.

Forensic mental health nurses deal with some particularly anti-social,

Table 21.1 Competency Framework 2000

Risk domain	Critically review the knowledge bases and demonstrate an understanding of issues and factors which underpin risk assessment. Perform an assessment of the risk both to and/or from client groups within forensic health and social care settings. Demonstrate a knowledge and understanding of theoretical factors which underpin risk management and contribute to strategies, and facilitate care delivery, which aims to minimize and manage risk of individual clients.
Professional, legal and ethical aspects of care domain	Demonstrate a developing knowledge base and level of professional competence. Undertake professional practice, taking account of legislation, national strategies and contemporary agenda's which impact upon forensic health and social care. Engage in ethical professional practice in accordance with professional standards and the specific characteristics and needs of forensic health and social care service provision. Apply knowledge and an understanding of theoretical factors, which underpin professional, legal and ethical issues of care.
Interpersonal domain	Actively engage with forensic health and social care users, professional colleagues and other disciplines in the performance of professional role and responsibilities. Demonstrate knowledge and understanding of theoretical factors which underpin interpersonal competencies.

Source: Adapted from NBS (2000)

dangerous, life-threatening behavioural problems, entrenched psychotic or offending behaviour and deep-rooted psychological problems. In the midst of all this they try to ensure an environment that is both therapeutic and safe.

Mental health nurses work with people for whom society has little regard and mentally disordered offenders are seen as:

- mentally ill;
- ccriminal; and
- in need of incarceration;

and are thus prone to considerable individual and institutional discrimination. As patients appear to get better they are often regarded as simply becoming more efficient as criminals. If they appear to denounce criminal behaviour they are often regarded as being in denial of their illness.

In 2001, Her Majesty's Prison Service published *The Responsible Prisoner: An Exploration of the Extent to which Prison Removes Responsibility Unnecessarily and An Invitation to Change* (Morgan et al, 2001), which sums up (p 6) the practice dilemma: 'if you can give more responsibility, then more responsible behaviour is likely to result. And if you deny responsibility to people you cannot blame them for behaving irresponsibly.'

References

Barker, P. J. (1995) *Healing Lives, Mending Minds*, University of Newcastle: Professorial Inaugural Lecture.

Barker, P. J. (1997) *Assessment in Psychiatric and Mental Health Nursing*, Cheltenham: Stanley Thornes.

Benson, L. & Ducanis, A. (1995) Nurses' perceptions of their role and role conflicts, *Rehabilitation Nurse*, 20(4), 204–11.

Burrow, S. (1993a) Therapy versus custody, *Nursing Times*, 87(39), 64–6.

Burrow, S. (1993b) The role conflict of the forensic nurse, *Senior Nurse*, 13(5), 20–5.

Burrow, S. (1993c) An outline of the role of the forensic nurse, *British Journal of Nursing*, 2(18), 899–904.

Byrt, R. (1993) Moral minefield, *Nursing Times*, 89(8), 63–6.

Dale, C. (2001) Interpersonal relationships: staff development, awareness and monitoring issues, in C. Dale, T. Thompson & P. Woods (eds), *Forensic Mental Health: Issues in Practice*, Edinburgh: Bailliere Tindall/RCN, 127–38.

Department of Health (1998) *Modernising Mental Health Services: Safe, Sound and Supportive*, London: HMSO.

Department of Health (1999) *National Service Framework for Mental Health: Modern Standards and Service Models*, London: HMSO.

Dickes, R. (1975) Technical considerations of the therapeutic and working alliance, *International Journal of Psychoanalytical Psychotherapy*, 4, 1–24.

Dimond, B. (1998) How can nurses avoid negligence claims? *British Journal of Nursing*, 7(6), 306.

English National Board (1989) *Project 2000 – A New Preparation for Practice, Guidelines and Criteria for Course Development and the Formation of Collaborative Links Between Approved Training Institutions Within the National Health Service and Centres of Higher Education*, London: ENB.

Fulton, Y. (1997) Nurses views on empowerment: a critical social theory perspective, *Journal of Advanced Nursing*, 26, 529–36.

Goffman, E. (1961) *Asylums*, Handsworth: Penguin.

Hart, D. A. (2000) *Working with People with Mental Health Problems who Require Specialist Levels of Security or Intervention*, Cleveland: Tees and North East Yorkshire NHS Trust.

Humphreys, M. & McClelland, N. (2001) Therapeutic dilemmas in forensic practice, in N. McClelland, M. Humphreys, L. Conlon & T. Hillis (eds), *Forensic Nursing and Mental Disorder in Clinical Practice*, Oxford: Butterworth Heinemann, 39–41.

Kirby, S. D. (2001) Educating practitioners for forensic health and social care, in G. Landsberg & A. Smiley (eds), *Forensic Mental Health: Working with the Mentally Ill Offender*, Kingston, NJ: Civic Research Institute, 45.1–45.10.

Kirby, S. D. & Cross, D. J. (2002) Socially constructed narrative intervention: a foundation for therapeutic alliances, in A. Kettles, P. Woods & M. Collins (eds), *Forensic Mental Health Nursing: Future Directions for Treatment*, London: Jessica Kingsley, 187–205.

Kirby, S. D. & Maguire, N. A. (1997) Forensic psychiatric nursing, in B. Thomas, S. Hardy & P. Cutting (eds), *Stuart & Sundeen's Mental Health Nursing: Principles and Practice (UK Edition)*, London: Mosby, 395–409.

Macleod Clark, J. & Maben, J. (1998) Health promotion: perceptions of Project 2000 educated nurses, *Health Education Research*, 13(2), 185–96.

Montgomery, J. (1997) *Health Care Law*, Oxford: Oxford University Press.

Moore, B. (1996) *Risk Assessment: A Practitioners Guide to Predicting Harmful Behaviour*, London: Whiting and Birch Ltd.

Morgan, R., Owers, A. & Shaw, S. (2001) *The Responsible Prisoner: An Exploration of the Extent to which Prison Removes Responsibility Unnecessarily and an Invitation to Change*, London: HM Prison Service.

Murphy, B. (1993) Attitudes towards the mentally ill in Ireland, *Irish Journal of Psychological Medicine*, 10(2), 26–38.

National Board for Nursing, Midwifery and Health Visiting for Scotland (2000) *Continuing Professional Development Portfolio: A Route to Enhanced Competence in Forensic Mental Health Nursing*, Edinburgh: NBS.

Niskala, H. (1987) Conflicting convictions: nurses in forensic settings, *Psychiatric Nursing*, 28(2), 10–14.

Northern Centre for Mental Health (2000) *A Competence-based Exit Profile for Pre-Registration Mental Health Nursing*, Durham: Northern Centre for Mental Health/ The Northern and Yorkshire Regional Education and Workforce Development Sub-group for Mental Health/University of Teesside.

Ogle, B. (1990) What is forensic correctional nursing?., *The Florida Nurse*, 38(6), 12.

Repper, J., Ford, R. & Cooke, A. (1994) How can nurses build trusting relationships with people who have severe and long term mental health problems? Experiences of case managers and their clients, *Journal of Advanced Nursing*, 19, 1096–104.

Safran, J. D., McMain, S. & Crocker, P. (1990) Therapeutic alliance rupture as a therapy event for empirical investigation, *Psychotherapy*, 27, 155–65.

Sainsbury Centre for Mental Health (2000) *The Capable Practitioner: Report for the National Service Workforce Action Team*, London: Sainsbury Centre for Mental Health.

Speedy, S. (1999) The therapeutic alliance, in M. Clinton and S. Nelson (eds), *Advanced Practice in Mental Health Nursing*, Oxford: Blackwell Science.

Sullivan, P. (1998) Therapeutic interaction and mental health nursing, *Nursing Standard*, 12(45), 39–42.

Tarbuck, P., Topping-Morris, B. & Burnard, P. (1999) Preface, in P. Tarbuck, B. Topping-Morris & P. Burnard (eds), *Forensic Mental Health Nursing: Strategy and Implementation*, London: Whurr Publishers, xv–xvi.

Tendler, S. (1995) Psychiatric nurse helps police distinguish the mentally ill, *The Times*, 17/01/95.

United Kingdom Central Council for Nursing, Midwifery and Health Visiting (1998) *Code of Professional Conduct*, London: UKCC.

Watson, C. & Kirby, S. D. (2000) A two nation perspective on issues of practice and provision for professionals caring for mentally disordered offenders, in D. Robinson & A. Kettles (eds), *Forensic Nursing and Multidisciplinary Care of the Mentally Disordered Offender*, London: Jessica Kingsley Publishers, 51–62.

Williams, P. & Dale, C. (2001) The application of values in working with patients in forensic mental health settings, in C. Dale, T. Thompson & P. Woods (eds), *Forensic Mental Health: Issues in Practice*, Edinburgh: Bailliere Tindall/RCN, 139–150.

Other recommended resources

Chaloner, C. & Coffey, M. (eds) (2000) *Forensic Mental Health Nursing: Current Approaches*, Oxford: Blackwell Science.

Dale, C., Thompson, T. & Woods, P. (eds) (2001) *Forensic Mental Health: Issues in Practice*, Edinburgh: Bailliere Tindall/RCN.

Gamble, C. & Brennan, G. (eds) (2000) *Working with Serious Mental Illness: A Manual for Clinical Practice*, Edinburgh: Bailliere Tindall/RCN.

Mason, T. & Mercer, D. (eds) (1998) *Critical Perspectives in Forensic Care: Inside Out*, Basingstoke: Macmillan, now Palgrave Macmillan.

Mason, T. & Mercer, D. (1999) *A Sociology of the Mentally Disordered Offender*, Harlow: Pearson Educational Ltd.

Mercer, D., Mason, T., McKeown, M. & McCann, G. (eds) (2000) *Forensic Mental Health Care: A Case Study Approach*, Edinburgh: Churchill Livingstone.

Ryan, T. (ed.) (1999) *Managing Crisis and Risk in Mental Health Nursing*, Cheltenham: Stanley Thornes (Publishers) Ltd.

United Kingdom Central Council for Nursing, Midwifery and Health Visiting/University of Central Lancashire (1999) *Nursing in Secure Environments*, London: UKCC.

Webb, D. & Harris, R. (eds) (1999) *Mentally Disordered Offenders: Managing People Nobody Owns*, London: Routledge.

CHAPTER 22

Acute In-patient Setting

GORDON MITCHELL, CHRIS STANBURY AND SHEILA ARNOLD

Indicative Benchmark Statements

▓ Ability to assess the impact of culture, race, gender and lifestyle on the needs of mental health service users and their carers

▓ Recognition of the prodromal signs of mental illness

▓ Application of basic principles from the psychodynamic, behavioural, social and humanistic conceptual models of mental health interventions

▓ Participation in the provision of evidence-based family intervention programmes for service users with severe mental illness

▓ Critical awareness of own competence and needs for future mental health nursing professional development

Introduction

When exploring the possible causes as to why a client may be admitted to an acute in-patient unit, the reader, particularly those who are student nurses, should explore the models of mental disorder as these link to the biopsychosocial assessment that is required. Therefore, this chapter will discuss the role of the mental health nurse working in this area, drawing on the example of a recently published report and conclude with an exploration of the possible biopsychosocial causes of the main mental disorders and examine just a few of the possible therapeutic nursing interventions that could be used.

The role of the newly qualified nurse in an acute in-patient setting

The purpose of an adult acute psychiatric inpatient service is to provide a high standard of humane treatment and care in a safe and therapeutic setting for service users in the most acute and vulnerable stage of their illness. (DoH, 2002a, p 5)

The Department of Health has set a clear agenda for the modernization of in-patient services to achieve that purpose. The registered practitioner who will work in acute in-patient services will need to be aware of the governance agenda, the contemporary context and the realities of the practice environment in which they will be working. In addition to the theoretical understanding of mental illness and the ability to apply evidence-based nursing interventions, practitioners need to be clear about the skills and competencies they will need, to function, and how to meet the challenge of the current developments in acute services (DoH, 2000).

Contemporary context

Both the Sainsbury (Sainsbury Centre, 1998) and the Standing Nursing and Midwifery Advisory Committee (DoH, 1999b) Reports highlight the negative experiences of users of acute psychiatric in-patient services. Concerns were expressed relating to personal safety, poor environments, lack of information, absence of planning and negotiation of care, lack of therapeutic interventions and restricted access to staff. Most importantly service users described feeling ignored, bored and isolated with nothing constructive to do.

It was reported that in-patient areas often had low profiles with poor investment and lack of clear leadership whereas those working in community settings were prioritized. There were often recruitment problems and high turnover of staff. The report Fitness for Practice (UKCC, 1999) found evidence that, at registration, nurses lacked the practical skills required and this too impacted on acute in-patient areas that traditionally recruited new practitioners. In addition there were changing demands on services with an increasing complexity of clinical presentations involving more dual diagnosis and personality issues. Acuteness of problems and levels of risk were often experienced as higher due to a more restricted number of beds being available.

The National Service Framework for Mental Health (DoH, 1999a) set out the expected standards for mental health service delivery but did not focus specifically on the problems in acute in-patient services. These services however are a core part of the whole system of mental health care and by 2000 several practice initiatives were being developed to address these concerns.

An example – practice development

In Autumn 2000 the Northern, Yorkshire and Trent NHS Regional Offices, in partnership with the Northern Centre for Mental Health and the Leicester

Centre for Best Practice, launched the Acute Care Collaborative Project in response to the problems of in-patient care. Across those regions 37 in-patient (pilot) sites were involved in the 15 month project. The overall aim of the project was to improve the service users' experience of in-patient care and achieve better outcomes of care. A multi-stakeholder reference group had formulated 26 standards of care, which focused on the admission, stay and discharge processes, as elements of a service user journey through the mental health system.

The Institute of Healthcare Improvement's collaborative model (Institute of Healthcare, 2002) was the change vehicle used to implement practice improvements to achieve the identified standards. This model focuses on supporting clinical teams to make small incremental changes based on a cycle of 'plan', 'do', 'study', 'act' – very similar to an action-learning approach. It also emphasizes the importance of shared learning and shared contribution, not only between service users and professionals but also between professionals of different disciplines and across different organizations.

The project initially involved the service users 'mapping out' experiences of their journeys through the pilot services to identify where change was needed in relation to the performance – against the care standards. Local initiatives were then planned to address these identified problems. Impact of change was measured by collecting quantitative data from case note audit and qualitative data from semi-structured interviews with service users themed around the set standards. Examples of good practice and ideas for change were shared between all the project teams at quarterly learning events. The overall outcomes of the collaborative project were significant in the number of improvements made and the demonstrable positive impact on care (Dale et al, 2002).

Key issues were addressed through this project that are relevant to the practitioner in the acute in-patient area. Primarily, that it is the partnership with service user and carers which effects greatest change because of the sharing of perspectives and ideas. It is the skill of collaboration that is necessary (Dale et al, 2002). Collaboration across the whole care community is crucial to move towards a seamless service. Robust pre-admission and pre-discharge planning were identified as major influences on the effectiveness of the patient experience of in-patient services because the purpose of the in-patient stay was clear and the follow through into community care was an integral part of the overall plan. The ability to work with other care providers and to maintain effective communication are key skills that need to be acquired. Implementing care pathways is a systematic method of ensuring effective planning that can further enhance the service user experience.

The project also highlighted the need for positive therapeutic engagement and recommended that systems and practices in in-patient work needed reorganization. Then, Dodds and Bowles (2001) in their study of in-patient refocusing in Bradford identified similar issues in the cultural and structural change that have to be implemented to facilitate practitioners to work therapeutically with service users. This not only means that nurses need a toolbox of therapeutic skills but that they are able to manage change effectively and use initiative to support reshaping of services. Reshaping meant, at times, challenging conventional approaches, e.g., the observation of patients identified as high risk. Some teams were beginning to explore how change to more therapeutic engagement could change the way patients are observed on a day-to-day basis. This has been implemented most successfully within the Bradford work (Bowles et al, 2002).

Another important outcome was the improved risk management methodologies adopted across the project sites. The population within in-patient services is in the most vulnerable stage of illness and therefore at greatest risk. The implementation of evidence-based and comprehensive risk management programmes and the use of relevant assessment tools are key competencies for the in-patient practitioner. This is consistent with the care co-ordination approach (DoH, 2000) which promotes effective communication, information sharing and partnership working. Those teams in organizations where care co-ordination was effectively implemented more readily achieved risk and care planning standards. The 'Acute Care Collaborative Project' is one example of how services will need to respond to the challenges in in-patient care and the project outcomes highlighted some of the key skills and competencies required by practitioners in those services.

Ongoing modernization and governance agendas

The NHS Plan (DoH, 2000) outlined the modernization agenda with the aim to redesign and restructure services and practice across the health service. The focus of redesign is the service user and the aim to improve their experience of care.

The policy implementation guide for acute in-patient provision (DoH, 2002a) details the expectations and standards of a modern acute in-patient service. The centrality of the service user, a clear therapeutic focus for in-patient care and the enhanced profile of services are fundamental to this guidance. Further guidance detailing the development of dual diagnosis (DoH, 2002b) and women's mental health services (DoH, 2002c) is also expected to impact greatly on the delivery of care within the in-patient service.

Nurses will be at the forefront of the change required to implement that guidance, they will need to be both competent and empowered to own and take forward the modernization agenda. They will require an understanding of the context of change and have the skills to use the preceptorship, mentorship and clinical supervision available to guide them. Positive clinical leadership and clear modern matron roles, together with structures and processes and the external networks facilitated by National Institute for Mental Health in England (NIMHE) (DoH, 2001a) should support the acute in-patient practitioner. That practitioner will, however, require all the fundamental skills and competencies discussed to work accountably within those structures and be able to maintain the clarity of purpose of acute in-patient services as initially defined.

Patients on admission should be assessed holistically including a biopsychosocial appraisal of their mental state. For example, a patient who is admitted with Clinical Depression may want to know how their prescribed medication works. By adopting a biological or disease perspective, you can inform them in laymen's terms of basic biochemical reactions.

When taking a psychological perspective the practitioner can explore the cognitive theory that suggests that the mental habits whereby self-blaming entails exaggerating the dark side of events, and a pessimistic view on life causes irrational beliefs and distorted attitudes towards oneself, which perpetuates the depression (Beck, 1976).

We are further conscious that without placing presenting problems within their correct cultural context people, particularly from potentially vulnerable groups may experience discrimination and oppression through misdiagnosis and inappropriate treatment. Such has been the extent of misdiagnosis in the past that some localities have seen the creation of specific black mental health teams to provide prorate care to people from ethnic minorities and, as a secondary activity, education and enlightenment to white practitioners lacking a multi-cultural dimension to their own practice. Finally if a black client is admitted with psychosis can his social and cultural background affect his diagnoses and presentation of his/her symptoms? That is why an understanding of the models of mental disorder is essential to undertake a holistic assessment. The authors accept the models discussed below are not specific to acute in-patient, but can be related to any client who has a mental health problem.

Models for mental disorder

When exploring models of mental disorder the reader must be aware that they can be split into three main sections: the biological; the psychological; and the social models.

Biological model

The biological (or disease) model believes that mental health problems are a consequence of biological or physical changes with a client's brain, but sometimes within other part of the client's body. Therefore, the main focus of this model is the exploration of the chemical changes within the brain and how this can affect clients' perception and thought processes.

The main tenets of the biological or disease model are:

- that mental pathology is linked and accompanied by physical pathology;
- different mental illnesses can be classified as different mental disorders, which each have common characteristics;
- a mental illness is biologically disadvantageous; and
- when exploring the causes of physical and mental pathology in mental illness are all explicable in terms of physical illness (Adapted from Tyrer & Steinberg, 1999, p 10).

Psychological model

When exploring the psychological model it us useful to further divide it into the *Behavioural*, *Cognitive* and *Psychodynamic* approaches.

The *Behavioural* approach differs dramatically from the biological, psychodynamic and social models/approaches in that the symptoms, that are manifested in the client's behaviour, are considered to be the disorder. As Eysenck (1965, cited in Tyrer & Steinberg, 1999) explained, learning theory does not believe in the 'unconscious' causes of mental illness, neurotic symptoms are just learned behaviour. Remove the symptoms and you remove the neurosis.

The main tenets of the behavioural approach are:

- a client's symptoms and behaviour are the main features of mental illness;
- the science of learning theory can explain the origin and persistence of the symptoms of behaviour; and
- by using a learning theory approach the therapist can remove maladaptive symptoms of behaviour and therefore cure the disorder (Adapted from Tyrer & Steinberg, 1999, p 55).

The *Cognitive* approach was first devised by Beck (1976) for the treatment of anxiety and depression. The main principle of this approach is that mental disorder is founded in errors or biases in the way a person thinks and the way the person responds (through stimuli) to their thought processes, creates the mental disorder.

The main tenets of the cognitive approach are:

- a client's perception of their world is determined by their thinking or cognition;
- cognition influences the client's symptoms, behaviour and attitudes;
- dysfunctional cognition creates mental illness; and
- if the client's mental illness is to improve major changes to the cognition need to be made (Adapted from Tyrer & Steinberg, 1999, p 75).

When you mention the *psychodynamic* approach people usually think of Freud, however Jung and Adler were also important in the development of the psychodynamic approach. Supporters of this approach range from dynamic psychotherapy (in which the client can be seen weekly for a few weeks or months) to psychoanalysis (in which the client could be seen daily for several years).

The main tenets of the psychodynamic approach are:

- the focus is the way the person feels;
- there are many ways in which a person's feelings can be influenced and we are often not aware of them;
- the therapist needs to use a technically structured approach to tap into the person's unconscious feelings;
- important feelings can be seen as emotional reactions to the therapist (Transference);
- also important are the therapist's reactions to the client (Countertransference);
- the therapist has to be objective and not judgmental;
- troubling feelings, inconsistencies and irrational feelings underline emotional disorders; and
- unconscious processes influence all relationships (e.g., nurse and patient) without either necessarily knowing why (Adapted from Tyrer & Steinberg, 1999, p 34).

Social model

The social model is based on the fundamental premise that the wider influences of social forces are seen to be the main influence or cause of mental distress. An example of this can be seen in the work of Holmes and Rahe (1967) who devised a Social Readjustment Rating Scale in an attempt to quantify the severity of a particular life event by the amount of change it produces in the client. This was an attempt by social theorists to demonstrate that they were scientific in their approach to the causes of mental illness.

The main tenets of the social model are:

- a person's class, occupational status and social role are important social forces in a person's mental disorder;
- a life event that can appear to be independent can trigger a mental disorder; and
- social influences can cause a person with a mental disorder to remain disordered (Adapted from Tyrer & Steinberg, 1999, p 87).

Therefore from these briefly discussed models the reader should be able to see from which philosophical direction many health care professions (and professionals) approach the assessment and care of a client with a mental disorder. This chapter will continue to explore some of the combination of

psychoeducational, pharmacotherapeutic, psychotherapeutic and social interventions that could be utilized for a client who may be diagnosed as having
a schizophrenic, depressive or bipolar disorder.

Working with clients and their families within acute in-patient care

Managing the experience of clients who find themselves within the acute
mental health setting involves the management and co-ordination of the
processes of admission, stay and discharge planning. The nurses' knowledge
and skills in engagement, partnership, collaboration and therapeutic working
influence the experience of the client and their family or carers (Gournay,
1995; Repper & Perkins, 1996). The process involves a holistic and individualized approach to the treatment and care of the client experiencing mental
distress (Barker, 1997). The period of time the client spends in in-patient care
offers the nurse a unique opportunity for intensive, continuous, consistent
and therapeutic interaction with them and their families. Within this section
interventions for people with schizophrenia, depression and bipolar disorders
will be explored within the context of, and with the emphasis being placed
upon, biopsychosocial approaches acknowledging contemporary literature,
health policy and empirical research.

In 1999 a report from the Standing Nursing and Midwifery Advisory
Committee acknowledged the significant contribution made by nurses caring
for clients in the acute mental health setting. They saw the practice of nursing as one of the most challenging responsibilities in the new National
Health Service but reported that nurses', clients' and carers' experience of
admission to in-patient wards had become increasingly custodial, with greater
risks and limited therapeutic activity. Contemporary discourses in mental
health care identify particular attitudes and strategies required by the nurse
when working with clients who experience long-term mental health problems
(Repper & Perkins, 1996) a particular demand of the nurse working in acute
in-patient care services. These include, handling conflict and crisis, moving
at the client's pace, being optimistic and facilitating hope. Developing trust,
being stable and predictable can also help in the development of a therapeutic alliance.

They identified a number of skill areas important to acute mental health
nursing. These included formal methods of assessment for measuring
and recording systematically the symptoms, social functioning needs, risks and
medication side effects. The utilization of methods that include the client
and carers' perspectives in the planning, delivery and evaluation of their care
(Leese et al, 1998) within a care planning framework that facilitates communication among disciplines and across care settings, implementation and
management strategies that respond to issues of risk, client and family psychosocial interventions, and the management of medication regimes, including

the detection and alleviation of side-effects. The following sections will explore the therapeutic work of nurses within the acute mental health setting.

Somatic/physical interventions

Psychopharmacotherapy is the use of psychoactive drugs to treat symptoms of mental illness and is indicated for many mental illnesses. The role of the nurse in the care of the client (and family) when supporting psychopharmacotherapy, is focused upon two main themes: nursing knowledge and nursing interventions utilized when working with clients and their family or carers (Carpenter & Sabaraini, 1996). Knowledge and understanding of the neuro anatomy and physiology should also include knowledge and understanding of neurochemistry and brain function; the medical neurological models of mental illness; mode of action of drugs and side-effects (Bennet et al, 1995; Rycroft-Malone et al, 2000). This should also embrace an understanding of the classification of psychoactive drugs; their modes of action and drug regimes in the treatment of specified mental illness; general drug side effects; drug specific side effects; risk assessment and management of psychopharmacotherapeutic regimes (De la Cour, 1995).

The nurse's practice should demonstrate an awareness of the concepts of non-compliance or non-adherence and how medical-professional and client-family accounts are integrated in the care planning process (Kemp et al, 1996; Perkins & Repper, 1999; Smith et al, 1999). This will include the exploration of the ethical, legal and moral dimensions of clinical practice in relation to compliance, adherence, concordance, paternalism, insight, advocacy and empowerment (Holm, 1993). Contemporary discourses in the literature advocate a concordant approach, which would require the nurse to engage the client (and family) in a negotiated decision-making process (Gardener et al, 1999; Gray et al, 2002) facilitating their empowerment in psychopharmacotherapeutic regimes.

An examination of the issues surrounding the nurse's role in mental illness assessment (Barker, 1997) and management strategies should include exploration of the use of specific tools in the assessment, monitoring and evaluation of illness management. This will involve the identification and use of specific tools in exploration of the potential or actuation of adverse physical side-effects (Day et al, 1995; De la Cour, 1995) and the psychological and social consequences of medical treatment. The nurse will implement physical, psychological and social assessment strategies and interventions when working with the client (Brasfield, 1991; Goldstein, 1995), taking into account the multiple perspectives of clients, families and professionals and the complexity of biopsychosocial phenomena (Agnes et al, 2002; Akiskal et al, 2001; Barrowclough & Tarrier, 1997; Campbell, 2003).

When working with clients and their families during psychopharmacotherapy the nurse will need to effectively engage the client in their care and the development of a therapeutic relationship will be essential for any ongoing therapeutic activity. The nurse should seek to understand the client's perspective, their experience of their mental distress/mental illness and how this can be acknowledged in the client's assessment (Coultier et al, 1999; Hayward et al, 1995; Kemp et al, 1996). For example, the nurse's use of self-assessment strategies and tools, information and psychoeducation, counselling and individual therapy (Campbell, 2003; Goldstein, 1995; Gournay, 2000) in care planning.

The nurse will promote the client's ability to self-monitor and manage their illness through the development and maintenance of coping/management strategies, for example, the symptoms of their illness and their psychosocial responses/experiences to illness. The nurse needs to utilize knowledge of psychopharmacotherapeutic management of mental illness including the client's medical presentation, the features of the illness, specific drug regimes (e.g., the clinical presentations of schizophrenia, depression and bipolar disorder) in order to promote positive client outcomes. It will also be important to understand the nature of any presenting adverse physical and psychosocial side-effects and consequences so that the nurse can develop assessment and intervention strategies including the client's perspective of possible or potential risk assessment and management strategies (Ryan, 1999), (e.g., self-medication). If information materials are to be used to support clients' involvement in treatment decisions, they must contain relevant, research-based data in a form that is acceptable and useful to the client (Coultier et al, 1999; Perry et al, 1999).

A commitment to working with the family and carers and taking on board their perspectives and experiences and their current and previous contribution to the client's care during psychopharmacotherapy is essential (Gournay, 2000). This should include the family/carers' perspective of the assessment of needs, how any organization of interviews with the client should be organized, the use of psychoeducation (understanding of illness/distress and biopsychosocial interventions), an exploration of illness management strategies, the development of problem-solving and coping strategies in order to support the client (Fadden, 1998a, b). Therefore, it will be necessary for the nurse to develop knowledge and skills in engaging families in the decision-making process within all aspects of the care package (Barrowclough & Tarrier, 1997; Lam, 1991). This will involve enhancing their knowledge and skills in dealing with crisis or relapse (Birchwood et al, 1998), in early intervention strategies including areas such as risk and/monitoring as well as the development of risk management strategies (Bowles et al, 2002; Dodds & Bowles, 2001; Ryan, 1999).

Within the acute care setting the nurse will be involved in supporting the client undergoing electroconvulsive therapy in the treatment of mental illness. The role of the nurse in the care of the client leading up to and during this procedure is important (Challiner & Griffiths, 2000; Dawson, 1997; Gass, 1998). This will involve integrating the national and local policies and procedures for the administration of procedure into the nursing practices (DoH, 1999a, b, 2000, 2001b, 2002a, b, c, d). Also the nurse will need to understand the national and local policies and procedures informing 'special observations' or physical containment of the client and the role of the nurse in care delivery (Bowles et al, 2003; Dodds & Bowles, 2001; Gournay et al, 1998).

The nurse working within acute care environments will have to demonstrate understanding and use of effective therapeutic skills and clinical leadership involving comprehensive and individualized assessment strategies, crisis management, symptom stabilization and medication management (DoH, 2002a, b, c). This will include the promotion of client self-management, reintegration of the client in the community and connection with the community support systems. The nurse will need to develop an understanding of multidisciplinary and integrated team working, for example, exploring the nature of 'team' relationships, multidisciplinary working (DoH, 2000). Also they will need to appreciate their influence upon the practices and processes during psychopharmacotherapy, engagement in decision-making, interpersonal strategies, leadership, advocacy, empowerment and working in complex mental health and social care systems.

Therapeutic milieu

Therapeutic milieu refers to a health promoting environment for clients in which the environment itself is used as an instrument for treatment. There are unstructured and structured aspects to the environment involving careful structuring of the social and physical aspects of the acute setting so that every interaction and activity is therapeutic for the client (DoH, 1999, 2002b; Echternacht, 2001; Gournay et al, 1998). This will include organizing and facilitating client meetings, recreational, social and therapeutic groups and providing planned activities such as arts, crafts and outings. The nurse will play a role in the determining, reinforcing and monitoring of the environment's rules, structure and boundaries. This may also involve caring for acutely ill clients who may require assistance in maintaining an orientation to reality, determining adequate staff to client ratios that afford adequate time to interact with clients in the ward and provide a physical environment that is safe, attractive, comfortable and functional. The unstructured aspects of milieu are the interactions that take place between the nurse and the client (Echternacht, 2001) and will involve an understanding of brief, unplanned nurse–client encounters that occur in the ward and how to respond to them. This requires the nurse to understand the application of psychotherapeutic knowledge, skills and principles to the brief clinical encounters that occur spontaneously in the ward setting (Echternacht, 2001; Peplau, 1988).

Psychological intervention

Psychological intervention involves the engagement of clients in therapeutic activity ranging from therapeutic conversation to more formal structured 'talking' therapy (Barker, 1999). Forming the therapeutic alliance is the central component used in the management of client phenomena. Most mental illnesses involve some type of disturbance in the client's emotional life. Psychological interventions aimed at the client phenomena can take many forms ranging from psychodynamic (Barker, 1999), Cognitive Behavioural Therapy (Hawton et al, 1989) through interpersonal therapy (Klerman et al, 1984), motivational interviewing (Miller & Rollnick, 2003) to solution focused or narrative therapies (Milner & O'Bryne, 2002) as well as counselling and supportive activities (DoH, 2001c). Zubin (1989) explores the issues examining the suiting of therapeutic interventions to the scientific models of aetiology used to understand the client's mental illness and the matching of interventions.

Social interventions

The impact of serious mental illness on the social and coping skills of the client and family provide challenges for the nurse in devising not only individualized psychological interventions but also social care. The nurse's role is in supporting the development of social, recreational, occupational and vocational activities within the client's care package. Some discussion on the knowledge and skill of the nurse in the promotion of recovery can be found in the Department of Health document *The Journey to Recovery: The Government's Vision for Mental Health* (DoH, 2001b). Successful aftercare functioning requires:

- attention to or management of the client's environment;
- a supportive quality and satisfactory living situation;
- the mental health and social well being of the client is influenced by environment and family/peers;
- occupational and recreational activities add organization and structure to the client's life style;
- problem solving and increasing positive and open communication; and
- interpersonal relationships, social networks, social skills, activities of daily living, social support/help.

Schizophrenia

Admission

In the assessment and management of acute episodes of schizophrenia the nurse working within the acute care setting will utilize assessment strategies

(Fox & Conroy, 2000; Gamble & Brennan, 2000) to gain information on the client's past and present medication regimes, symptom and risk assessment (Cochrane-Brink et al, 2000; Nimeus et al, 2000; Ryan, 1999; Walsh et al, 1999), psychological wellbeing, social functioning, support systems and family communication/problem solving strategies. Assessment tools used may vary but some are demonstrating their utility in care planning and therapeutic targeting. They range from global assessment of psychiatric illness, health or functioning to more specific assessment of client or family phenomena. For example the Global Assessment of Functioning Scale (GSF) is an overall measure of the client's functioning whereas the Brief Psychiatric Rating Scale (Overall & Gorman, 1962) is used to assess the severity of a range of psychiatric symptoms. Evaluation scales such as the Modified Scale for the Assessment of Negative Symptoms (SANS) (quoted in Birchwood & Tarrier, 1994, p 12) or the Positive and Negative Syndrome Scale for Schizophrenia (Kay et al, 1988) are used to assess changes in negative symptoms over the period of treatment or to determine the presence of schizophrenic symptoms. The Quality of Life Scale (Heinrichs et al, 1984) is used to assess changes in the client's quality of life over the treatment phase, the higher the score the greater the improvement in interpersonal functioning (Franklin et al, 1986; O'Boyle, 1994; Oliver et al, 1996). The Camberwell Family Interview (Leff and Vaughan, 1985) explores the experiences of the family and social/environmental emotional climate.

Therefore therapeutic approaches must be tailored to the client's presentation. For a client who experienced any manner of symptoms including disorder perceptions of reality, hallucinations and illusions, delusions, disordered thinking and emotional expression, the role of the nurse would be to facilitate individual cognitive behavioural interventions such as those proposed in the Cochrane review (Jones et al, 1998) to target specific symptom of schizophrenia. A disturbance in the regulation or control of affect (often seen in bipolar illness and cognitive disorders) may be present, as well as a number of other types of disturbance in emotional functioning (Brooker & Repper, 1998; Chadwick, 1997; Thomas, 1997). The more familiar the nurse is with the client's style of emotional expression, the better positioned they will be to make appropriate interventions in the therapeutic process (Chadwick, 1997).

The nurse will also play an important role in the stabilization of the client utilizing medication management strategies, the administration of conventional and atypical anti-psychotic drugs, and the optimiziation of neuroleptic treatment in psychotic illness (Pratt, 1998; Searle, 1998).

In-patient stay

After the intense psychotic symptoms have been controlled by medication and a combination of individual and supportive therapy and/or counselling have been used to stabilize the client (Gournaym, 1997; 2000). The nurse will focus on working with the client to enhance their coping, problem-solving and illness management skills (Birchwood & Tarrier, 1994).

The psychosocial interventions' (PSI) approach places emphasis on client education and understanding in order for them to participate in their care and possibly move towards self-management and recovery (Birchwood & Tarrier, 1994; Brooker & Repper, 1998; Gournay, 2000). Therefore, it is important that the nurse has assessed the client's level of intelligence or comprehension, memory function and any challenges and limitation that they may have. Having an understanding of the client's cognitive capabilities can help the nurse and client avoid unnecessary frustration and can ultimately (and hopefully) lead to the development of a more effective care delivery. Psychoeducational activities (Pekkala & Merinder, 2000) require techniques that take into account the client's ability in abstract thinking, self-observation and reality testing. Psychoeducational activities include specialized education techniques, which may make use of educational videos, reading materials, formal and informal and individual and group teaching strategies.

The nurse will use individual cognitive behavioural interventions to help the client establish links between their thoughts, feelings and actions with respect to the targeting of symptoms (Chadwick et al, 1996; Kingdon & Turkington, 1994). Or for the correction of the person's misconceptions, irrational beliefs and reasoning biases related to their presenting symptoms. The client may also be taught to use cognitive behavioural concepts to monitor their own thoughts, feelings and behaviours in order to promote alternative ways of coping with their illness. Behavioural disturbances include issues surrounding motivation, stamina, unpredictable behaviours, drive and low energy levels, for example, clients with schizophrenia and depression. Aloofness, awkwardness and passivity all combined can make the client difficult to engage with interpersonally and socially.

The nurse may use individual therapy to facilitate the development of the client's insight and control of their symptoms through education and support to cope with life stressors and to recognize stress responses (relapse signatures) and situations and develop coping strategies (Bellack et al, 1989; McNally & Goldberg, 1997; Martin, 2000). For the nurse, utilizing supportive therapy as an ongoing helping strategy involves active listening, demonstrating empathy, using appropriate reassurance, reinforcement of patient health promoting initiatives and supporting and facilitating problem solving in times of crisis. Family Work or Interventions involves the nurse in working with the client's family and/or carers implementing psychoeducational strategies and communication and problem solving enhancement (Barrowclough & Tarrier, 1997; Birchwood & Tarrier, 1994).

Within the care package, planning and interventions for the development of the client's self-management and recovery skills are paramount as they learn about their illness and its treatment. Care packages should also focus on interventions working on socialization and vocational skills (Crowther et al, 2000; Pilling et al, 2000) to promote social adjustment and improved quality of life.

It has been demonstrated that supportive, guidance and directive approaches are effective in promoting social and vocational functioning (Gournay, 2000; Harmon & Traatnack, 1992).

Family work/intervention (Anderson & Adams, 1996; Barrowclough & Tarrier, 1997; Lam, 1991; Pharoah et al, 1999) is a key component of psychosocial intervention and an important part of the client care management in improving the emotion climate to reduce stress, enhance coping skills and prevent relapse (Fadden, 1998a, b). It is based on the concept of 'Expressed Emotion' (Smith & Birchwood, 1993), which suggests that critical or over-involvement/protective attitudes from the family are predictive of relapse and re-hospitalization (Birchwood et al, 1998).

Discharge planning

The client's in-patient stay has established a baseline assessment and treatment for the maintenance phase to supported the longer term recovery phase of the illness. The most intense symptoms of schizophrenia have been controlled or stabilized with medication but there may be milder persistent symptoms. The foundation of family working that has been initiated within the in-patient setting (Barrowclough & Tarrier, 1997; Fadden, 1998a, b) is an important part of discharge planning also. The nurse working in the acute in-patient ward develops the foundations of the client's individualized care package that can be built upon through the care co-ordination process (DoH, 2000) as they move back into the community (Armstrong, 1998). During the process of on-going care the nurse needs to facilitate a flexible treatment and psychosocial care package in which the client can experience, the often inevitable, relapses of mental illness without losing the continuity of the recovery process (DoH, 2001b).

Depression

Admission

The acute treatment of depression involves establishing a correct diagnosis and applying clear evidence-based and goal-directed principles (Agnes et al, 2002; APA, 1994; WHO, 1992). The goals of in-patient treatment and care will focus on the achievement of a remission of symptoms through psychopharmacotherapy and psychosocial interventions in order to improve the client's quality of life, and prevent relapse or recurrence of depression.

In the acute phase the nurse will carry out a biopsychosocial assessment of the client, establish a therapeutic alliance, support psychopharmacological treatment, choose and implement specific psychosocial interventions to achieve therapeutic goals and meet the client needs (Sharkey, 2002). Whatever treatment a client will receive will be dependent upon their presentation of depression and will possibly involve a combination of anti-depressant medication and psychotherapeutic intervention. Psychosocial assessment and intervention strategies can be implemented during the client's acute in-patient stay to manage the acute episode and promote recovery from depression. Walsh (1998) identifies an initial phase which he refers to as the 'major depressive episode' where the interventions techniques will focus on ego-supportive interventions and crisis intervention.

Assessment will involve the identification of symptoms and their severity and the assessment of risk (Ryan, 1999; Sharkey, 1997). A strong indicator of suicide risk in the acute stage of depression is hopelessness and the nursing assessment of risk should include inquiry into the client's plans and hopes for the future. Initial management of suicidal thoughts can include distraction techniques (physical activity, talking about their concerns), keeping a list of reasons for living and having access to someone during crisis. The assessment of physical wellbeing and the recognition and investigation of physical ill-health are also important as co-morbid medical conditions may require medical attention.

There are a number of global and specific assessment tools the nurse can utilize in the care of clients experiencing depression including instruments such as; the General Health Questionnaire (Goldberg & Williams, 1988); Beck's Depression Inventory (Beck et al, 1961); Inventory for Depressive Symptomology (Rush et al, 1986); Brief Depression Rating Scale (Kellner, 1986); Beck Hopelessness Scale (Beck et al, 1974) and Suicide Intent Scale (Beck et al, 1975), and the Nurses' Observation Scale for Inpatient Evaluation (Honigfeld, 1976).

Psychopharmacotherapy is often the first treatment to be administered. The psychoeducational activities promoting the client's understanding of anti-depressants, dosage, mode of action and side effects and monitoring the client's response, i.e. symptom control or remission, will start at a level that takes into account their depressive symptoms. Side effects are the most common reason for a client prematurely stopping medications. Most side effects are mild and transient, but clients should be informed about any serious side effects so they know what to watch for and what to do should they occur. Inquiry into side effects should be an on-going aspect of assessment. Adherence to prescribed medication is often important in the treatment of depression but it should be recognized that it can take between two and four weeks before clients begin to respond to the drugs.

In-patient stay

Psychoeducation is the organization of opportunities to discuss the causes of depression, the signs and symptoms, options for treatment or care, risks and benefits of anti-depressant treatment including possible side effects and expectations of response. Through better understanding of their experience of depression and its expected course, clients may become more involved and feel more in control in the care-planning and decision-making process. The nurse will continue to implement psychoeducational activities throughout the client's in-patient stay in order to build upon their understanding of the nature and course of action of the medication regime, symptom and side effect monitoring and management, and to promote adherence to medical treatment. The nurse may encourage the client to keep a diary of their experiences, engage them in therapeutic conversation, setting realistic goals and working at the client's pace throughout the stabilization phase of their illness.

The nursing interventions should take into account that medication can sometimes improve the severity of lack of energy or initiative, poor concentration, psychomotor slowing and suicidal or delusional thoughts that may have caused extreme dysfunction in daily living and impeded movement towards mental health or recovery. Clients should also be helped to identify their target symptoms or 'individual experiences' in order that they may monitor or gauge the effectiveness of medication. Monitoring for suicidal ideation and risk involves developing a suicide precaution plan that can indicate actions needed by both the client and nurse (Morgan, 1998; Ryan, 1999).

The need for structure, physical activity, regular nutritional meals, regular support and encouragement from the nurse and significant others is also part of the care package (Barker, 1992). To keep things simple (manageable) with the addition of a regular, predictable, sequential care package that works towards recovery can impart a sense of simplicity and order thereby promoting hope and behavioural change. There is a need for organization when working with the depressed client who may often be living in disarray, due to the illness and therefore their approach to treatment and life activities in general may be haphazard and chaotic. They need help in sorting out their internal emotional lives, interpersonal relationships and day-to-day living, as well as developing an individual approach to illness management and recovery (Barker, 1992).

The nurse should help or assist and support the client in formulating treatment priorities, dealing initially with symptoms, conditions, and behaviours that are life threatening and then progressing on to developing such attitudes and skills that will support long-term recovery and emotional growth. The nurse will need to help the client address any losses and in order to get well the client needs to find meaning in their life, realistic goals and perhaps new relationships (Klerman et al, 1984). The nurse will guide the client in the completion of a daily mood chart, encourage them to become active, e.g., have a brief walk and do one pleasurable activity each day, and recommend self-help workbooks for depression (Barker, 1993; Paterson & Bilsker, 2002).

Psychotherapy has been found to be an effective intervention for depression for motivated clients. The evidence of efficacy is greatest for structured, time-limited psychotherapies (Mago & Crits-Christoph, 1999; Quick, 1998), including cognitive behavioural therapy (Hawton et al, 1989) interpersonal therapy (Klerman et al, 1984) and problem-solving therapy (Mynors-Wallis et al, 2000). Walsh (1998) identifies a second phase termed 'dysthymic' where the interventions focus on interpersonal therapy and cognitive behavioural approaches. The goal of cognitive behavioural intervention is to develop better coping strategies by uncovering dysfunctional, distorted (or negative) thinking and supplanting it with more adaptive, rational thinking (Hawton et al, 1989). Medication may be useful in controlling the most severe, disabling and life-threatening symptoms. Teasdale et al (2002) also reinforces the nurses' use of 'mindfulness-based cognitive therapy', which places an emphasis on prevention of relapse or recurrence of major depression.

Discharge planning

The aim in discharge planning is to build upon the progress made during in-patient stay and work towards the treatment, prevention or management of recurrent depressive episodes (Mago, 1999). The nurse's focus will be on improving long-term outcomes for the client who is at risk of life-long and multiple recurrences which may be chronic and unremitting (Fava, 2002). There is an expectation that medication and interpersonal therapy will continue for six to nine months for clients who have experienced a major episode of depression and possibly longer for clients who are at risk of multiple episodes or relapse (Gortner et al, 1998; Reynolds et al, 1999). Walsh (1998) also point out the importance of establishing and developing community/social links as a buffer to stressful life events and the promotion of mental health and prevention of relapse into depression.

Bipolar disorder

Admission

In the acute in-patient unit the nurse is presented with an opportunity to facilitate the care co-ordination of the client with bipolar disorder commencing with biopsychosocial assessment of their unique experience and presentation of mood disorders including the family perspective (Dore & Romans, 2001). The nurse will collate data in their history of symptoms of mania, depression or mixed mood phases, the course of their illness, risks and recovery. The assessment should include recognition and identification of the acute phase and presence of depressive, hypomanic and manic features and the nature of disruption to psychosocial functioning and impairment to their quality of life. Also whether the client has a mixed or rapid-cycling state, psychotic features, risk of suicide, self-harm or aggression, substance use, social, financial and sexual risk-taking behaviours and the presence of cognitive or functional impairment, including current problems, mood, medication regime, suicide risk assessment and possible substance use.

Working comprehensively to diagnose and treat bipolar disorder is important in order to reduce the time a client may spend disordered before receiving a correct diagnosis and effective treatment (Sachs et al, 2000). The principle is that early diagnosis, effective treatment and finding the right medications can help the client avoid suicide, substance use, marital and work problems, treatment difficulties and incorrect, inappropriate or partial treatment.

The nurse will utilize evidence-based assessment tools; self-report strategies and diagnostic criteria. The Beck-Rafaelson Mania Scale and the Hamilton Depression Scale (Beck et al, 1979), which is sensitive to changes occurring during treatment, it has been found to be a particularly appropriate tool for nurses to use as a therapeutic evaluation instrument (Barker, 1997). The nurse can also educate and guide the client's use of a simple mood diary and course of illness chart to provide a longitudinal view of their symptoms and the course of their illness.

In-patient stay

The nurse's role during the acute phase of the illness involves supporting the stabilization of the mood, ensuring safety and understanding the client's pattern of mood symptoms and is critical to successful illness management. The nursing interventions include supporting psychopharmacotherapy and helping the client establish healthy social and biological rhythms.

During the continuation phase the nurse will support and monitor the client's continued use of diaries or charts to record mood for information to help the client and multidisciplinary team to understand their experience of bipolar disorder and bring together information such as mood state, medication levels and stressful events (Solomon et al, 1995). This information can inform decisions about the nature and level of intervention, i.e., medication regimes, diet, sleep, exercise, daily activities and life events. The nurse's understanding and skill in the delivery of psychosocial interventions including psychoeducational strategies, psychological therapies and psychosocial rehabilitation in the acute setting are crucial to positive client outcomes (Otto, 2002; Pollack, 1995). These include educating and supporting the client in the management of their experience of bipolar disorder by using a combination of strategies (Kusumakar et al, 1997), i.e., medication management, psychotherapy, personalized strategies and identifying support systems. Throughout the client's in-patient stay the nurse will continue to promote development of the client's insight into their experience of bipolar disorder and support the development of self/illness management, adherence to medication (Peralta & Cuesta, 1998) coping and problem-solving skills. The nurse will helping clients to explore their personal history, develop collaborative partnerships with professionals, set goals, manage medication, build a support system and develop strategies in order to maintain a healthy lifestyle, manage stress and cope with the illness when symptoms develop.

The nurse's establishment of a therapeutic alliance will utilize interpersonal and communication strategies for management of the client's bipolar presentation, for example, fluctuating mood swings, increase in energy levels, decreased need for sleep and possible psychotic symptoms such as hallucinations and delusions. The nurse may need to anticipate and intervene in the client's interactions with others, as they may become intrusive and inappropriate, with playful or pleasant mood changing abruptly to anger, irritation and verbal abusiveness. The client may also become involved in compulsive, risking activities and sexual behaviours (Ryan, 1999).

The continuity of contact time available to the nurse and client in the acute setting offers an opportunity to work collaboratively towards realistic, tangible and attainable goals in the long-term management of the client's illness. The nurse can instil hope and optimism promoting the client's coping and problem-solving skills, raise their esteem and alter their perception to help comprehend their illness and effectively self-manage it (Gournay, 1995). As with depression the nurse needs to maintain empathy, understanding and support for the client. Sometimes low self-esteem, guilt and fear are underlying dynamics for the symptoms of mania. Counselling must be supportive and empathic as well as directive and confrontative to help the client maintain a level of normality and social functioning as well as achieving recovery from debilitating episodes of the illness.

Discharge planning

At the time of discharge the nurse has a number of roles and functions in helping the client build upon the stabilization of symptoms and promotion of illness management strategies developed during the client's in-patient stay. This preventive and maintenance phase is where treatment planning consolidates the gains and focuses on the long-term prevention and management of future episodes. The plan will be to promote or contribute to the establishment of the client's long term stabilization and growth through education in relapse prevention/management and planning for optimal client functioning and care provision. For example, the nurse can assist the client and family members in the recognition of the early signs of relapse (relapse signatures) or situations where it may be necessary to adjust their medication or seek help. The nurse has had an opportunity to know a great deal about the client's mental state and coping strategies and to gain information about the role and experience of the family and to work in partnership with them, listening to their views and supporting them as necessary.

During the client's in-patient stay the nurse will have had opportunity to engage the family in the care planning process and will need to take into account that they also may need help or advice. A Sainsbury Centre survey ascertained the personal experience of families living with a person with bipolar disorder and found they often suffered some form of stress, anxiety or depression themselves from living with a person with bipolar disorder (Sainsbury Centre for Mental Health, 1994). The survey also Identified what was important to them and included access to professional services, 24 hours a day and seven days a week, information about the illness, opportunities to learn personal coping strategies, regular updates from professionals and more education about bipolar disorder.

The discharge planning should build upon the foundations established during in-patient care and will need to take into account the client and family's continual need for information about bipolar disorder, early detection and management of episodes and the formal and informal services available.

The nurse will inform the client and family of, and liaise with, the formal and informal services and support in the community, including day centres, day hospitals, drop-in or social clubs, therapy centres, sheltered work facilities, self-help groups and organizations.

Conclusion

Working with clients involves the nurse using a number of assessment and therapeutic interventions when trying to make combined therapy work, as discussed in this chapter. Although the focus of some debate, a number of excellent studies comparing psychotherapy or medications alone versus combination therapy have reported two important findings. First, the combination of psychotherapy and medication is better than either treatment alone (primarily in severely ill or chronic patients) and second, biological symptoms (e.g., sleep disturbance, agitation) generally respond better to medications, whereas psychological and interpersonal deficits are more effectively treated by psychotherapy (Barlow et al, 2000; Dewan & Pies, 2001; Keller et al, 2000). Therefore, the acute admission nurse needs to ensure that they keep themselves up-to-date with the latest discussions on assessment and interventions so that they can offer the best possible care to this vulnerable client group.

References

Agnes, T., Oetter, H. & Lam, R. W. (2002) Treatment of depression in primary care: part 1: principles of acute treatment, *British Columbia Medical Association*, 44(9), 473–8.

Akiskal, H., Huntouche, S., Bourgeois, M. L., Azorin, J. M., Sechter, D., Allilaire, J. F., Chatenet-Duchene, L. & Lancrenon, S. (2001) Toward a refined phenomenology of mania: combining clinician-assessment and self-report in the French EPIMAN study, *Journal of Affective Disorders*, 67, 89–96.

American Psychiatric Association (1994) *Diagnostic and Statistical Manual of Mental Disorders IV (DSM IV)*, Washington: American Psychiatric Association.

Anderson, J. & Adams, C. (1996) Family interventions in schizophrenia, *British Medical Journal*, 313(7056), 505–6.

Armstrong, E. (1998) The primary/secondary care interface, in C. Brooker & J. Repper (1998), *Serious Mental Health Problems in the Community: Policy, Practice and Research*, London: Balliere Tindall, Ch 5.

Barker, P. J. (1992) *Severe Depression: The Practitioners Guide*, London: Chapman & Hall.

Barker, P. J. (1993) *A Self-Help Guide to Managing Depression*, Cheltenham: Stanley Thornes.

Barker, P. J. (1997) *Assessment in Psychiatric and Mental Health Nursing: In Search of the Whole Person*, London: Stanley Thornes.

Barker, P. J. (ed) (1999) *Talking Cures: a Guide to the Psychotherapies for Health Care Professionals*, London: Nursing Times Books.

Barlow, D. H., Gorman, J. M., Shear, M. K. & Woods, S. W. (2000) Cognitive-behavioural therapy, imipramine, or their combination for panic disorder: a randomised controlled trial, *Journal of the American Medical Association*, 283(19), 2529–36.

Barrowclough, C. & Tarrier, N. (1997) *Families of Schizophrenic Patients: Cognitive Behavioural Interventions*, London: Stanley Thornes.

Beck, A. T., Weissman, A., Lester, D. & Trexler, L. (1974) The measurement of pessimism: the hopelessness scale, *Journal of Consulting and Clinical Psychology*, 42, 861–61.

Beck, A. T., Kovacs, M. & Weissman, A. (1979) Assessment of suicidal intention: The scale for suicidal ideation, *Journal of Consulting and Clinical Psychology*, 47, 2, 343–52.

Beck, A. T. (1976) *Cognitive Therapy and the Emotional Disorders*, New York: International Universities Press.

Beck, A. T., Ward, C. H. & Mendelson, M. et al (1961) An inventory for measuring depression, *Archives of General Psychiatry*, 4, 561–71.

Beck, A. T., Rush, A. J., Shaw, E. E. & Emery, G. (1979) *Cognitive Therapy of Depression: A Treatment Manual*, New York: Guilford Press.

Bellack, A., Morrison, R. & Mueser, D. (1989) Social problem solving in schizophrenia, *Schizophrenia Bulletin*, 18(1), 101–16.

Bennett, J., Done, J., Harrison-Read, P. & Hunt, B. (1995) Development of the rating scale/checklist to assess the side effects of antipsychotics by community psychiatric nurses, in C. Brooker & E. White (eds), *Community Psychiatric Nursing: A Research Perspective. Vol. 3*, London: Chapman and Hall.

Bhugra, D., Leff, J., Mallett, R., Der, G., Corridan, B. & Rudge, S. (1997) Incidence and outcome of schizophrenia in Whites, African Caribbeans and Asians in London, *Psychological Medicine*, 27, 791–8.

Birchwood, M. & Jackson, C. (2001) *Schizophrenia*, Hove, East Sussex: Psychology Press Ltd.

Birchwood, M. & Tarrier, N. (eds) (1994) *Psychological Management of Schizophrenia*, London: Wiley.

Birchwood, M., Smith, J., Macmillan, F. & McGovern, D. (1998) Early intervention in psychotic relapse, in C. Brooker & J. Repper (eds), *Serious Mental Health Problems in the Community: Policy, Practice and Research*, London: Balliere Tindall, ch 10.

Bowles, N., Dodds, P., Hackney, D., Sunderland, C. & Thomas, P. (2002) Formal observations and engagement: a discussion paper, *Journal of Psychiatric and Mental Health Nursing*, 9, 255–60.

Bowles, N., Dodds, P., Hackney, D. & Sunderland, C. (2003) Beyond observations, *Openmind*, 119, 18–19.

Brasfield, K. H. (1991) Practical psychopharmacologic consideration in depression, *Nursing Clinics of North America*, 26(3), 651–63.

British Psychological Society (2000) *Recent Advances in Understanding Mental Illness and Psychotic Experiences*, London: BPS.

Brooker, C. & Repper, J. (1998) *Serious Mental Health Problems in the Community, Policy, Practice and Research*, London: Balliere Tindall.

Campbell, P. (2003) Talking about my medication, *Openmind*, 119, 16–17.

Carpenter, J. & Sabaraini, S. (1996) Involving service users and carers in the care programme approach, *Journal of Mental Health*, 5(5), 483–8.

Chadwick, P. (1997) *Schizophrenia: The Positive Perspective*, London: Routledge.

Chadwick, P., Birchwood, M. & Trower, P. (1996) *Cognitive Therapy for Delusions, Voices and Paranoia*, London: Wiley.

Challiner, V. & Griffiths, P. (2000) Electro-convulsive therapy: a review of the literature, *Journal of Psychiatric and Mental Health Nursing*, 7, 191–8.

Cohcrane-Brink, K., Lofchy, J. & Sakinofsky, I. (2000) Clinical rating scales in suicide risk assessment, *General Hospital Psychiatry*, 22, 445–51.

Coultier, A., Entwistle, V. & Gilbert, D. (1999) Sharing decisions with patients: is the information good enough? *British Medical Journal*, 318, 318–22.

Crowther, R., Bond, G., Huxley, P. & Marshall, M. (2000) Vocational rehabilitation for people with severe mental disorder (protocol), *The Cochrane Library*, Issue 3, Oxford.

Dale, M., Dempsey, K., Ellis, J., O'Hare, J., Stanbury, C. & Stoddart, Y. (2002) *Getting Better – Together: Reflections on the Mental Health Collaborative*, Durham: Northern Centre for Mental Health.

Dawson, P. J. (1997) A personal reflection on the nature of somatic treatments and the implications for mental health nursing, *Journal of Advanced Nursing*, 26, 744–50.

Day, J. C., Wood, G., Dewey, M. & Bentall, R. P. (1995) A self-rating scale for measuring neuroleptic side-effects; validation in a group of schizophrenic patients, *British Journal of Psychiatry*, 166, 650–3.

De la Cour, J. (1995) Neuroleptic Malignant Syndrome: Do we know enough? *Journal of Advanced Nursing*, 21, 897–904.

Department of Health (1999a) *National Service Framework for Mental Health. Modern Standards and Service Models*, London: HMSO.

Department of Health (1999b) *Standing Nursing and Midwifery Advisory Committee SNMAC: Mental Health Nursing: Addressing Acute Concerns*, London: HMSO.

Department of Health (2000) *Effective Care Co-ordination in Mental Health Services – Modernising the Care Programme Approach. A Policy Booklet*, London: HMSO.

Department of Health (2001a) *The National Institute for Mental Health in England: Role and Function*, London: HMSO.

Department of Health (2001b) *The Journey to Recovery: The Government's Vision for Mental Health*, London: HMSO.

Department of Health (2001c) *Treatment Choice in Psychological Therapies and Counselling: Evidence Based Clinical Guideline*, London: HMSO.

Department of Health (2002a) *Mental Health Policy Implementation Guide – Adult Acute Inpatient Care Provision*, London: HMSO.

Department of Health (2002b) *Mental Health Policy Implementation Guide – Dual Diagnosis Good Practice Guide*, London: HMSO.

Department of Health (2002c) *Women's Mental Health: Into the Mainstream. Strategic Development of Mental Health Care for Women*, London: HMSO.

Department of Health (2002d) *Choosing Talking Therapies*, London: HMSO.

Dewan, M. J. & Pies, R. W. (2001) *The Difficult-To-Treat Psychiatric Patient*, Washington: American Psychiatric Publishing Inc.

Dodds, P. & Bowles, N. (2001) Dismantling formal observation and refocusing nursing activity in acute in-patient psychiatry – a case study, *Journal of Mental Health and Psychiatric Nursing*, 8, 183–8.

Dore, G. & Romans, S. E. (2001) Impact of bipolar affective disorder on family and partners, *Journal of Affective Disorders*, 67, 147–58.

Echternacht, M. R. (2001) Fluid group: concept and clinical application in the therapeutic milieu, *Journal of the American Psychiatric Nurses Association*, April 7, 39–44.

Egan, G. (2002) *The Skilled Helper*, (7th edn), Pacific Grove, CA: Brooks/Cole.

Fadden, G. (1998a) Family intervention in psychosis, *Journal of Mental Health*, 72, 115–22.

Fadden, G. (1998b) Family intervention, in C. Brooker & J. Repper (eds), *Serious Mental Health Problems in the Community: Policy, Practice and Research*, London: Balliere Tindall. ch 8.

Fava, M. (2002) Improving outcomes in the long-term treatment of depression: giving patients a choice, *Program and Abstracts of the American Psychiatric Association 155th Annual Meeting*; 18–23 May, Philadelphia, PA: ISS, 29.

Fox, J. & Conroy, P. (2000) Assessing clients' needs: the semi-structured interview, in C. Gamble & G. Brennan (eds), *Working with Serious Mental Illness*, London: Balliere Tindall.

Franklin J., Simmons J., Solovitz, B., Clemons, J. & Miller, G. (1986) Assessing quality of life of the mentally ill, *Evaluation and the Health Professions*, 9(3), 376–88.

Gamble, C. & Brennan, G. (eds) (2000) Assessments: a rationale and glossary of tools, in *Working with Serious Mental Illness*, London: Balliere Tindall.

Gardener, R., Owen, L. & Thompson, S. (1999) Compliance: the need for a fresh approach, *Mental Health Nursing*, 19(5), 18–22.

Gass, J. P. (1998) The knowledge and attitudes of mental health nurses to electro-convulsive therapy, *Journal of Advanced Nursing*, 27, 83–90.

Goldberg, D. & Williams, P. (1988) *A User's Guide to the General Health Questionnaire*, Windsor: NFER-Nelson.

Goldstein, M. (1995) Psychoeducation and relapse prevention, *International Clinical Psychopharrmacology*, Suppl. 5, 59–69.

Gortner, E. T., Gollan, J. K. & Dobson, K. S. et al (1998) Cognitive behavioural treatment for depression: relapse prevention, *Journal of Consulting and Clinical Psychology*, 66, 377–84.

Gournay, K. (1995) Mental health nurses working purposefully with people with serious and enduring mental illness: an international perspective, *International Journal of Nursing Studies*, 32(4), 341–52.

Gournay, K. (2000) Role of the community psychiatric nurse in the management of schizophrenia, *Advances in Psychiatric Treatment*, 6, 243–51.

Gournay, K., Birley, J. & Bennett, D. (1998) Therapeutic interventions and milieu in psychiatry in the NHS between 1948 and 1998, *Journal of Mental Health*, 7(3), 261–72.

Gournay, K., Ward, M., Wright, S. & Thornicroft, G. (1998) Crisis in the captial, *Mental Health Practice*, 1(5), 10–15.

Gray, R., Wykes, T. & Gournay, K. (2002) From compliance to concordance: a review of the literature on interventions to enhance compliance with antipsychotic medication, *Journal of Psychiatric and Mental Health Nursing*, 9, 277–84.

Hammen, C. (1997) *Depression*, Hove, East Sussex: Psychology Press.

Harmon, R. B. & Traatnack, S. A. (1992) Teaching hospitalised patients with serious persistent mental illness, *Journal of Psychosocial Nursing*, 143, 1551–6.

Hawton, K., Salkovskis, P. M., Kirk, J. & Clark, D. M. (1989) *Cognitive Behavioural Therapy for Psychiatric Problems: A Practical Guide*, London: Oxford Medical Publications.

Hayward, P., Chan, N., Kemp, R., Youle, S. & David, A. (1995) Medication self-management: a preliminary report on an intervention to improve medication compliance, *Journal of Mental Health*, 4, 511–17.

Heinrichs, D. W., Hanlon, T. E. & Carpenter, W. T. (1984) The quality of life scale: an instrument for rating the schizophrenic deficit syndrome, *Schizophrenia Bulletin*, 10, 388–98.

Holm, S. (1993) What is wrong with compliance? *Journal of Medical Ethics*, 19,108–10.

Holmes, T. H. & Rahe, R. H. (1967) The social readjustment rating scale, *Journal of Psychosomatic Research*, 11, 213–18.

Honigfeld, G. (1976) NOSIE: Nurses' observation scale for in-patient evaluation, in G. Honigfeld (ed.), *ACDEU Assessment Manual for Psychopharmacology*, Rockville, MD: National Institute of Mental Health.

Institute of Healthcare (2002) *Improvement Leader's Guide to Process Mapping, Analysis and Redesign*, London: Department of Health.

Jones, C., Cormac, I., Mota, J. & Campbell, C. (1998) *Cognitive Behaviour Therapy for Schizophrenia*, The Cochrane Library.

Kay, S. R., Opler, L. A. & Lindenmayer, J. P. (1988) Reliability and validity of the positive and negative syndrome scale for schizophrenics, *Psychiatry Research*, 23, 99–110.

Keller, M. B., McCullough, J. P., Klein, D. N. et al (2000) A comparison of Nefazodone, the cognitive behavioural-analysis system of psychotherapy, and their combination for the treatment of chronic depression, *New England Journal of Medicine*, 342(20), 1462–70.

Kellner, R. (1986) The brief depression rating scale, in N. Sartorius & T. A. Bans (eds), *Assessment for Depression*, New York: Springer Verlag.

Kemp, R., Hayward, P., Applewhaite, G., Everitt, B. & David, A. (1996) Compliance therapy in psychotic patients: randomised controlled trial, *British Medical Journal*, 312(10), 345–9.

Kingdon, D. G. & Turkington, D. (1994) *Cognitive-Behavioural Therapy of Schizophrenia*, Hove: The Guilford Press.

Klerman, G. L., Weissman, M. M., Rounsaville, B. J. & Chevron, E. S. (1984) *Interpersonal Psychotherapy of Depression*, USA: Basic Books.

Kusumakar, V., Yatham, L. N., Haslam, D. R. S., Parikh, S. V., Matte, R., Sharma, V., Silverstone, P. H., Kutcher, S. P. & Kennedy, S. (1997) The foundations of effective management of bipolar disorder, *Canadian Journal of Psychiatry*, 42, Suppl 2, 69S–73S.

Lam, D. (1991) Psychosocial family intervention in schizophrenia: a review of empirical studies, *Psychological Medicine*, 21, 423–41.

Leese, M., Johnson, S., Slade, M., Parkman, S., Kelly, M., Phelan, M. & Thornicroft, G. (1998) User perspective on needs and satisfaction with mental health services: PRISM psychosis study, *British Journal of Psychiatry*, 173, 409–15.

Leff, J. & Vaughan, C. (1985) *Expressed Emotions in Families: Its Significance for Mental Illness*, New York: Guildford Press.

Mago, R. & Crits-Christoph, P. (1999) Prevention of recurrent depression with cognitive behavioral therapy, *Archives of General Psychiatry*, 56(5), 479.

Martin, P. (2000) Hearing voices and listening to those that hear them, *Journal of Psychiatric and Mental Health Nursing*, 7, 135–41.

McNally, S. & Goldberg, J. (1997) Natural cognitive coping strategies in schizophrenia, *British Journal of Medical Psychology*, 70, 157–9.

Miller, W. R. & Rollnick, S. (2003) *Motivational Interviewing*, (2nd edn), London: Guilford Press.

Milner, J. & O'Bryne, P. (2002) *Brief Counselling: Narratives and Solutions*, Basingstoke: Palgrave Macmillan.

Mitchell, G. (1997) Depression in elderly people, *Elderly Care*, 9(1), 12–15.

Morgan, S. (1998) The assessment and management of risk, in C. Brooker & J. Repper (eds), *Serious Mental Health Problems in the Community: Policy, Practice and Research*, London: Balliere Tindall, ch 12.

Mynors-Wallis, L. M., Gath, K. H., Day, A. et al (2000) Randomised controlled trial of problem solving treatment, antidepressant medication, and combined treatment for major depression in primary care, *British Medical Journal*, 320, 26–30.

NHS Centre for Reviews and Dissemination (2000) Psychosocial Interventions for schizophrenia, *Effective Health Care*, 6(3), 1–8, York: University of York.

Nimeus, A., Alsen, M. & Traskmas-Benz, L. (2000) The suicide assessment scale: an instrument assessing suicide risk of suicide attempters, *European Psychiatry*, 15, 416–23.

O'Boyle, C. (1994) The schedule for the evaluation of individual quality of life, *International Journal of Mental Health*, 23(3), 3–23.

Oliver, N., Carson, J., Missenden, K., Towey, A., Dunn, L., Collins, E. & Holloway, F. (1996) Assessing the quality of life of the long-term mentally ill: a comparative study of two measures, *International Journal of Methods in Psychiatric Research*, 6, 161–6.

Otto, M. W. (2002) Update on psychosocial treatments of bipolar disorder, *Program and Abstracts of the American Psychiatric Association 155th Annual Meeting*, 18–23 May, Philadelphia: PA.

Overall, J. & Gorman, D. (1962) The brief psychiatric rating scale, *Psychological Reports*, 10, 799–812.

Paterson, R. & Bilsker, D. (2002) *Self-Care Depression Programme: Patient Guide*, Vancouver: Vancouver University of British Columbia, online at: http://www.mheccu.ubc.ca/publications/scdp/patientguide.pdf

Pekkala, E. & Merinder, L. (2000) Psychoeducational interventions for schizophrenia and other severe mental illness (Cochrane Review), *The Cochrane Library*, Issue 3, Oxford.

Peplau, H. E. (1988) *Interpersonal Relations in Nursing*, Basingstoke: Macmillan, now Palgrave Macmillan.

Peralta, V. & Cuesta, M. J. (1998) Lack of insight in mood disorders, *Journal of Affective Disorders*, 49, 55–8.

Perkins, R. & Repper, J. (1999) Compliance or informed choice? *Journal of Mental Health*, 8(2), 117–29.

Perry, A., Tarrier, N., Morris, R., McCarthy, E. & Limb, K. (1999) Randomised controlled trial of efficacy of teaching patients with bipolar disorder to identify early symptoms of relapse and obtain treatment, *British Medical Journal*, 318, 149–53.

Pharoah, F., Mari, J. & Striener, D. (1999) Family intervention for schizophrenia (Cochrane Review), *The Cochrane Library*, Issue 3, Oxford.

Pilling, S., Orbach, G., Connaughton, J., Nicol, M. & Bebbington, P. (2000) *Social Skills Programmes for Schizophrenia* (Cochrane Review), *The Cochrane Library*, Issue 3, Oxford.

Pollack, L. E. (1995) Treatments of in-patients with bipolar disorders: a role for self-management groups, *Journal of Psychosocial Nursing*, 31(1), 11–16.

Pratt, P. (1998) The administration and monitoring of neuroleptic medication, in C. Brooker & J. Repper (eds), *Serious Mental Health Problems in the Community: Policy, Practice and Research*, London: Balliere Tindall, ch 11.

Quick, E. (1998) Doing what works in brief and intermittent therapy, *Journal of Mental Health*, 7(5), 527–33.

Repper, R. E. & Perkins, J. M. (1996) *Working Alongside People with Long-term Mental Health Problems*, London: Chapman & Hall.

Reynolds, C. F., Frank, E., Perel, J. M. et al (1999) Nortriptyline and interpersonal psychotherapy as maintenance therapies for recurrent major depression: a randomised controlled trial in patients older than 59 years, *Journal of American Medical Association*, 281, 39–45.

Rush, A. J., Giles, D. E., Schlesser, M. S. et al (1986) The inventory for depressive symptomology (IDS): preliminary findings, *Psychiatry Research*, 18, 65–87.

Ryan, T. (1999) *Managing Crisis and Risk in Mental Health Nursing*, Cheltenham: Stanley Thornes.

Rycroft-Malone, J., Lattes, S., Yerrell, P. & Shaw, D. (2000) Nursing and medication, *Nursing Standard*, 14(50), 35–9.

Sachs, G. S., Printz, D. J., Kahn, D. A., Carpenter, D. & Docherty, J. P. (2000) *The Expert Consensus Guideline Series: Medication Treatment of Bipolar Disorder*, A Postgraduate Medicine Special Report. April 2000. The McGraw-Hill Companies, Inc.

Sainsbury Centre for Mental Health (1994) *Perspectives on Manic Depression*, London: Sainsbury Centre for Mental Health.

Sainsbury Centre for Mental Health (1998) *Acute Problems. A Survey of the Quality of Care in Acute Psychiatric Wards*, London: Sainsbury Centre for Mental Health.

Searle, G. (1998) Optimising neuroleptic treatment in psychotic illness, *Psychiatric Bulletin*, 22, 548–51.

Sharkey, V. B. (1997) Sexuality, sexual abuse: Ommisions in admissions?, *Journal of Advanced Nursing*, 25, 1025–32.

Sharkey, V. B. (2002) Perspectives of collaboration/non-collaboration in a mental health in-patient setting, *Journal of Psychiatric and Mental Health Nursing*, 9, 49–55.

Smith, J. & Birchwood, M. (1993) The needs of high and low expressed emotion families: a normative approach, *Social Psychiatry & Psychiatric Medicine*, 28, 11–16.

Smith, J., Hughes, I. & Budd, R. (1999) Non-compliance with anti-psychotic depot medication: user's views on advantages and disadvantages, *Journal of Mental Health*, 8(3), 287–96.

Solomon, D. A., Keitner, G. I., Miller, I. W. et al (1995) Course of illness and maintenance treatment for patients with bipolar disorder, *Journal of Clinical Psychiatry*, 5(1), 105–13.

Speedy, S. (1999) The therapeutic alliance, in M. Clinton & S. Nelson (eds), *Advanced Practice in Mental Health Nursing*, Oxford: Blackwell Science, ch 4.

Teasdale, J. D., Segal, Z. V., Williams, J. M. et al (2002) Prevention of relapse/recurrence in major depression by mindfulness-based cognitive therapy, *Journal of Consulting and Clinical Psychology*, 68, 615–23.

Thomas, P. (1997) *The Dialectics of Schizophrenia*, London: Free Association Books.

Tyrer, P. & Steinberg, D. (1999) *Models for Mental Disorder*, (3rd edn), Chichester: John Wiley & Sons.

United Kingdom Central Council (1999) *Fitness for Practice: the Report of the UKCC Commission for Nursing and Midwifery Education*, London: UKCC.

Walsh, J. (1998) The clinical case management of clients with major depression, *Journal of Case Management*, 7(2), 53–61.

Walsh, E., Harvey, K., White, I., Fraser, J., Higgitt, A. & Murray, R. (2001) Suicidal behaviour in psychosis: Prevalence and predictors from a randomised controlled trial of case management: Report from the UK700 trial, *British Journal of Psychiatry*, 178, 255–60.

Watkins, P. (2001) *Mental Health Nursing: The Art of Compassionate Care*, London: Butterworth Heinemann.

World Health Organization (1992) *The ICD-10 Classification of Mental and Behavioural Disorders*, Geneva: WHO.

Wright, H. & Giddey, M. (eds) (1993) *Mental Health Nursing: From First Principles to Professional Practice*, Cheltenham: Stanley Thornes.

Zubin, J. (1989) Suiting therapeutic interventions to the scientific models of aetiology, *British Journal of Psychiatry*, 155, 5–14.

CHAPTER 23

Assertive Community Treatment with People Experiencing Serious Mental Illness

MIKE FLEET

Indicative Benchmark Statements

▓ Practice in accordance with an ethical and legal framework which ensures the primacy of patient and client interest and well-being, and respects confidentiality

▓ Facilitation of therapeutic co-operation with mental health service users and their carers, taking account of those nurses find difficult to engage

▓ The application of helping relationships as the cornerstone of their mental health nursing practice

▓ Retrieval and critical appraisal of mental health research and relevant evidence

▓ Create and utilize opportunities to promote the health and well-being of patients, clients and groups

Introduction

Assertive outreach is entrenched as part of UK Government policy (DoH, 1999, 2000, 2001). In essence assertive outreach is a way of engaging services with clients that cannot, or do not wish to, engage with services. Despite all the hype and political rhetoric assertive outreach is not a treatment in its own right; it is simply a vehicle by which evidence-informed treatment packages can be offered to clients. One major aspect of the assertive outreach movement is Assertive Community Treatment (hereafter referred to as ACT).

The historical perspective

The history of ACT is closely linked with the advent of the hegemony of neuroleptic medication but has definite links to the concept of biopsychosocial interventions. The 1950s saw the synthesis of chlorpromazine, enabling pharmaceutical intervention that enabled some clients to live lives closer to those of the general population. With the further advent of depot medication clients were enabled to leave hospital and not require frequent supervised administration of oral medication. In the 1960s this facilitated a move to de-hospitalization and de-institutionalization. Unfortunately this lead to failure in the USA owing to the disjointed healthcare system (Intagliata, 1982; Talbott et al, 1987). Various experiments were undertaken, with the common theme being the concept of a 'systems agent' to steer the client through the system. One such experiment was the 'Training in Community Living Program' (Stein & Test, 1980).

The 'Training in Community Living Program' developed in Madison, Wisconsin during the 1970s as an alternative to mental hospital treatment, is widely accepted as the first model of assertive community treatment. The programme aims were to enhance clients' ability to live in the community, decreasing time spent in institutions. Additionally the programme focused on decreasing symptoms and increasing both self-esteem and quality of life. These aims were met by the team assuming responsibility for helping the client to meet their needs, such as material essentials, and assist in the acquiring of the coping skills necessary to meet the demands of community living; and developing the motivation to persevere with the complexities of everyday life with freedom from pathologically dependent relationships. These aims were achieved through support and by the education of significant others. There was an expectation that the clinician would be assertive in delivering care and be responsible for the co-ordination of interagency care. Thus ensuring that care becomes client needs led as opposed to service led.

In order to meet these goals substantial human resources were committed to provide whatever assistance people needed in order to live in the community, e.g. assisting with securing accommodation, finding employment, budgeting, shopping, and personal care. Services were provided in two shifts, with one staff member being on call at night, seven days a week. The outcome of the programme being reduced readmission rates. The Training in Community Living Program eventually evolved into the Program of Assertive Community Treatment (PACT), a fairly standardized service, popular in the United States (Phillips et al, 2001).

Outside of the United States similar programmes included the Community Treatment Team model (Hoult et al, 1981) in Australia and the Daily Living Programme in the UK (Marks et al, 1994). Today ACT as a system of care, although not available universally to those who might benefit from it, is being promoted as standard practice globally; there are adaptations implemented in Europe, Canada and Australasia (Phillips et al, 2001).

ACT principles are being employed in several service areas. In the establishment and development of general community mental health teams and services targeting groups such as those with recent onset of illness, concurrent drug related problems and mental illness, the homeless, forensic or hard to engage clients (Burns, 2001). Burns (2001) goes on to suggest that the UK is awash with outreach programmes, from both the statutory as well as the voluntary sectors. Unfortunately, voluntary sector teams, although engaging well with clients and increasing user satisfaction, usually have very little influence over admission and discharge of their clients, with increased hospital bed costs and mixed clinical and social outcomes (Minghella et al, 2002).

Definition of ACT

There has been much confusion over terms in case management, of which ACT is a type. On the whole there is a continuum of case management between service brokerage and clinical case management. Between these two pure positions the role of the 'systems agent' differs.

In service brokerage the systems agent acts as an 'enabler', providing a co-ordinator function by brokering services. The agent is usually office based, focusing on the organization and its co-ordination on behalf of the client, acting as a referrer to other services, but providing little or no direct clinical service to the client. This, therefore, enables the systems agent to provide a co-ordination service for a large number of people.

On the other hand, the role of the systems agent in clinical case management, the clinical case manager, is concerned with all aspects of the client's physical and social environment: housing, psychiatric treatment, physical health care, financial benefits, transportation, families and social networks. On the whole clinical case management compares favourably with service brokerage (Marshall et al, 1995), depending upon the target client group. The brokerage model relies heavily on the motivation of the client to engage with a significant number of service agencies. The clinical case management model minimizes the number of agencies with which the client needs to engage. Thereby keeping lines of communication narrow and minimizing avoidable loss of contact between services and the client.

In order to differentiate between brokerage and clinical case management and, therefore, the role of the systems agents, Thornicroft (1991), considered 12 axes of case management functions. Owing to the multifaceted nature of the provision of mental health and social care, it is very rarely that a practice area can claim to be following, perfectly, a brokerage or clinical case management model. The use of the axes facilitates determination as to what extent a practice area could be said to be using a service brokerage or a clinical case management model. These axes consider elements of working practice including if there is individual rather than team management of a 'caseload', direct care versus brokerage, staff to client ratio and the point of contact between client and services, whether home or clinic for example.

There is a widening acceptance that clinical case management is synonymous with ACT (Burns, 1997), which is particularly problematic given that ACT is frequently compared and contrasted with variations of clinical case management. There is considerable variation between ACT programmes and some disagreement on the components that are critical to success (Mueser et al, 1998; Schaedle, 1999). However, services share common features:

- Services are targeted at the 'heavy service users', those people with serious mental illness.
- Treatment and support services are individualized and provided directly by the ACT team members rather than brokered to external agencies.
- 'Outreach' services are provided where problems occur, in the least restrictive setting possible; in the person's home or other community setting rather than in hospital or clinic settings.
- The staff to client ratio is small (between 1 to 10 and 1 to 15) with team members sharing responsibility for the individual clients.
- To be truly faithful to the ACT model, services are available 24 hours per day. It must be remembered that ACT originally began in the USA where the health care system is radically different from the UK. Given that the UK has a nationwide system of General Practitioners, Accident and Emergency departments, most with access to liaison psychiatry staff, and each providing a 24 hour service, the need for ACT teams in the UK to provide 24 hour services is open to debate. Should, in fact, political expediency be allowed to dictate services for which there is no clinical need?
- Clients are contacted frequently (usually more than weekly) and engagement is assertive, in which the client is contacted even if ambivalent or negative.
- Services are provided for as long as support or treatment is required.

The benefits of ACT

Assertive Community Treatment is one of the most well evaluated and documented non-medication mental health interventions. However, this evidence is mixed and dependent on the definitions of the terms ACT, case management or care management under consideration.

Several substantial reviews of ACT have been undertaken. The recent Cochrane Review (Marshall & Lockwood, 2001) concluded that compared to standard community care people allocated to ACT were:

- more likely to remain in contact with services;
- less likely to be admitted to hospital and when admitted spend less time in hospital;

- more likely to be living independently;
- more likely to have found employment; and
- more satisfied with the service they receive.

It also showed that ACT is a more attractive way of working for professionals There were no differences between ACT and control treatments on mental state or social functioning (Marshall & Lockwood, 2001). In contrast the Cochrane Review examining ACT in addition to other forms of case management for people with severe mental illness was less positive (Marshall et al, 2001). The review found that case management approximately doubled the rate of hospital admissions with little evidence of improvement in mental state, social functioning or quality of life. It concluded that: 'case management is . . . of questionable value . . . it is doubtful whether it should be offered by community psychiatric services. It is hard to see how policy makers who subscribe to an evidence-based approach can justify retaining case management as "the cornerstone" of community mental health care.'

While Cochrane reviews are very useful, and highly regarded in terms of 'hard evidence', they do have very stringent criteria for those research activities included in the review. Ziguras and Stuart (2000) undertook a meta-analysis of controlled trials examining the effectiveness of case management over 20 years and had a more liberal approach to study inclusion than the Cochrane Review. Ziguras and Stuart examined 44 studies, nine of which directly compared ACT with clinical case management and 35 compared ACT *or* clinical case management with 'standard' treatment. Both types of case management were found to:

- reduce family burden;
- reduce the overall cost of care;
- reduce symptoms;
- increase client contact with services and reduce dropout rates; and
- improve social functioning.

Improved satisfaction with services and quality of life has also been found by Huxley and Warner (1992). Ziguras and Stuart (2000) found that, while clinical case management increased the frequency of hospitalization, it decreased the total number of hospital days. The obvious inference being, increased contact between professionals and clients resulted in the earlier detection of serious relapse, hence the increased admission rate, with subsequent reduced duration of stay.

There is little doubt that ACT is helpful in reducing hospitalization, improving housing stability, and possibly contributes to modest improvements in quality of life and symptomatology. However, the research evidence does not make clear what elements of ACT contribute to improvements or whether or not improvements are sustained over time once ACT services are withdrawn (Mueser et al, 1998). Successful ACT programmes described in the literature have often been implemented as part of well-resourced and planned integrated services. For example, Hambridge and Rosen (1994) described a reduction of 62 per cent in bed occupancy by clients referred to a newly developed team in Sydney, Australia. This service was also part of an integrated programme that included supervised accommodation and residential rehabilitation, a transitional work programme, two community mental health centres with 24-hour mobile crisis services and living skills centres.

On the whole a purist approach to ACT appears only possible if the setting is exactly the same as for the original Wisconsin team. ACT must invariably be adapted to the specific needs of communities, geographical settings and adapted to the presence, or absence, of additional services. Very little research has been undertaken examining how ACT fits in to a wider integrated service, such as is the norm in the UK.

The UK has been slower to adopt ACT. Results of a recent random controlled trial of ACT in the UK have been less impressive than elsewhere. Burns et al (1999) compared to standard case management (case load between 1 to 30 and 1 to 35) and to intensive case management (case load between 1 to 10 and 1 to 15) at four sites. They reported no significant gains in clinical or social functioning in either group at one or two years, and no significant difference in hospital use between groups. However, the study was flawed in the respect of medical input and control, some sites had single consultant responsibility for all the clients in the research group while in other areas the responsibility was spread across several consultants. A recent study (Jones, 2002), suggests that it is not resources such as the low staff to client ratio that is effective, 'but rather a cohesive, focussed team approach.'

Case Study 23.1   Frankie

Frankie had a diagnosis of paranoid schizophrenia. He had a long history of contact with the mental health services, including several admissions after being involved in violent incidents, on more than one occasion threatening a flatmate and others with a knife. Each violent incident had been preceded by abstinence from medication, including depot medication.

After his last admission Frankie was prescribed Clozapine, which he was eager to take to improve the symptoms of his illness. Unfortunately, owing to his chaotic lifestyle and forgetfulness, Frankie was unable to administer his medication unsupervised. By offering daily visits, including weekends, it was possible for Frankie to self-administer his Clozapine and remain well. Naturally, this could not always be done by the Keyworker, they have days off, annual leave, and God forbid, sick days. By developing a cohesive team approach, Frankie could be visited by people with whom he had developed a relationship, even though not at the depth he had developed with his keyworker.

A later study (Burns et al, 2000) examining effects of caseload size concluded that: 'UK standard care contains many of the characteristics of assertive outreach services and differences in outcome may require that greater attention be paid to delivering evidence-based interventions.'

Model fidelity

There is some evidence that programmes more faithful to the ACT model have superior outcomes (McGrew et al, 1994; McHugo et al, 1999; Teague et al, 1998). A measure of model fidelity has been developed, the Dartmouth Assertive Community Treatment Scale (Teague et al, 1998). This measure considers several factors which are indicative of high fidelity in an ACT team, factors categorized into staffing/resources, organizational and services.

Staffing and resources: small, shared caseload (ten or fewer clients per case manager with 90 per cent or more of clients having contact with more than one staff member in a given week. Team meetings at least four times per week. There is a practicing team leader, leading a team operating at 95 per cent or more staffing levels with less than 20 per cent staff turnover in two years. In addition, there is a psychiatrist, substance abuse specialist and vocational specialist on staff.

Organizationally there should be explicit admission criteria and a low intake rate. The team has full responsibility for treatment services, crisis services (24 hr coverage) and hospital admissions (initiating 95 per cent of admissions). The team also has responsibility for discharge planning (planning jointly 95 per cent of discharges) and no time limit on services.

The services themselves should be in vivo (80 per cent of service time in the community) with a no dropout policy (95 per cent retention over 12 months) with assertive engagement. The services should be as much as is needed (2 hours or more per week) with frequent contact (on average four or more times per week). Working with the client's support system and offering individualized substance abuse treatment and dual disorder treatment groups. Ideally service users are employed as members of the treatment team.

Most programmes that would claim to be ACT services deviate from these specifications in some way. Burns et al (2001) suggest that a significant influence of national culture is evident both in the acceptability of case management and in approaches to researching and undertaking case management. While these specifications are important, authors disagree on the relative importance of different components (McGrew & Bond, 1995; Schaedle & Epstein, 2000). For example, 24 hour care by a dedicated team may be an expensive luxury and duplication of service when alternative crisis services are available. In early implementations of ACT avoidance of office or clinic visits was pursued pedantically, however avoidance of office visits may be better thought of as an outcome of assertive outreach, rather than an end in itself. The need to have one team member as a co-ordinator and a team approach are often considered important structural elements of ACT programmes (McGrew & Bond, 1995).

Target client group

From its conception ACT has targeted those perceived as having the most intractable symptoms of serious mental illness, the highest level of functional impairment and hence a big drain on in-patient and community resources; the 'heavy service user'. Kent et al (1995) describe the heavy service user as the 10 to 30 per cent of clients who use 50 to 80 per cent of resources. While primarily aimed at the 'difficult to engage' client, some teams accept referrals from general practitioners and even self-referral. Why then is 'engagement' important?

The goal of engagement is to form a trusting relationship or working alliance that will enable the worker to support the client through treatment. Engagement in treatment may take place if the client sees that affiliation with the team can be of benefit. There are a number of interventions that may aid the process of engagement: practical assistance, empathic interviewing (Miller & Rollnick, 1991), crisis intervention, forming an alliance with the family or other social network members; and ensuring that legal constraints are sensible (Sainsbury Centre for Mental Health, 1998). The relationship is initially built on helping the client to achieve ends that he or she identifies as important.

Why then do clients not engage with services? There can be several factors including: poor past history of service contact, personality disorder, racism, dual diagnosis and/or lack of trust. And, why do services not engage with clients? Again there are several factors including dual diagnosis, personality disorder, past history and services not being available.

Evidence-based interventions in ACT

ACT is not a treatment in its own right, but rather a vehicle by which evidence-informed treatment packages can be offered to clients. Treatment packages could include such approaches as psychosocial interventions and/or medication management. Psychosocial interventions are not merely a collection of tools and skills to employ with those experiencing serious and enduring mental health problems. These interventions demand of the practitioner an attitude that places the client or the carer at the centre of all interventions, developing and maintaining a collaborative partnership, a real partnership as opposed to merely giving lip-service to the concept. There are several assumptions upon which psychosocial interventions are based and several components of these interventions. While psychosocial interventions is an umbrella term, a cognitive–behavioural orientation is the pole that supports the umbrella.

The assumptions of psychosocial interventions include:

- acceptance of a stress/vulnerability model for symptoms;
- medication is an accepted therapy;

- development of a positive working alliance between the therapist and the client and/or family;
- most, if not all, intervention sessions held at the client's home;
- emphasis on psychoeducation;
- cognitive–behavioural orientation with emphasis on practical day-to-day issues;
- interventions maintained over a period of time or in the context of an ongoing service; and
- service users are coping to their best possible level given their current resources.

While the components of psychosocial interventions are:

- engagement;
- assessment;
- psychoeducation;
- social skills training;
- coping strategy enhancement;
- cognitive–behaviour approaches to delusions and hallucinations;
- working with families; and
- medication adherence work.

Supporting the employment of psychosocial interventions is the use of neuroleptic medication. Medication is *the* major evidence-based practice. There is more evidence of the efficacy or otherwise of medication within mental health than any other intervention. Non-adherence to treatment regimes may be for many reasons, one of which may be simply the complexity of the regime. A major factor within ACT is the ability and resources to maintain daily supervised medication as well as the development of a collaborative relationship to enable the worker to support the client during psychopharmacological interventions.

Case Study 23.2   Jasper

Jasper, a middle-aged man of non-European origin, has had admissions to hospital on a twice-yearly basis for nearly ten years. Each admission was compulsory, under a section of the Mental Health Act (1983). During hospital admissions Jasper would develop a relationship with his keyworker from the CMHT. On discharge from hospital he would then refuse contact with his keyworker, or when he did allow contact he was mute and aloof.

During a formal admission to hospital he was referred to an ACT team. During in-reach sessions Jasper, again, developed a relationship with Hector, his keyworker from the ACT team. During this 'honeymoon' period Hector discovered information from Jasper that he had an interest in fishing that he had never been able to fulfil and it would be difficult to fulfil in a large urban conurbation. Hector offered to take Jasper and his friend on a fishing trip to the coast. This trip enabled Jasper and Hector to engage at a more human level than the simple professional level previously encountered. This relationship was further developed by *in vivo* collaborative working, allowing Hector to spend time with Jasper discussing early warning signs of relapse in his illness. This discussion facilitated Hector in offering pharmacological intervention at an early and effective time. Where this intervention did not work, the relationship enabled Jasper to initiate his own hospital admission, on a non-compulsory basis with the result of increased self-esteem for Jasper and admissions of a much shorter duration.

Ethical issues in ACT

The nature of ACT work brings to the fore many ethical considerations and dilemmas. Conflicts can arise between autonomy and beneficence; between beneficence and nonmaleficence, and between nonmaleficence to the individual and nonmaleficence to the community (Stovall, 2001).

Autonomy has been defined as: 'the capacity to think, decide and act on the basis of such thought and decision freely and independently and without let or hindrance' (Gillon, 1985). Respect for autonomy involves regarding clients as persons entitled to the same basic rights as everyone else; the right to know, the right to privacy and the right to receive care and treatment (Thompson et al, 1994). Autonomy refers to an individual's ability to reach his or her own decisions and requires practitioners to respect those decisions. However, this respect can come into conflict when considering the roles and duties that society expects and demands of mental health professionals. Respect for autonomy and the right to consent or refuse treatment is a widely accepted value in health care. While clients have the right to have any proposed treatment including risks and alternatives clearly explained to them, this is only possible if the client is in sufficient appropriate contact with services to have these elements explained.

Beneficence implies the duty to do good and maximize good. It obliges that professionals help clients by promoting and safeguarding their health and welfare. Therefore, placing a burden on professionals to utilize evidence-informed interventions to decrease the harm that mental illness can cause. The concept of beneficence obliges the professional in ACT Teams to maximize good, respect for autonomy obliges the professionals to support the client's decisions. However an individual can only be truly autonomous if they have the fullest of information. ACT teams can provide this information only if they can be in contact with a client. The information a client needs to make an informed decision changes over time and with the change in circumstances. Only by being in regular contact can the team and the individual assess what information a client needs to know to make an informed decision.

Ethical problems are common to mental health care generally but are more problematic in ACT owing to the persistence of assertive outreach. ACT is more intrusive than hospital or clinic-based services in which people may exercise their autonomy by deciding to disengage from services, or not to attend appointments. Control over medication and finances are often of immense concern to people with serious mental illness, the same as anyone else, and problems can result in hospitalization or homelessness (Stovall, 2001).

ACT can impinge on the autonomy of clients. The American experience, the Program of Assertive Community Treatment (PACT) in the US has faced considerable opposition from anti-psychiatry groups. One group compares PACT with the Trojan horse: 'This "wraparound" service, as it's sometimes called, looks pretty on the outside, but inside you can find a lot of "medication militia" hiding out' (Support Coalition International, 2001).

In ACT work the emphasis can be upon medication compliance and symptom monitoring. While these are fundamental evidence-based practices, this emphasis can give rise to a paternalistic approach to care (Spindel & Nugent, 2001). When the biomedical formulation of problems becomes the sole focus of ACT, benevolent paternalism can be viewed as malevolent. The concept of non-maleficence imposes the duty to do no harm or to minimize harm. This requires that the professional refrains from doing anything that could be detrimental to others. But does this merely cover non-maleficence to the client or does it extend to the community as a whole? Are the two mutually exclusive?

Psychiatry can be (and has been) seen to have a social control function (Lakeman & Curzon, 1997), in ACT services this can create tension between the team's allegiance to the client, their family and to wider society. One tacit goal of psychiatric treatment is to minimize the risks posed to society by the client's behaviour. It is likely that those referred to ACT teams are more likely to pose a risk to themselves or others when relapsed, have tenuous community tenure, be unemployed, have had multiple admissions to hospital and experience social exclusion. Solomon et al (1994) suggest that case management could degenerate into providing merely a monitoring service rather than rehabilitation and thereby increase re-hospitalization.

There is a suggestion of boundary setting as a feature of ACT (Neale & Rosenheck, 2000). This boundary setting needs to be balanced with the provision of care; professionals balancing societal, familial and client demands and interests in their day-to-day work.

As we have seen, assertive outreach, a major feature of ACT, is high on the political agenda. The resources, both human and time, necessary to engage those clients labelled as 'difficult to engage' are available to an ACT Team. However, engagement is merely a vehicle by which evidence-based interventions can made available to clients. While engagement is a worthy goal, it is a fairly short-term goal. Without the long-term goal of delivering evidence-based interventions to the client, engagement could be viewed as a waste of resources.

The right to consent to, or refuse, treatment is a basic value in health care, and a basic human right. In order to ensure that consent is truly informed a number of issues have to be considered such as the benefits and costs of any intervention and what may happen if the intervention is not undertaken. Without this knowledge the client cannot give informed consent. Surely, without this knowledge the client cannot give informed refusal.

Conclusion

ACT is a well-evaluated mental health intervention and the benefits are well-documented, such as benefits to individual clients with improved quality of life and reduced hospital stays and the benefits to service structures by reducing in-patient costs and benefits to workers with an increased satisfaction in their working practice. The success or failure of ACT will depend to a large degree on the target client group. A primary function of ACT is assertive outreach.

The role of assertive outreach is to engage with clients. The primary role of engagement is to enable the worker to support the client through evidence-based interventions. Therefore there must be evidence-based interventions that can be offered to the target client. Is this possible? A resounding 'YES' in the case of serious mental illness, and a guarded 'probably not yet' in the case of personality disorder.

Despite the political agenda, assertive outreach and ACT are not treatments in their own right, they are merely vehicles by which evidence-based interventions can be *offered* to clients. This implies the client can accept, or decline, these interventions. Legally the client must give informed consent to undertake any interventions. Ethical considerations demand that for consent to be informed the client must be made aware of several elements. ACT offers the client the opportunity to be aware of these elements thus making the client's decision to accept *or* decline the interventions truly informed.

References

Burns, T. (1997) Case management, care management and care programming, *British Journal of Psychiatry*, 170, 393–5.

Burns, T. (2001) To outreach or not to outreach, *Journal of Forensic Psychiatry*, 12(1), 13–17.

Burns, T., Creed, F., Fahy, T., Thompson, S., Tyrer, P. & White, I. (1999). Intensive versus standard case management for severe psychotic illness: a randomised trial, UK 700 Group, *Lancet*, 353(9171), 2185–9.

Burns, T., Fiander, M., Kent, A., Ukoumunne, O. C., Byford, S., Fahy, T. & Kumar, K. R. (2000) Effects of caseload size on the process of care of patients with severe psychotic illness, Report from the UK 700 Trial, *British Journal of Psychiatry*, 177, 427–33.

Burns, T., Fioritti, A., Holloway, F., Malm, U. & Rossler, W. (2001) Case management and assertive community treatment in Europe, *Psychiatric Services*, 52(5), 631–6.

Department of Health (1999) *National Service Framework for Mental Health: Modern Standards and Service Models*, London: HMSO.

Department of Health (2000) *NHS Plan*, London: HMSO.

Department of Health (2001) *The Mental Health Policy Implementation Guide*, London: HMSO.

Gillon, R. (1985) *Philosophical Medical Ethics*, Chichester: John Wiley.

Hambridge, J. A. & Rosen, A. (1994) Assertive community treatment for the seriously mentally ill in suburban Sydney: a programme description and evaluation, *Australian & New Zealand Journal of Psychiatry*, 28(3), 438–45.

Hoult, J., Reynolds, I., Charbonneau-Powis, M., Coles, P. & Briggs, J. (1981) A controlled study of psychiatric hospital versus community treatment – the effect on relatives, *Australian & New Zealand Journal of Psychiatry*, 15(4), 323–8.

Huxley, P. & Warner, R. (1992) Case management, quality of life, and satisfaction with services of long-term psychiatric patients, *Hospital & Community Psychiatry*, 43(8), 799–802.

Intagliata, J. (1982) Improving the quality of community care for the chronically mentally disabled: the role of case management, *Schizophrenia Bulletin*, 8(4), 655–74.

Jones, A. (2002) Assertive community treatment: development of the team, selection of clients, and impact on length of hospital stay, *Journal of Psychiatric and Mental Health Nursing*, 9, 261–70.

Kent, S., Fogarty, M. & Yellowlees, P. (1995) A review of studies of heavy users of psychiatric services, *Psychiatric Services*, 46(12), 1247–53.

Lakeman, R. & Curzon, B. (1997) Society, disturbance and mental illness, in P. Barker & B. Davidson (eds), *Ethical Strife*, London: Arnold, 26–38.

Marks, I. M., Connolly, J., Muijen, M., Audini, B., McNamee, G. & Lawrence, R. E. (1994) Home-based versus hospital-based care for people with serious mental illness, *British Journal of Psychiatry*, 165, 179–94.

Marshall, M. & Lockwood, A. (2001) Assertive community treatment for people with severe mental disorders, *Cochrane Database Systematic Review*, 4.

Marshall, M., Lockwood, A. & Gath, D. (1995) Social services care management for long-term mental disorders: a randomised controlled trial. *Lancet*, 345(8947) 409–12.

Marshall, M., Gray, A., Lockwood, A. & Green, R. (2001) Case management for people with severe mental disorders, *Cochrane Database Systematic Review*, 4, online at: http://biomed.niss.co.uk/ovidweb.cgi

McGrew, J. H. & Bond, G. R. (1995) Critical ingredients of assertive community treatment: judgments of the experts, *Journal of Mental Health Administration*, 22(2), 113–25.

McGrew, J. H., Bond, G. R., Dietzen, L. & Salyers, M. (1994) measuring the fidelity of implementation of a mental health program model, *Journal of Consulting & Clinical Psychology*, 62(4), 670–8.

McHugo, G. J., Drake, R. E., Teague, G. B. & Xie, H. (1999) Fidelity to assertive community treatment and client outcomes in the new hampshire dual disorders study, *Psychiatric Services*, 50(6), 818–24.

Miller, W. & Rollnick, S. (1991) *Motivational Interviewing: Preparing People to Change Addictive Behaviour*, New York: Guilford Press.

Minghella, E., Gauntlett, N. & Ford, R. (2002) Assertive outreach: does it reach expectations? *Journal of Mental Health*, 11(1), 27–42.

Mueser, K. T., Bond, G. R., Drake, R. E. & Resnick, S. G. (1998) Models of community care for severe mental illness: a review of research on case management, *Schizophrenia Bulletin*, 24(1), 37–74.

Neale, M. S. & Rosenheck, R. A. (2000) Therapeutic limit setting in an assertive community treatment program, *Psychiatric Services*, 51, 499–505.

Phillips, S. D., Burns, B. J., Edgar, E. R., Mueser, K. T., Linkins, K. W., Rosenheck, R. A., Drake, R. E. & McDonel Herr, E. C. (2001) Moving assertive community treatment into standard practice, *Psychiatric Services*, 52(6), 771–9.

Sainsbury Centre for Mental Health (1998) *Keys to Engagement*, London: Sainsbury Centre for Mental Health.

Schaedle, R. W. (1999) Critical ingredients of intensive case management: judgements of researchers/administrators, program managers and case managers, *Dissertation Abstracts International*, 60(4A), 1331, University Microfilms International, US.

Schaedle, R. W. & Epstein, I. (2000) Specifying intensive case management: a multiple perspective approach, *Mental Health Service Research*, 2(2), 95–105.

Solomon, P., Draine, J. & Meyerson, A. (1994) Jail recidivism and receipt of community mental health services, *Hospital & Community Psychiatry*, 45(8), 793–7.

Spindel, P. & Nugent, J. (2001) The trouble with PACT: questioning the increasing use of assertive community treatment teams in community mental health, online at: http://www.akmhcweb.org/Articles/pact.htm

Stein, L. I. & Test, M. A. (1980) Alternative to mental hospital treatment: I. conceptual model, treatment program and clinical evaluation, *Archives of General Psychiatry*, 37(4), 392–7.

Stovall, J. (2001) Is assertive community treatment ethical care? *Harvard Review of Psychiatry*, 9(3), 139–43.

Support Coalition International (2001) Mental Health Workers Bring Psychiatric Drugs to your Home to Assure Compliance: Stop PACT! online at: http://www.mindfreedom.org/mindfreedom/ioc/workers.shtml

Talbott, J. A., Clark, G. H. J., Sharfstein, S. S. & Klein, J. (1987) Issues in developing standards governing psychiatric practice in community health centers, *Hospital and Community Psychiatry*, 38(11), 1198–202.

Teague, G. B., Bond, G. R. & Drake, R. E. (1998) Program fidelity in assertive community treatment: development and use of a measure, *American Journal of Orthopsychiatry*, 68(2), 216–32.

Thompson I. E., Melia, K. M. & Boyd, K. M. (1994) *Nursing Ethics*, (3rd edn), Edinburgh: Churchill Livingstone.

Thornicroft G. (1991) The concept of case management for long-term mental illness, *International Review of Psychiatry*, 3, 125–32.

Ziguras, S. J. & Stuart, G. W. (2000) A meta-analysis of the effectiveness of mental health case management over 20 years, *Psychiatric Services*, 51(11), 1410–21.

CHAPTER 24

Mental Health and Community Safety

DENIS A. HART AND STEPHAN D. KIRBY

Introduction

We have already seen in this text how concerns for community safety have grown over the years. This has been reflected both in the chapter on risk assessment and the last chapter on assertive outreach. This chapter looks at the origins of enforcement stemming from the mental health (Patients in the Community) Act (1995) (DoH, 1995) and carries the debate forward into the newly created Multi Agency Public Protection Panels (MAPPs).

Discharge from mental hospital was recognized as a priority area of concern under the Mental Health Act 1983 whereby anybody who had been previously detained under Section 3, 37, 47 or 48 must have an individual care plan drawn up with an identified key worker to ensure that it would be implemented. Section 117 actually: 'imposes a duty jointly on the health authority and the social services to provide after care services for as long as they were needed. The authorities should cooperate with voluntary agencies. However, there is no definition in the Act of what level of after care is required' (Brayne & Martin, 2001, p 312).

Under powers contained in Section 17 MHA 1983, a Doctor in charge can recall a patient on leave of absence. Detained patients who go Absent Without Leave (AWOL) can, under Section 18 be detained and returned to the hospital or:

- an approved social worker (ASW);
- hospital staff;
- the police; or
- any other person authorized by the hospital managers.

After care plans were purely voluntary until the Mental Health (Patients in the Community) Act 1995 (DoH, 1995). The new legislation introduced additional powers aimed at protecting the pubic, namely after care under supervision as a result of concerns about public safety. Such powers are obtained: 'on the application of the hospital, made to the Health Authority responsible for after care services. The local authority must be consulted and the application must include an after care plan which names the Doctor and the patients' supervisor after discharge' (Brayne & Martin, 2001, p 312). The discharged patient will be required by the hospital to co-operate with the treatment plan produced under Section 117, MHA 1983. Failure to cooperate could lead to compulsory readmission to hospital. The power to supervise the patient's aftercare is laid down by the amended MHA. Section 25 E(4)b considers whether it might be appropriate for him or her to be admitted to hospital for treatment and requires approval from a doctor and an ASW. The power lasts for 6 months and thereafter 6 months and then yearly (Section 25 G(2(a, b)). Section 66, MHA, allows a patient who objects to such a measure to apply for a review to the MHRT. It should be noted that such aftercare supervision *only* applies to those patients who are not subject to guardianship.

The main advantages of after care under supervision are:

- It provides some guarantee that discharged patients will receive the help they need once in the community.
- It enables professionals to be alert to the whereabouts and activities of people who may still pose a risk to others.
- The patients has an identified person, the supervisor, to seek out help.

The problem areas centre around:

- a lack of suitable accommodation and support services in the community; and
- diverting attention from under resourced support services and placing the blame on the person rather than the system.

Furedi (1997, p 4) has argued that the: 'evaluation of everything from the perspective of safety is a defining characteristic of contemporary society'. The origin of this seems to lie in the *Health Service Guidelines for the Introduction of Supervision Registers* (DoH, 1994) which required all health authorities to have: 'Registers which identify and provide information on patients who are likely to be at risk of committing serious violence'. Bean (2002, p 32) echoes these views: 'Community safety is fast becoming a catch-all term', and goes on to point out that: 'some patients who commit very serious harm do so in circumstances which are unpredictable'. Bean goes on to (p 33) make a crucial observation: 'A key principle of English Law is that the law should only be involved after the crime has been committed, and it has always been uneasy about moving from that retributive base to deal with assessments of what people are rather than what they have done.'

As mental hospitals closed there was always the likelihood that society would continue to hold fears, both rational and irrational, that those discharged would pose a threat to the community. In anticipation the Government introduced in 1990, the Care Programme Approach (CPA) (DoH, 1990). Kemshall (2002, p 97) explains:

> that CPA emphasised assessment, a care/treatment plan, an allocated key worker for each case and regular reviews of progress. The CPA represented an acknowledgement that the principles of community care following hospital closures required tighter structures and systems for their delivery.

However, many inquiring reports suggested care in the community was failing and the lack of adequate resources fuelled such a view. The National Association for the Care and Resettlement of Offenders (NACRO) (1998), pinpointed eight key issues emerging from inquiry reports:

- a lack of co-ordination and poor communication between those providing care, support, management and treatment;
- insufficient resources both in hospital provision and in community support services;
- the need for special supervision arrangement;
- poor information sharing and recording;
- inadequate and unreliable assessment of risk and violent behaviour;
- lack of co-operation between agencies;
- patients rights required greater attention;
- legislation required attention, in particular for supervision on discharge and for compulsory treatment and supervision in the community.

In spite of the tightening up which occurred in the Mental Health (Patients in the Community) Act 1995, Grounds (1996) observed that risk and protection began to dominate the mental health policy agenda. As Kemshall (2002, p 99) noted: 'responsibility for risk is firmly individual, either of the worker or patient – worker for failing to manage it effectively, or of the patient for failing to comply with risk management strategies'.

Mental health nurses are currently being bombarded with mixed messages, for, on the one hand: 'the success of a cohesive and productive multi-professional team should be measured in relation to how well the user has been involved in the consultation process' (Payne, 2000, p 237), which echoes part of the *National Service Framework* (DoH, 2001). While on the other hand, the proposed Community Care Order: 'fits into that general scheme of things including the racial and political climate of the times, where toughness, surveillance and increasing controls are the watchword' (Bean, 2002, p 73).

There have been three key thrusts driving current practice, creating MAPPs and the revision of mental health legislation:

- the development of compulsory community care;
- preoccupation with mentally disordered offenders; and
- the development of the notion of preventative detention for high risk cases.

Although MAPPs have been only established recently their legitimacy lies in provisions initiated by the *Health Service Guidelines for the Introduction of Supervision Registers* (DoH, 1994). The *Guidelines* say that:

> disclosure to other agencies may be either with the patients consent, or, without consent if disclosure can be justified in the public interest. The provider unit must be able to justify such disclosures, taking full account of the view of the Consultant Psychiatrist responsible for the care of the patient (Responsible Medical Officer – RMO). It is rare for the Police to be given access. The provider unit may also bring the case to the newly formed Public Protection Panels who could decide to provide surveillance or some other programme for the patient. (Bean, 2002, p 66)

Bean (2002, p 156) adds that:

> the demands for public safety are now so strong that we have been accustomed to legislation which would have been unthinkable a few generations ago . . . We have the Sex Offenders Act requiring selected sex offenders to register with the police and we have Public Protection Panels – who consider these sex offenders, and other offenders brought to its notice, who its members consider dangerous – staffed by representatives of the police, the probation service and the local authority.

The proposed mental health legislation goes further down this road as assertive outreach takes in a compulsory element in the form of the proposed Community Care Order while further measures are aimed at dealing with the 'untreatable'. The Home Secretary wishes to provide protection from those: 'severely personality disordered individuals' who 'have a propensity to commit the most serious sexual and violent acts'. Essentially the new legislation is expected to give courts: the power to order indefinite detention whether or not they have committed an offence. The implications of these trends for future practice is not consistent with empowerment, advocacy and involvement of service users which we have been encouraged to aspire to and hold dear as values.

Kemshall (2002, p 128) offers an effective summary:

> Welfare workers in the 21st Century find themselves part of a new residualism of welfarism within which risk plays a key part on resource allocation and in the framing of their professional practice and encounters with service users. Their professional world is characterised by key themes: fiscal prudence, rationing, risk assessment, targeting and responsibilisation of service users . . . the increasing residualism of welfare is mirrored in the distancing of workers from users, particularly in social care, combined with increasingly formal techniques of assessment to ensure appropriate and consistent targeting.

If we couple to this the need to prioritize control and supervision and we can see how slowly the 'total institution' (Goffman, 1961) environment offered by mental hospitals is being slowly transferred to those living and working in the community.

References

Bean, P. (2002) *Mental Disorder and Community Safety*, Basingstoke: Palgrave Macmillan.

Brayne, H. & Martin, G. (2001) *Law for Social Workers*, Oxford: Blackstone Press.

Department of Health (1990) *The Care Programme Approach for People with a Mental Illness*, London: HMSO.

Department of Health (1994) *Health Service Guidelines for the Introduction of Supervision Registers*, London: HMSO.

Department of Health (1995) *Mental Health (Patients in the Community) Act*, London: HMSO.

Department of Health (2001) *National Service Framework for Older People*, London: HMSO.

Furedi, F. (1997) *Culture of Fear: Risk Taking and the Morality of Law Expectation*, London: Cassell.

Goffman, E. (1961) *Asylums: Essays on the Social Situation of Mental Patients and Other Inmates*, London: Penguin.

Grounds, A. (1996) *Psychiatry and Public Protection*, Public Lecture, Annual Meeting, Mental Health Commission for Mental Health.

Kemshall, H. (2002) *Risk, Social Policy and Welfare*, Buckingham: Open University Press.

National Association for the Care and Resettlement of Offenders (1998) *Risks and Rights: Mentally Disordered Offenders and Public Protection: A Report by NACRO's Mental Health Advisory Committee*, London: NACRO.

Payne, M. (2000) *Team Working in Multi Professional Care*, Basingstoke: Macmillan Press, now Palgrave Macmillan.

PART IV

USING EFFECTIVE LEARNING TO DEVELOP REFLECTIVE PRACTICE

In this Part we change emphasis from examining the needs of patients and their carers and the provision of treatment modalities and instead focus upon you, as an effective learner, striving to develop critically reflective practice. Of central importance to your role is the recognition of the legal duties and responsibilities placed upon you. We will then go on to look at how you need to manage effectively your own workload, to learn from experience and develop enhanced competence. Finally we will look at the mental health task from the subjective point of view of three people who work in posts within the profession.

CHAPTER 25

Legal and Professional Issues in Mental Health Nursing Practice

GORDON MITCHELL

Indicative Benchmark Statements

▓ Participation in the application of mental health law and related legislation

▓ An appreciation of mental health service users and carers civil rights, consent to treatment and the utilization of powers of compulsion and detention

▓ Ability to act for mental health services users who lack capacity to make decisions for themselves

▓ Maintenance of comprehensive mental health nursing records

Introduction

The purpose of this chapter is not only to acquaint the reader with the fundamental knowledge of mental health legislation, but also to help them gain an insight into the complex world of medical law and its implications for mental health practice. The importance of knowing your role and responsibilities as an accountable practitioner can be seen in some recent figurers released by the NHS Litigation Authority, that 3254 claims in the year 1999–2000 costs the NHS £386 million. This figure is dwarfed by the annual estimates made by the National Audit Office for the expected future cost of settling outstanding negligence claims to be £4.4 billion (Fenn, 2002). Knowledge of the Mental Health Act (1983) is the cornerstone of all mental health practitioners especially since there has been a rise of 20,000 people who have been detained under the act in the 10-year period between 1990 to 2000 (Vass, 2001). Therefore this chapter will hopefully equip the mental health practitioner with knowledge and understanding of mental health and medical law and its implications for your practice.

Accountability

The development of nursing as an accountable profession is inextricably linked with the historical development of nursing. It could be argued that account-ability really began in 1919 with the passing of the Nurses Registration Act (Watson, 1995). For the first time this Act meant that registered nurses were legally accountable for their work and could be removed from the register for unprofessional behaviour.

In defining accountability, Law (1983) proposes that the qualified nurse should be answerable for his/her own practice, and to achieve this the nurse must be able to explain and defend the rational for their actions, which must be based on knowledge rather than tradition and routine. As Moloney (1986) further explains that when the nurse is answerable for their practice/actions, it places responsibility for the outcomes of nursing care directly on the practitioner. With the introduction of Clinical Governance the emphasis on knowledge, which should underpin practice, is even more important.

Therefore, to whom is the nurse accountable?

- the profession in general through their actions;
- colleagues through their employment contact and the Code of Professional Conduct;
- the patient by their 'duty of care';
- the employer by the signing of their employment contract;
- society in general as nurses are expected to act and behave in certain ways;
- the professional regulatory body, registering with them and following their Code of Professional Conduct;
- the law, either civil or criminal;
- the patient family/carer, by the way he/she speaks and treats them; and
- importantly to him/herself through their own moral codes.

The levels of accountability are not of equal importance, with some being more important than others and therefore conflict between them is certainly possible. One of the most important aspects of accountability for a mental health nurse (or any nurse for that matter) is their legal accountability to the law. Legal accountability is the prime form of accountability for every citizen, and nurses like all other professions, are personally accountable through the law for their actions or omissions. This form of accountability is channelled through the criminal and civil law. When exploring a nurse's legal account-ably the first issue that would be determined would be if the nurse has a 'duty of care' to the patient.

What is a duty of care?

A duty of care is not owed universally and a person bringing any action would have to prove, first, that a duty of care was owed to them personally; second, that the nurse was in breach of that duty and third, that they suffered harm as a consequence of that breach which was not so unforeseeable as to be regarded in civil or criminal law as to remote.

In the legal test case Donaghue (or M'Alister) v Stevenson (1932) see Case Study 25.1.

Case Study 25.1 Test case 1

A lady was served a glass of ginger beer, which was poured from an opaque glass bottle. When the remainder of the ginger beer was being poured into the glass the contents were seen to be contaminated with the decomposing remains of a dead snail. As a result of seeing the dead snail and the realization that she had consumed contaminated ginger beer the lady suffered from severe shock and diarrhoea and vomiting; she later died as a result of her injuries.

A claim for compensation by the lady, and later by her estate was lodged in the courts. Initially the claim was rejected and even on appeal the case was rejected. However on appeal to the House of Lords the claim for compensation for negligence against the manufacturer was upheld. The reason the majority of the Law Lords upheld the claim was as Lord Atkin (Donaghue (or M'Alister) v Stevenson (1932). This is explained the principle of common law negligence is to 'take reasonable care to avoid acts or omissions, which you can reasonably foresee, would be likely to injure your neighbour'.

Source: Donaghue (or M'Alister) v Stevenson (1932)

Therefore a duty of care can be said to exist if one can see one's actions are reasonably likely to cause harm to another person.

Negligence

In defining negligence an important principle that must be taken into consideration is the Bolam Test. This relates to negligence and the information given to patients and the legal test case is Bolam v. Friern Hospital Management Committee (1957). See Case Study 25.2.

Case Study 25.2 Test case 2

John Bolam was a patient at a mental hospital, and was diagnosed as suffering from a depressive disorder. He was advised by Dr de Bastarrechea, a Consultant attached to this hospital, to undergo Electro-Convulsive Therapy (ECT). Mr Bolam signed a consent form but was not alerted to the risk of fracture that can occur because of the convulsions this treatment induces.

Mr Bolam had the treatment but was not given any relaxant drugs. As a consequence he suffered a dislocation of the hip joints and fractures to the pelvis on both sides. Mr Bolam claimed
damages from Friern hospital, alleging that ECT without the prior administration of relaxant
drugs, or without restraining his convulsions manually, amounted to negligence.

Source: Bolam v. Friern Hospital Management Committee (1957) 1 WLR 582

Do you think that Bolam own his case and why?

When examining this case to determine whether negligence had been committed, the court had to decide if there was any negligence in the patient's
diagnosis or the decision to use ECT. This was not the case; it was only that
information that had been given to the patient was a matter of professional
judgement or skill had been questioned. Therefore what the court had to
decide was whether the information that was given to Mr Bolam was in accordance with the practice accepted by the body of medical opinion in 1954
when the proposed negligent act took place, not 1957 when the court case
took place. In making their judgement the court decided that the doctors
involved in this case had acted in accordance with the practice accepted as
proper by a responsible body of medical men skilled in that particular art
(McHale et al, 1997).

Therefore, the same principles would apply to a nurse accused of negligence. Therefore, an ordinary nurse professing to have the same skills would
judge them. What would happen if a nurse decided, with the approval and
training of their employer, to extend his/her skills to that which once
belonged to a doctor? Importantly, since the nurse has the approval and the
appropriate training by their employer they would be covered by vicarious liability and their employer would be liable for any damages awarded against the
nurse. However, if a nurse performs a skill without their employer's permission or training then it could be argued that they are not covered by vicarious liability and would be personally liable for any damages.

Consent

The requirement in English law for consent to be obtained before treatment
commences is an important principle that constrains the power of health care
professionals. Within English law 'Tort' of 'trespass to the person' is committed when there is direct intentional application of force upon a person.
The major defence against Tort is consent. Therefore, if the patient gives
consent for contact to occur then the treatment can be lawfully given in the
majority of cases. Consent can be obtained either orally or written; both are
equally valid. Also there can be implied or expressed consent, as it is when a

patient presents themselves to their doctor for examination and acquiesces in the suggested routine.

For consent to be valid it must be:

- free, the patient must not be subject to any pressure or coercion or the consent could become invalid;
- real/understanding, the patient must know what they are consenting to; and
- competent, the patient must be old enough to consent and be mentally competent.

Therefore, if a competent adult refuses in no uncertain terms, for example, a blood transfusion, despite knowing that it is required to save their life and is aware of the risks, then unless it can be proved that their lack of consent is due to undue influence by some other person, treatment cannot be lawfully given. An example of this important principle can be seen in the test case Malett v Shulman (1990).

What about the unconscious patent?

We can examine two test cases; the first one, Marshall v Curry (1933). In this case a surgeon while performing an operation for the repair of a hernia, removed the patient's testicle. The patient sought damages for battery as he argued that he did not give consent for the testicle to be removed. The surgeon argued that the removal of the testicle was essential because if he had done nothing the life of the patient would have been imperilled as the testicle was diseased.

In the second case, Murry v McMurchy (1949), the doctor had discovered during a Caesarean section that the condition of the patient's uterus would have made it hazardous for her to go through another pregnancy. Although it was not essential for another procedure to be carried out immediately the doctor tied the patients Fallopian tubes. The patient also sought damages for battery (Mason and McCall Smith, 1994).

In the first case the courts took the view that the doctor had acted in the best interest of the patient by 'protecting the patient's health and possibly his life'. Therefore the removal of the testicle was necessary and it would not have been reasonable to postpone the procedure until another date. In the second case the patient won her case as the court took the view that it was not un-reasonable to postpone the tying of the patients Fallopian tubes and obtain consent from the patient (Mason and McCall Smith, 1994).

However, one of the most important test cases in relation to consent to treatment that came to the courts was Sidaway v Bethlem Royal Hospital (1985), see Case Study 25.3.

> **Case Study 25.3   Test case 3**
>
> Amy Sidaway suffered from persistent pain to her neck and shoulder and was advised by the surgeon to have an operation on her spinal column to relieve the pain. The surgeon warned her of the possibility of disturbing a nerve root and the possible consequences of doing so but did not mention the possibility of damage to the spinal cord. Even though he would be operating within 3 millimetres of it.
>
> Amy consented to the operation. However during the operation she suffered an injury to her spinal cord which resulted in her being severely disabled. Amy sued the surgeon and the hospital. Amy argued that the surgeon had been in breach of his duty of care owed to her by not warning her of all the possible risks inherent in the operation. Therefore she was not able to give her informed consent to the operation. Amy however, did not suggest that the operation was carried out negligently. The case was complicated by the fact that the doctor who performed the operation had died by the time the case came to trial.
>
> *Source*: Mason and McCall Smith (1994)

Do you think Amy won her case and why?

This case went on appeal to the House of Lords where they had to decide whether the failure to advise Amy of the risk of injury to the spinal cord was negligent. In rejecting Amy's case the Law Lords used the Bolam principles (as discussed earlier) in formulating their judgement. As Lord Scarman suggested 'the Bolam principle may be used to rule that a doctor is not negligent if he acts in accordance with a practice that is accepted at that time by a responsible body of medical opinion'. Therefore, the law imposes the duty of care, but the standard of care is a matter of medical judgement and medical judgement should determine whether there exists a duty to warn of risk and its scope. Furthermore, Lord Diplock argued that the public would be badly served if the law only restricted the doctor to long-established, well-tried methods of treatment only.

These principles have been called the 'prudent doctor' or 'reasonable doctor' test. This allows the doctor to give information to the patient to obtain their consent as long as it is of professional medical standard, i.e. the information, which other doctors would have given to the patient. This is in contrast to the 'prudent patient' test that was rejected in the Sidaway case. This test, which is used in some states in the United States of America, believes that doctor must disclose all the 'material risks' involved in the procedure.

Competency

One of the main legal/ethical and professional issues that affects mental health practice is competency. Hoggett (1996) proposes that even if the person who has a mental health disorder gives his/her valid consent for a course of drug treatment or ECT he/she may withdraw their consent at any time even if the treatment has not been completed. Mason and McCall Smith (1994) go on to explain that the treatment that can be given to patients who withdraw or refuse to give their consent is limited even for involuntary patients and is proscribed by statute. Importantly the statute excludes treatments of an unrelated physical condition.

In defining the 'competent patient' as 'one who has provided a knowledgeable consent to treatment' Kennedy and Grubb (1994, p 127) propose that the doctor has an obligation to educate the patient and to ascertain whether they have understood the facts. If they do not then the doctor does not have informed consent. An example of this legal/ethical dilemma can be seen in the example below taken from Kennedy and Grubb (1994).

A 49-year-old lady, who understood the purpose of ECT, was informed that there was a 1 in 3000 chance of dying from the treatment. The lady replied 'I hope I am the one.' Therefore was this lady competent to give her consent and how much understanding must there be in order for the patient to be viewed as competent?

The layperson might think that because a person has a mental health problem/disorder does that make them incompetent and therefore their consent is not required? Furthermore, if a person is detained under the Mental Health Act (1983) (DoH, 1983), can treatment for a physical treatment be enforced? To answer these questions we need to once again examine some case law to helps us through these difficult questions, especially since case law is more limited in this area (see Case Study 25.4).

Case Study 25.4   Test case 4

In Re v 'C' (Adult refuses medical treatment) (1994), 'C' was a patient at Broadmoor Hospital. He was diagnosed with paranoid schizophrenia and he expressed grandiose delusions of being an internationally renowned doctor. 'C' developed a dangerous gangrenous infection in his leg and his surgeon believed that his leg should be amputated in order to save his life. The surgeon argued that his chances of survival without an amputation were no more than 15 per cent.

'C' refused to give his consent for the operation, arguing that he would rather die with two feet than live with one. He also believed that he might survive with the help of God, the doctors and the nurses and if he did die then his foot would not cause his death. Eventually the surgeon persuaded 'C' to accept more conservative treatment and the danger of death was averted with no need for an amputation.

However the surgeon warned that his leg might still deteriorate and he might still require an amputation. Therefore 'C' instructed his solicitor to go to court to seek a declaration from the court that no amputation should take place without his written consent. The courts therefore had to decide whether his capacity to give consent was reduced by his mental illness since he did not adequately understand the nature, purpose and effect of the proposed amputation, which would render his refusal to give consent invalid.

Source: McHale et al (1997)

Do you think 'C' won his case and why?

In coming to a judgment the judge rejected the traditional 'minimal competence' test that is used, in that the patient has an understanding of the nature and effect of the proposed treatment. Instead he used a psychiatrist's analysis of understanding, in that the patient does:

- comprehend and retain the information;
- believe it; and
- weigh up the balance to arrive at a choice.

In granting an injunction to prevent the hospital amputating 'C's' leg the judge decided the patient did understand the relevant information and that there was no direct link between his refusal and his persecutory delusions. As the judge said 'I am satisfied that he has understood and retained the relevant treatment information and he has arrived at a clear choice' (Senshy, 2002). Senshy (2002) further makes the point that refusal by a mentally competent person to give their consent or not is an absolute right even if the reason for this is irrational. However, this is not a universally accepted viewpoint as argued by Moorhead and Turkington (2002) when they point out that an irrational reason for the refusal of treatment indicates that their ability to weigh evidence is impaired.

Another example where the courts do not always agree with medical opinion is in the case of R v 'H' (1992) where a deputy judge refused to grant an order forcing a woman who was suspected of having a brain tumour to have a CT scan. Even though she had a diagnosis of schizophrenia the judge ruled that there was no distinction between diagnosis and therapeutic procedures, therefore the patient had the right to refuse treatment.

Who can give consent?

It is important to note that no one is in a position to give consent on another adult's behalf, except for parental responsibility (McHale et al, 1997). If a patient is unable to give their valid consent the courts usually take the decision based on the premise that as long as the treatment is in the best interests of the patient and this is judged so by a responsible body of medical opinion then treatment can be given.

An example of this can be seen in test case 5 'F' v West Berkshire Health Authority (1989) (see Case Study 25.5).

Case Study 25.5 Test case 5

In this case a women ('F') had serious learning difficulties. Although her chronological age was 36 she had an assessed mental age of five and her verbal capacity was that of a two-year-old.

She was a voluntary in-patient and had been there for over 20 years. During this time she had formed a sexual relationship with a male patient and the doctor in charge of her care was concerned that she might become pregnant. In fact both her mother and the team of health care professions believed that pregnancy would be a disaster for her and thought it best for her to be sterilised.

As she was unable to give her consent for the operation to take place a declaration was sought from the courts that the operation would be lawful. The House of Lords held that it had no power to consent on her behalf, but they did consider whether it would be lawful for the operation to be given without 'F's' consent.

Source: McHale et al (1997)

What do you think the Law Lords ruled and why?

In making their judgment the Law Lords ruled that the operation would be lawful as the doctors were acting in the patients best interests. Lord Brandon argued that in his opinion the doctor can lawfully operate or give treatment to adult patients who are incapable of consenting providing that the operation or treatment will be in the best interests of the patient. In defining what 'the best interest' of the patient is, he proposes that the operation or treatment must be carried out in order to either to save lives or to ensure improvement or prevent deterioration in the patient's physical or mental health. However the question that must be asked is whether the Law Lords were right to give decision-making powers to doctors rather than to family members. Lord Brandon once again answers this question by saying that it is necessary that, on occasions, another person (with appropriate qualifications) should take such decisions, if the patient is unable to give or refuse their consent.

Mental Health Act (1983)

It is not expected of a student nurse to know every section and paragraph of the Mental Health Act, however, there is a fundamental level of knowledge required when any patient is detained in hospital. Table 25.1 cotains some of the sections of the Act that you should know.

For more detailed information please read Hoggett's 1996 book *Mental Health Law*.

Table 25.1   Some sections of the Mental Health Act (1983)

Section Number	Definition	Duration	Application	Appeal
2	Admission for assessment	28 days	Two medical recommendations and approved social worker or next of kin	Within 14 days
3	Admission for treatment	6 months then may be renewed for a further 6 months then yearly	Two medical recommendations and approved social worker or next of kin	Anytime within the 6 months
4	Emergency admission for assessment	72 hours	One medical recommendation and approved social worker or next of kin	No
5(2)	Doctors holding powers for patients already in hospital	72 hours	One medical recommendation	No
5(4)	Nurses holding powers for patients already in hospital	6 hours	Registered mental health nurse or registered nurse in learning disabilities (1st Level)	No

Source: Adapted from Hoggett (1996)

Part IV of Mental Health Act (1983) consent to treatment

Under the provision of Part IV of the Mental Health Act (1983) (DoH, 1983), those patients who are detained under long-term detention provisions can, in certain circumstances, be given compulsory treatment. For those patients Part IV covers all possible treatments, in both emergency and non-emergency situations.

The role of the nurse

Under the provision of Sections 57 and 58 the independent registered medical practitioner, in determining whether the treatment should proceed, must consult with a nurse and another health care professional who has been professionally connected with the patient's medical treatment. However there is no requirement for the independent registered medical practitioner to actually record the other health care professionals' opinions. A disagreement is unusual but it is advisable that the nurse should ensure that the advice they gave is recorded clearly and comprehensively in the nursing records.

What would happen if a patient had to have emergency physical treatment?

Think about this situation. Paul is severely depressed and has been detained under Section 3 Mental Health Act (1983) (DoH, 1983) for two months, as he was suicidal and had previously tried to commit suicide. One morning he complains of severe stomach pains. He was diagnosed as suffering from appendicitis and was transferred to a General Hospital. On examination it was recommended that an operation to remove his appendix be performed immediately. On being told this Paul said he would not give his consent for the operation. What do you think is the legal position in this case?

Part IV of the Act is seen as applying to treatment of mental illness. In that case its provisions are irrelevant in Paul's situation. Alternatively, it could be argued that under Section 62 of the Act the words 'any treatment' can be treatment for physical disorders. If the purpose is to save life, then section 62-(1) (a) could be argued covers this situation. However this is not a universally accepted opinion, especially when you consider R v 'C' (1994) as discussed earlier. Therefore the doctor would have to decide if Section 62 was not applicable therefore they would have to act under the rules of common law in acting in the bests interests of the patient as we discussed in test case 5 'F' v West Berkshire Health Authority (1989). Of course the doctor would have to be able to justify their decision to the court if the patient brought a civil case of trespass against them.

Psychiatry and criminal law

The psychiatrist can be asked to be involved in criminal law at a number of points within a criminal trial. These can be to:

- provide evidence to the court of the accused person's mental state;
- assist the court in the exercise of its sentencing power; and
- provide evidence on the mental state of a witness.

An example of this can be seen in the case of R v Weightman (1991) when the accused had confessed to the police that she had murdered her young child. The defence sought to use psychiatric evidence to the affect that the accused suffered from a histrionic personality disorder, which inclined her to make theatrical statements. Therefore the validity of her confession should be questioned.

Do you think the defence was allowed to use this evidence and why?

The court ruled against the defence, arguing that evidence, which disclosed anything less than a mental disorder, was not relevant. Also an important aspect in English law is that the jury on the basis of its own experience of human nature rather than on the basis of psychiatric insight would determine reliability of the confession. The Court of Appeal went on to warn, 'the fact that an expert witness has impressive scientific qualifications does not, by that alone, make his opinion on matters of human nature and behaviour within the limits of normality any more helpful than that of the jurors themselves: but there is a danger that they think it does' (Mason & McCall Smith, 1994, p 403). When looking at what mental disorder is the courts would use the four specific forms of mental disorder as described in the Mental Health Act (1983) (DoH, 1983), these are:

- mental illness;
- severe mental impairment;
- psychopathic disorder; and
- mental impairment.

Insanity

If an accused is using a defence of insanity then this does not, in itself, qualify as a defence to a criminal charge in English Law. The court would use the McNaghten (or M'Naughten) rules as these lay down the basic test for acquittal on the grounds of insanity. The McNaghten rules originate in a judgment from the House of Lords in 1843 in the case of Daniel McNaughten who had been charged with the shooting of the Prime Minister's secretary in the belief that the secretary was the Prime Minister himself. In this case the defence lodged a defence of insanity. The court ruled that for someone to plead insanity then they must 'be labouring under such a defect of reason, from disease of the mind as not to know: The nature and quality of the act he/she was doing or, if they did know it; That he/she did not know what he/she was doing was wrong' Adapted from Mason and McCall Smith (1994, pp 408–9)

There has been much criticism of the McNaghten rules, in that, why should Victorian concepts influence modern day psychiatric practice. Furthermore what constitutes a 'disease' of the mind? In the case of 'R' v Kemp (1957) the courts ruled that arteriosclerosis (hardening of the arteries) was a disease of the mind and therefore, could be used as a defence to a criminal charge. Another criticism of the rules has been significance of the term 'wrong'. Mason and McCall Smith (1994) pose the question of 'does the accused person have to know that his act is morally wrong or do they have to know it is legally wrong' (Mason & McCall Smith, 1994, p 409). This could lead to a defence of insanity being denied to an accused who heard voices commanding him to commit a crime and, although he knew this crime was illegal, thought that the voice came from God and acted accordingly.

If an accused person's plea of insanity was accepted, under the Criminal Procedures Act (1991), any defendant who was found 'not guilty by reason of insanity' as laid down by the Trial of Lunatics Act (1883), a restriction order would be placed on them indefinitely, and they would be placed in a hospital (usually secure) specified by the Home Secretary.

Unfitness to plead

The basis of the plea is an inability to understand proceedings and to defend oneself. The Criminal Procedure (Insanity and Unfitness to Plead) Act 1991 allows for a trial of the facts in order that the jury may decide whether the accused actually committed the offence in question. Before 1991 there would have been no trial and the accused would be sent to hospital under a restriction order.

Sentencing mentally disordered offenders under the Mental Health Act (1983)

Under Section 37: this hospital order depends on clinical evidence that the offender suffers from a mental disorder for which compulsory treatment in hospital is appropriate. About 600 orders are made by the courts in England annually. Discharge is at the discretion of the consultant or the Mental Health Review Tribunal.

Under Section 41: the judge can impose an order restricting discharge indefinitely. There are about 250 cases a year that are handed over to psychiatrists for treatment and the Home Secretary for discharge. If the treatment is ineffective there is no option for the patient to be sent to prison.

Under Section 48: any person who is remanded in custody by a magistrates court can be transferred to hospital. If they are awaiting trial in the crown court, the Home Secretary must have a report from two doctors that the prisoner is suffering from a mental illness or severe mental impairment. The doctors must also agree on the type of mental illness or impairment the prisoner is suffering from.

It is important to note that before a patient is transferred to a hospital from the courts or prison the court has to be given evidence that there is a bed available within the stated time. The person who gives this assurance is the doctor who will be responsible for the patient or the hospital manager.

Conclusion

The purpose of this chapter was to demonstrate that a satisfactory knowledge of the Mental Health Act, although essential, is insufficient to practice as a mental health practitioner. This chapter therefore has given examples from case law to demonstrate that because a person has a mental health problem or disorder their consent is required for physical treatment, if required, and may not be covered under the Mental Health Act. With nurses being asked by the Government and employers to extend and expand their clinical skills, knowledge of this legal and professional minefield is even more essential. Therefore, it is essential that when nurses undertake an extended role that they are adequately trained to do so and work within the limits of their competence.

References

Bolam v Frien Barnet Hospital Management Committee (1957) 1 WLR 582.

Department of Health (1983) *Mental Health Act 1983*, London: HMSO.

Donoghue v Stevenson (1932) AC 562.

F v West Berkshire Health Authority (1989) 2 All E.R. 545, (1990) 2 A.C.1, (1989) 2 W.L.R. 938, (1989) 2 F.L.R. 476.

Fenn, P. (2002) Counting the cost of medical negligence, *British Medical Journal*, 325(7358), 233–5.

Hoggett, B. (1996) *Mental Health Law*, (4th edn), London: Sweet and Maxwell.

Kennedy, I. & Grubb, A. (1994) *Medical Law*, (2nd edn), London: Butterworth.

Law, G. M. (1983) Providing a framework, *Nursing Times*, 79, 34–6.

Malett v Shulman (1990) 67 DLR (4th) 321 (Ont CA).

Marshall v Curry (1933) 3 DLR 260.

Mason, J. K. & McCall Smith, R. A. (1994) *Law and Medical Ethics* (4th edn), London: Butterworth.

McHale, J,. Fox, M., and Murphy, J. (1997), *Heath Care Law,* London: Sweet and Maxwell.

Moloney, M. M. (1986) The extended role of the nurse, *Care of the Critically Ill*, 9, 30–4.

Moorhead, S. & Turkington, D. (2002) Role of emotional capacity in consent should be clarified, *British Medical Journal* 325(7371), 1039.

Murrey v McMurchy (1949) 2 DLR 442.

R v C (refusal of medical treatment) (1994) 1 F.L.R. 31.

R v H (Mental Patient) (1992) 8 B.M.L.R.71.

R v Kemp (1957) 1QB 399, (1956) 3 All ER 249.

R v Weightman (1991) Crim LR 204.

Sensky, T. (2002) Withdrawal of life sustaining treatment, *British Medical Journal*, 325, 175–6.

Sidaway v Board of Governors of the Bethlem Royal Hospital and the Maudsley Hospital (1985) AC 871.

Vass, A. (2001) Detentions under the Mental Health Act rise by 20,000 over 10 years, *British Medical Journal*, 323(7322), 1148.

Watson, R. (1995) *Accountability in Nursing Practice*, London: Chapman and Hall.

CHAPTER 26

Management Issues in Practice

JAMES T. WATSON

Indicative Benchmark Statements

▨ A commitment to the guidance from the National Institute for Clinical Excellence to ensure efficiency and cost effectiveness of services

▨ Contribution to the range of administrative duties which are essential to effective case management

▨ Maintenance of comprehensive mental health nursing records

▨ Ability to provide support and supervision to mental health and social care non-specialist and support staff

▨ Report writing in multidisciplinary and multi-agency mental health and social care context

▨ Participation in peer supervision strategies and learning sets

---

Introduction

The term 'management' seems to generate different ideas to people who come in contact with it. Management in the Health Service seems to be reserved for those in charge of wards, departments and above. However, the inter-related activities of 'planning', 'organizing', 'leading' and 'controlling' carried out by managers can, and often are, used by people at lower levels in the organization. While the activities are listed separately, it is often the case that work involves the use of a number of these activities at the same time, which seems to make the managers' job more complex.

Management activities include:

- Planning: Deciding in advance, what to do, how to do it and who should do it;
- Organizing: Co-ordinating resources;

- Leading: Directing and guiding others; and
- Controlling: Measurement and correction of others' behaviour.

The purpose of this chapter is to utilize these interrelated activities in relation to working in the practice setting within the in the Health Service.

Planning and organizing

Planning is a complex and comprehensive process and is important as it contributes to success and control over the future (Du Brin, 2003). It can be seen to offset the effect of uncertainty of change, focus attention on organizational goals, make operations more economical and aid the process of control and output of quality.

Dixon (1997) suggests that planning can be seen as deciding what to do in advance, how to do the particular task, when to do it and who should do it. The most common example of planning seen in any department is what is referred to as 'planning the off duty'. This activity has a major contribution to the welfare of the patient/client through the planning of human and budget resources. Planning at this level is classified as operational planning, it is highly detailed and covers a short time span.

To facilitate planning of the off duty it is necessary to use the planning process model for a summary of the stages linked to the off-duty development. Managers experienced in this activity often mentally work through the stages. However, they still utilize the same process. The planning cycle related to developing the off-duty comprises:

- *Objectives*. What is the purpose of the planning?
  - to facilitate the effective and efficient use of resources;
  - to deliver a high quality care; and
  - to ensure fairness of working conditions to staff.
- *Internal appraisal*: Collection of data concerning factors influencing the off duty
  - workload and factors affecting this;
  - staff available;
  - staff skill mix;
  - social consideration of staff;
  - normal working rotas;
  - staff personalities;
  - budget available.
- *External appraisal*: (Where appropriate)
  - availability of staff from agencies;
  - influence of seasons on health needs;
  - evaluate alternatives to meet the objectives;
  - identify problem areas;

- develop alternative solutions;
- Problem areas: too many alternatives, not enough time to evaluate them all, degree of uncertainty in forecasting dues to of factors such as sickness
- *Formulate plans:* Taking into consideration all the factors plan out the off duty for x weeks using the matrix off duty structure (staff and working hours)
- *Evaluation:*
  - Have the objectives been achieved?
  - What problems were identified?
  - How were the problems dealt with and what are the implications for the future?

Using the data to plan the off-duty can generate a number of management issues. The costing of staff, the number of staff and skill mix all relate to the dependencies for care of patients, the education/training needs of staff and the effectiveness of working practices. Such information is vital for the maintenance and improvement of care.

Planning of the off-duty often includes organizing, in terms of how staff should work. Vertical structures are often used to reflect the way staff are organized to give care. Vertical structures with hierarchical levels may suggest that work allocation is filtered down while group listings may indicate a team approach, which is a more commonly used structure in the NHS, even though there may be a hierarchical structure within the teams.

In organizing, authority, responsibility and delegation are required (Daft, 2003). Although Dixon (1997) suggests that while authority can be delegated, responsibility remains the province of the manager. The off-duty identifies those who have authority delegated to them. In the case of team leaders, authority is the formal right, through one's position in the organization, to make decisions and issue orders. However, team leaders, may have a certain amount of accountability, authority and responsibility linked to their position as qualified professionals.

Organization through delegation requires the manager or team leader to be aware of a variety of factors relating to the individuals, task.

Factors in delegating tasks

- Has the individual the skills to carry out the task or will supervision and training be required?
- Is the task within the scope of the individual's work?
- Is the individual adequately motivated for the task?
- Give the individual the authority and responsibility for the task.
- Provide appropriate feedback of activity and results.
- Reward the individual's performance.

These factors need to be taken into consideration by both the manger and the team leader if the objectives for caring for the patient are to be achieved.

Leading

Leading in the NHS has become one of the main drivers for change in the way care is delivered. Initiatives to develop leadership qualities in NHS staff can be seen in many areas, for example the Leading an Empowered Organization (LEO) programmes. The manager's power to lead differs from that of a leader who is not a manager. The status of the manager is one of legal authority within the organization and has the power to reward or punish. Such power often results in leadership creating compliance behaviour in the followers, owing to fear of punishment, or indeed the benefits of rewards.

Power to influence behaviour of others can also come from other sources, for example personality (*referent*), and expertise (*expert skill/knowledge*). While managers may adopt approaches based on other power sources, they still operate from the position of a manager. Leadership without legal status, relies much more on the other power bases such as position, expertise and personality. These Leaders are often more supportive, motivated, have a vision of future changes and can relate to the others in the team. The power base of the manager is often a hindrance to the leader activity.

An alternative approach to leadership is through leadership styles. This is the way managers use their authority. These styles are influenced by a variety of factors such as the manager's past experience in other organizations, social, education background, personality and the organizational structure and culture of their present environment.

Leadership styles

- *Autocratic style*: Displays behaviour that centralizes authority, relies on legitimate reward and coercive power to influence behaviour of others.
- *Democratic style*: Displays behaviour that gives responsibility to others, encourages participation, and support while using referent power to influence behaviour of others.

Managers do often have a leadership role but that is often influenced by the organization culture and structure as well as their status. The modernization of the NHS is being developed to transform the NHS and create a culture of learning and multiagency working, which is demonstrated by multi-professional teams and the collaboration of professional expertise.

It would seem, therefore, that the leadership approach would need to 'fit' the above NHS changes. The emphasis on working together implies the need for team leadership. Situational leadership focuses on 'leadership in the situations' (Northouse, 2001). The assumption being that each situation is different and demands a different kind of leadership. This implies that managers need to have the ability to adapt their style from a 'directive' to a 'consultative' dimension as situations change. To determine the needs of the situation the manager must assess the individual from two perspectives, the person's motivation and their ability, this suggests that over a period of time the leadership style should change as the individual become more motivated and more skilled. Situational leadership focuses on individuals within the team, and the problems of application may change as team size increases.

Daft (2003) suggests that two types of leadership have an impact on bringing about change in the organization: 'The charismatic' and 'The transformational' leader. In the context of NHS change the characteristics of such leadership styles would appear to fit. Approaches of this nature support the concept of empowering people in organizations and appear to link in with the aspects of the philosophy of the LEO programmes.

Charismatic and transformation leadership styles

- *Charismatic Leadership*: Leads by inspiring others, expresses strong values, demonstrates competence and confidence, arouses motivation, high expectations for followers. This leadership style uses referent power to facilitate others to follow.
- *Transformational Leadership*: Also driven by referent power, but demonstrates the ability to bring about innovation and change through transforming the way followers think about problems, values and beliefs regarding work and the organization to bring about a more cohesive organization perspective. Leading change through the organizational culture and structure

Leading within the boundaries of a management role may need to take into consideration rules, regulations and loyalties that may influence the style managers would prefer to take as apposed to that which they do take. However, the NHS report, *Managing for Excellence* (DoH, 2002), would seem to address these issues by changing the culture of management within the NHS.

The need to enable managers to develop leadership skills and be able to adapt this role in different situations in addition to facilitate others to take on a pure leadership role would seem to fit in to the new organizational culture within the NHS.

Controlling

Controlling is a term that is often interpreted in a negative way, however in terms of the organization's purpose, some degree of control over what takes place and who does it and what they use to complete it is essential for the organization to active its purpose. This gives us three areas in which to consider this management activity: 'human behaviour', 'processes' and 'resources'. Often these areas are combined in different strategies within the organization.

Human behaviour from an authoritarian approach can be controlled, or as others may suggest from a democratic approach, influenced, by a variety of factors in the organization that can be seen as 'formal' and/or 'informal'.

Factors that influence behaviour

Formal

- Policy;
- procedures;
- rules and regulations;
- leadership; and
- organizational structure.

Informal

- Organizational culture; and
- group norms.

In the NHS, a strategy for formally influencing behaviour can be seen through the introduction of clinical governance and informally, through changing the organizational culture.

The main driving force for such change in the NHS comes from a political source influenced by factors such as 'demographic changes', 'technological changes', 'public expectations' and 'professional concerns of better standards of care'. The creation of clinical governance was to provide NHS organizations with a framework upon which to build a single coherent local programme for quality improvement.

Clinical governance is an umbrella term for a number of co-ordinated strategies designed to improve the quality of care. The key components are 'safety', 'culture', 'quality improvement and maintenance', 'organizational accountability' and 'professional accountability'. The latter leads to a link with personal development processes in the organization and the functions of professional bodies in maintaining standards and regulations for registration.

Quality improvement is often used to encompass those activities that reflect the processes that are carried out when providing a service to the patient or to others who are part of the service provision, such as doctors, nurses, or physiotherapists – all who are involved in delivering the care.

Quality of care delivery can be enhanced through managers influencing staff behaviour relating to professional development by means of appraisal systems. This is a means by which the organization can enhance and develop the skills and knowledge of the workforce to support its purpose. The concept of an individual appraisal system is based on the 'Management by objectives' approach. Individuals, with their manager, identify and negotiate their professional needs, which are then compared to the overall organization objectives. The desired needs are set out as personal objectives, along with the action required to achieve them.

Finally a list of actions, and the necessary evidence that proves achievement over a specific time period, is agreed. This has the benefit of empowering the individual with the responsibility for their own professional development with support from the manager and at the same time it ensures that the organization obtains the professional knowledge and skills to achieve its objectives.

Clinical supervision is a framework which, McSherry et al (2002) suggest, enables the identification and exploration of issues regarding the quality of care delivered and the identification of further professional development to enhance an individual's competence. They go on to suggest that robust systems and process are needed for it to be effective.

The concept of clinical supervision is driven by the need for the professional to reflect (and then problem solve) on their own practice with a group or peer, and is related to the professional group norms and values. Any such approach to the framework could be perceived as a manager's tool as part of the formal monitoring system to measure performance rather than the professional having the responsibility and being accountable for enhancing the quality of care through for their own development of competencies. As the framework for clinical supervision requires time, work rescheduling, and a climate of openness and respect for it to function, it falls to the manager to enable the framework to be developed through the management of resources.

Clinical governance is the link pin to quality improvement. The overall responsibly for this framework is the Chief Executive of the Trust. The framework for its introduction is developed at Trust level and is supported by a clinical lead (usually a senior clinician). Subcommittees may be set up to deal with various aspects of quality such as risk management, clinical standards development and audit, on which they report to the lead clinician their progress.

Each Trust is supported through its clinical governance processes by the National Institute for Clinical Excellence (NICE) guidelines, which have developed national standards and guidelines, and also the Commission for Health Improvement (CHI), which performs a monitoring and evaluation function.

At the practice level clinical governance is used with clear links to clinical supervision and the appraisal system and McSherry and Pearce (2002) suggest a sequence of events that can link both activities together. Identifying poor practice through observation and reflection can be achieved through clinical supervision, while reviewing strengths, weaknesses, opportunities and threats (SWOT Analysis) relating to the professional and the environment and developing the personal development plan can be achieved through the personal development review. With its focus on maintaining and improving standards of care, clinical governance requires feedback from the recipient and user as an essential part of the process.

Recipient and user evaluation of services

Quality improvement can be approached through data collection from the various stakeholders of health care, primarily those who receive it – the patient, and those who use or deliver it – the health carers and health professionals and finally those who purchase it – the hospital Trusts. Feedback from different groups will undoubtedly vary in their focus on what they consider to be good quality.

The NHS has developed structures within the approach to quality to enhance and measure standards of quality through feedback. The National Institute for Clinical Excellence (NICE) regularly carries out spot checks on new arrangements, develops new clinical guidelines, appraises new technologies and promotes clinical audit. Also the Commissions for Health Improvement (CHI) conduct local and national reviews of implementation of NICE guidelines, monitor the quality of care through performance strategies and listen to the experiences of patient and ensure their complaints are dealt with effectively and timely.

There is now more emphasis for feedback from patients to assist in the improvement of the quality of care delivered, so the idea of the 'expert patient' was introduced by the NHS. Assumptions were made that patients with long-standing or chronic diseases could offer valuable insight and experience to healthcare professionals in the care of other such patients. Therefore offering alternative approaches and treatments to patients and improving the professionals understanding of these conditions and patient needs, thereby improves the quality of care.

Patient satisfaction surveys offer another form of feedback to the continued care improvement agenda. Ovretveit (1992) offers some insight into the flaws of such an approach by suggesting that the clients' perception of a service may be influenced by what they want from the service, what they realistically expect the service to provide and what the client thinks they need. Perceptions of this nature may be influenced by other peoples' opinions of their experience, media presentation of health care, and publications released by the NHS. All this will be used to compare the care they receive on which they base the feedback of their experience. Suggestion boxes throughout the Trust, as a means of collecting opinions from both the patient and staff and offering suggestions for the improvement of care provided and resource to support the care, are invaluable provided the people are aware of such a system.

As Total Quality Management, the present approach to quality improvement, is about 'getting it right first time' by ensuring quality at every level in the organization and the focus is of customer care (Clark & Copcutt, 1997) then it is important that feedback from all users and providers of the services be utilized to enable the service to be improved, thereby improving quality of care.

Data collection and its uses

Feedback from any source is considered valuable when development or improvement of processes is involved. The data may be collected using a number of tools. The tools are designed to collect specific forms of data for a particular purpose. Others are designed to collect data present from its source such as form completion in a particular process. This data may be quantitative (facts) or qualitative (opinions) in nature. However, analysis and interpretation of the data is required to enable the manager to carry out the activities of planning, leading, co-ordinating and controlling and to contribute to the achievement of the organization's objectives.

Data collection tools

- Questionnaires;
- interviews;
- discussions;
- observation and field notes;
- case history;
- documentary evidence; and
- diaries.

Each of the activities encompassed within management contribute to the collection of data through the various tools. The data are then analysed and may demonstrate patterns and relationships, which can then be used to inform decision making that ultimately affects the present and the future activities. The data can also be used to develop reports and proposals to improve the quality of the organisation's purpose and objectives. A report of data collection, which may be an investigation or enquiry, often falls on the manager to compile. The subject of the report and data collected are often linked to the activities managers are involved in, 'planning', 'organizing', 'leading' and 'controlling'. Reports are developed with the following considerations; 'what the report is about', and 'to whom it is intended', 'their level of knowledge', 'the use of the report' and 'the focus of the report'.

In general, reports have a common structure, although there are small variations in their headings dependant upon the author, they also differ slightly with the proposal structure. A suggested report structure is given below. In some cases reports are presented in the shape of a form, which is pre-structured with differing sections for information to be entered by the person completing the report.

Suggested formal report structure

- Title page;
- Table of contents;
- Terms of reference;
- Procedures;
- Findings;
- Conclusions;
- Recommendations;
- Appendices; and
- Bibliography.

This structure starts with the *Title*, informing the reader of who wrote the report, where it came from, what it is about and when it was written. The *Contents* are a guide to the structure of the report in terms of the sequence of the content which is set out in sections and appropriate subsections linked to page numbers. The *Terms of Reference* indicate why the report was necessary and any relevant information to support this in addition to the objectives the report intends to achieve. The *Procedure* informs the reader of the way in which the report was compiled, and the strategies used to collect the data, the analysis of the data, a broad indication of the content and how it is presented. The *Findings* convey the results of the analysis, and are dependent on the type of data and the way they have been analysed. The *Conclusions* are a short summary indicating what the report has found. This section should contain no new information, and should lead the reader to the next stage of the report. The *Recommendations* are based on the Conclusions and should be linked to the data collection and the analysis of the report. They should influence the reader towards accepting the fact that the actions that are recommended are appropriate and viable. The *Appendices* deal with relevant material that would normally detract from the report and it is also common to include a *Bibliographic* source of other information and any references used to compile the report.

There are a number of ways in which the report can be developed to create an impact on its reader. Heller & Hindle (1998) suggest making the report interesting, using numbered paragraphs to make cross referencing easier, using headings and sub-headings for related themes. Jay (1995) suggests using a plain English style, using metaphors to explain ideas, and avoiding jargon and clichés. Presentation of the data in the report can be made more understandable through the use of tables, diagrams and the use of colour to emphasize important aspects of data.

In the present climate of quality improvement, changing the way work is done is becoming more important. The approach taken to achieve this is through a strategy of process mapping by a team of people who are involved in the practical aspect of work, supported by a project manger. The NHS Modernization Agency offers support for this strategy through the documents *Process Mapping, Analysis and Redesign* (NHSMA, 2001a) and *Twenty-Seven Principles for Service Redesign* (NHSMA, 2001b).

A selected service, which encompasses a number of tasks such as patient admission, is broken down into separate processes. Each process is then reviewed and evaluated in terms of people involved and resources used. This results in the process being redesigned to make the work more efficient and effective, consequently improving the quality.

Redesigning of work offers the opportunity for the redefinition of work boundaries, increasing education and training for skill development and motivating staff to become more involved and willing to accept changes within the organization. This approach, and the implementation of clinical governance through a multi-professional approach, also has an influence on the organizational culture. Handy (1993) implies that culture is concerned with beliefs about the way people work and the underlying norms and values related to work. In the present environment there is a move towards encouraging members of the NHS to learn from experience, delivering care through the support and expertise of multi-professional teams. This approach to changing behaviour, informally, supports the development of the new organizational culture referred to as 'the organization with a memory' (Department of Health, 2000) in which the drive towards a new learning culture is to remove and replace the older and redundant 'blame culture'.

Conclusion

Although management is often seen by students as something nurses do not do, the examples used in this chapter (off-duty development, working in teams, monitoring care delivery), are a common part of nursing life. It is hoped that nurses will see the relevance of management and its activities; 'planning', 'organizing', 'leading' and 'controlling', in their every day working life when care is to be delivered to patients.

References

Clark, E. J. & Copcutt, L. (1997) *Management for Nurses and Health Care Professionals*, Edinburgh: Churchill Livingstone.

Daft, R. L. (2003) *Management*, (6th edn), Ohio: South Western Thompson Learning.

Department of Health (2000) *The Organisation with a Memory*, London: HMSO.

Department of Health (2002) *Managing for Excellence*, London: HMSO.

Dixon, R. (1997) *The Management Task*, (2nd edn), Oxford: Butterworth Heinemann.

Du Brin, A. J. (2003) *Essentials of Management*, (6th edn), Ohio: South Western Thompson Learning.

Handy, C. (1999) *Understanding Originations*, Harmondsworth: Penguin.

Heller, R. & Hindle, T. (1998) *Essential Manager's Handbook*, London: Dorling Kindersley.

Jay, R. (1995) *How to Write Proposals and Reports that Get Results*, London: Pitman.

McSherry, R. & Pearce, P. (2002) *Clinical Governance: A Guide to Implementation for Health Care Professionals*, Oxford: Blackwell Sciences.

McSherry, R., Kell, J. & Pearce, P. (2002) Clinical supervision and clinical governance, *Nursing Times*, 23(98), 30–2.

National Health Service Modernisation Agency (2001a) *Improvement Leaders Guide To Process Mapping, Analysis and Redesign*, London: HMSO.

National Health Service Modernisation Agency (2001b) *Twenty-Seven Principles for Service Redesign*, London: HMSO.

Northouse, P. G. (2001) *Leadership Theory and Practice*, (2nd edn), London: Sage.

Ovretveit, J. (1992) *Health Service Quality*, Oxford: Blackwell Sciences.

CHAPTER 27

Facilitating Multi-disciplinary Relationships and Practice

MAGGIE HADLAND

Indicative Benchmark Statements

- Awareness of the need to share mental health nursing information with other agencies involved in maintaining public safety

- Identification of the main roles and tasks of the mental health and social care team

- Participation in mental health multidisciplinary team working

- Assertiveness, conflict management and problem solving skills within the multi-disciplinary mental health and social care team

- identification of strategies to enhance staff preservation and prevent individual and team burnout

---

Introduction

In mental health, multi-professional working is the order of the day. This chapter looks at why we need to work collaboratively, and at some of the factors that can influence multi-professional team working. First, the development of professional roles and identities are considered, and how this leads to differing perspectives on the client. Then we will look at self-presentation, and how the perception process influences relationships with others. It describes how groups and teams work and why they don't always work, as well as suggesting some problem-solving strategies. Finally, we look at dealing with conflict, and assertiveness is examined as the key to using interpersonal skills effectively.

Multi-professional practice

Why is a chapter on relationships between health care professionals needed in a textbook on mental health? The answer is that good mental health practice is all about working effectively with others in order to provide seamless care for the client. 'Collaboration [is the] key issue in the direction of all health and community services' (Spratley & Pietroni, 1996 p 255).

The need for increased co-operation between agencies that provide health and social care was first addressed by the enquiry into the death of Maria Colwell in 1974 (Spratley & Pietroni, 1996) and subsequent reports all highlight the lack of interdisciplinary communication. A review of the role of professional knowledge and the social hierarchy of professions has been enshrined in the government initiatives that stress collaborative working, such as the Children Act 1988 (Home Office, 1988) and the Community Care Act (DHSS, 1989). There is increased emphasis on greater democracy (including service user involvement) and less emphasis on the traditional professional hierarchies and their specific areas of knowledge and skill. In the light of a move towards providing more seamless and integrated care, and where service users are increasingly voicing negative opinions of the quality of care they receive, collaborative working must be addressed in a more formal way.

These changes in philosophy (reflected in government strategies and legislation) were often put into practice in a piecemeal and poorly considered fashion. Professionals from a range of disciplines were thrown together and told: 'You are a multidisciplinary team, work together!' and no attempt was made to prepare people to take this new philosophy on board. In in-patient settings, there is frequently only lip service paid to the idea of MDT working – the concept of the 'ward round' still underlines the fact that the head of the MDT is the consultant, and often all the decisions pertaining to a patient are solely his.

Jones (1986) identifies that a great deal of stress comes from the separations of structure and administration, but also points out that higher stress levels are associated with working in an area of unclear role differentiation. This is echoed by Huntington (cited in Spratley & Pietroni, 1996), who argues that being accountable to varying authorities can create conflict for different practitioners, and that all will have their own hierarchies, pay structures, and professional identities. These difficulties are often expressed as personality clashes, but may be simply an expression of differences in working terms, conditions and practices.

Difficulties in inter-agency working are centred on the following areas:

- conflicts; revalues and procedures;
- resource and agency control problems;
- social defences; and
- loss of control.

These difficulties stem from the differences in occupational culture in which each profession is socialized. Occupational culture is made up of the following aspects:

- the specific aim, task and mission of the occupation;
- the focus and orientation of the profession;
- the ideological and knowledge base;
- status and prestige;
- a particular orientation towards patients/clients; and
- a particular orientation towards other professionals.

Let's take a closer look at some of these aspects in relation to doctors, nurses, and social workers. Doctors are undoubtedly the most powerful professional group in health care – WHY?

- Doctors tend to be recruited from the more powerful social groups, and medical schools demand higher entry qualifications than for other health professionals.
- Medicine, like the other professions, has a lengthy and intensive training process that ensures a strong sense of professional identity – only qualified people are admitted to the profession and allowed to call themselves 'Doctor'.
- Once qualified, doctors have a legal monopoly on the process of diagnosis, the prescription of drugs, performing surgical procedures and admitting to and discharging patients from hospital (with some exceptions now such as the triage nurse in A&E, nurse prescribing and minor ops and endoscopies).
- Gender is still an issue – there are still more male doctors and female nurses than the other way around – mirroring the less powerful position of women in society.
- Financial and status rewards are higher for doctors than for other health professionals (Adapted from Brooking, 1991 cited in Mackay, 1995).

Nurses continue to pay a supportive role in spite of changes in nurse education and new attitudes – the power differential in the multidisciplinary team continues to be weighted in favour of the medical staff (Marshall, 1991 cited in Johnson, 1993). Consider the fact that nurses are required to carry out medically prescribed treatments, but doctors do not carry out nursing treatments. Historically, the pre-eminence of science and the scientific approach has resulted in medicine being dominant in health care (Spratley and Pietroni, 1996). Medicine is seen as concerned with finding answers to disease and its cure, while nursing has traditionally been concerned with 'caring'. Unfortunately, curing is seen as more important than caring, and we put greater and greater expectations on medicine's ability to cure us – even of mortality itself!

The differences between health professionals can be compared to the way that people are socialized into tribal behaviours: the term 'tribalism' is used to explain the differences in orientation to the patient/client and to other professional groups. Each profession acts like a tribe, with its own normative systems and set of values. Like tribal society, each profession defines deviant behaviour and imposes sanctions on non-conforming members: consider the negative values surrounding members of one profession taking on board some of the philosophies and ways of working of another profession! Members of the professional 'tribe' are nurtured in ways that emphasizes their differences from other professional groups, and once admitted to full membership of the tribe, there are rules and regulations, leadership and a clear pecking order.

Some suggestions for better multi-professional working

- exposure to and collaboration with the 'out group';
- ideally early in training and continued through professional life; and
- a greater understanding of the different roles and skills that each health professional has to offer (first suggested by Sir Roy Griffiths (Griffiths, 1988 in a letter to the Secretary of State) (Adapted from Jones, 1986).

The work of Spratley and Pietroni (1996) looks at the differing perspectives that different health professionals hold, both towards the client and towards each other. Stokes (1995, cited in Obholzer and Roberts) draws parallels between the type of training and the often unconscious assumptions that each professional then brings to the client and the team.

Doctors are educated in the medical model with its emphasis on the diagnosis and cure of disease. Initially dependent on those with more knowledge, the lengthy training teaches them to work as autonomous professionals who have to shoulder solitary responsibility and make difficult decisions on their own. The model of work in which they are socialized is that of the consultant and junior doctors doing the ward round: old habits therefore 'die hard' and this is the model of team relationships they tend to adhere to. This can make them seem determined to 'rule' at all costs, especially if there are worries about the clients' well being, which could rebound on them.

Nurses are traditionally trained in the medical model to complement the doctors role, they are also hampered by a popular image of nurses as either 'angels of mercy' or a scantily uniformed temptress who would be more at home on page 3 of the tabloid press! Times are changing, and graduate training and new attitudes has resulted in nurses becoming more autonomous and more likely to challenge the status quo. The emphasis is still on care rather than cure, although the nurse practitioner and nurse consultant roles are starting to make a difference. Nursing management is strongly hierarchical and bureaucratic, and nurses are socialized much more into obeying the rules than their medical colleagues. They are developed through training as much more team players than the medical staff, which means that they find it more difficult to make decisions alone.

Social workers do not have an illness model, but see the client in terms of function and dysfunction, and how they fit into systems – whether the family or wider society. The focus is on social care and statutory responses to the conflicting needs of their disparate clients. An over-emphasis on justice and fairness can result in the belief that it is society that is the problem, not the client. Historically social workers suffer from a lack of professional status, and the image of the interfering 'do-gooder'. They have to work within a rigid structure and set of bureaucratic rules, largely as a result of the many inquiries that have centred round social work negligence (Spratley and Pietroni, 1996).

Language also differs from profession to profession, sometimes leading to misunderstandings and hampering joint working. The same words may have very different meanings, e.g. 'community care' may mean different things to different professionals, 'risk management' means one thing to a mental health professional and something altogether different to the manager of a medical unit. Pietroni's work with trainees in medicine, nursing and social work found that negative stereotypes of the other professions were already operating (Pietroni, 1992).

So where do these negative stereotyped ideas about other professionals come from? In order to understand this, we must look at psychological and sociological theories that try to explain how we perceive other people, and how we wish to be perceived.

Self-presentation

We talk about 'making a good impression'. Whether we like to admit it or not, we worry about what other people think of us. Think about the last time you went for an interview – did you just drag on the first clothes that came to hand, or did you think about what to wear? The chances are you thought long and hard about the sort of impression you wanted to make.

Think about the following situations:

- first day at work;
- meeting your boyfriend or girlfriends' parents for the first time;
- going for a night out with friends;
- a rock concert;
- your best friend's wedding;
- a meal out in a posh restaurant.

Would you wear the same clothes for each occasion? Would you behave differently for each occasion? Most people would try to change their image to fit with what they thought was appropriate for the situation – in other words, we manipulate our image to present ourselves in the best possible light. Leary (1996) suggests there are three reasons why human beings are so concerned with *self-presentation*:

- *Interpersonal influence*: Self-presentation is a way of influencing how people respond to us. Poor self-presentation may mean that we won't get the job we want, make friends or find a partner. Human beings want to be liked – a survey conducted by Leary (1996) suggested that qualities such as friendly, intelligent, attractive and fun were the desired impressions they wanted others to have about them: being thought of as boring, conceited and stupid were the impressions people did not want to make. Furthermore, men and women differed only very slightly in the qualities they identified (men rated athleticism as a highly desirable quality). Jones and Pitman (1982) link self-presentation with power, in other words, people can influence the behaviour of others by presenting themselves in a particular way.
- *Personal identity*: Our sense of who we are is formed by the impressions we make on other people. 'What will they think of me?' is often the agonized cry that follows an episode of which we are ashamed – to behave badly in front of others reflects on our sense of who we believe ourselves to be. Self-presentation can also help us to acquire the behaviours we need to be able to enact a new role (Goffman, 1959) – as a student, presenting one's self as a competent nurse is important to develop that identity. If people behave towards you as if you were a competent professional, then you start to believe it. Jones (1964) describes this as the process of signification. It seems that self-presentation plays such an important part in identity formation that we learn to be concerned about what others think from a very early age (Leary, 1996).
- *Emotional regulation*: Our self-esteem can be affected by imagining what others think of us. Being liked and feeling approved of by others helps to bolster self-esteem and reduce negative feelings. Successful impression management may be a way of improving how we feel (Baumgardner et al, 1989). Self-disclosure also helps to reduce negative emotions and increase positive ones, and self-disclosure is closely related to self-presentation (Leary, 1996).

It has been suggested that self-presentation was initially important for survival (Baumeister and Leary, 1994 cited in Leary, 1996). In order to ensure that people were included in protective social groups, humans may have evolved a motivation for nurturing supportive social relationships and co-operative behaviour. Those whose self-presentation skills made them more socially acceptable to the clan would be more likely to find a mate and pass on their genes.

Socially, self-presentation plays a large part in co-operative behaviour. If everybody just behaved the way they wanted to, with no thought for others, social regulation would be impossible and chaos would result! Goffman (1959) made the point that social interaction would be more difficult if we didn't construct and project social identities. Knowing something about someone also makes it easier to predict behaviour in a given situation.

Argyle (1994) reports that we tend to use three categories to form impressions of others:

- *personality traits* such as how intelligent or sociable we appear to be;
- *physical characteristics* like attractiveness and height; and
- *social and occupational roles* tell us about someone's social status, wealth, eligibility, and so on.

Think about the last time you went to a party or social gathering where you knew nobody. How did you decide which person to go and speak to? What questions did you ask initially to help you form an impression of the person? How closely did your predictions about the person match what you found out? First impressions are important in determining our decision to continue relating to that person, and we make an effort to find evidence that supports our initial assessment (Schermerhorn et al, 2000).

Perception and attribution

This is concerned with how we use information about others to make judgements about them. Jones and Davis (1965) and Jones and McGillis (1976) maintain that we pay attention to the clues about another person which are most likely to give us information about that person's character, and we pay less attention to the clues that suggest the person is behaving in that way because of external demands (this is *correspondent inference theory*). How would we find out what sort of a person the boss was? Just seeing him or her performing their usual role would not give us much information – those behaviours would be what was expected in that situation, and are more likely to be externally motivated (Heider, 1958). But if we saw them crying with distraught relatives, playing with their small children in the park, or found we shared a similar interest, we might infer quite different things about them. Jones and McGillis (1976) point out that we pay attention to the behaviours that we feel are freely chosen: that is, behaviours not determined by occupational role. We learn more about an individual by noting behaviours that have low social desirability (in other words, behaviours that are not intended to promote the status of the individual).

Attribution theory

Heider (1958) maintains that when we perceive an action, we must decide whether it is the result of *internal attributes*, i.e., the personal characteristics of the individual, or *external attributes*, i.e., something outside the person such as the situation. Duncan (1976) tested this theory by looking at inter-racial violence. He showed white American college students a film of an argument between two people that escalated until one person pushed the other. The film had four variations:

- black person pushes white person;
- white person pushes black person;
- black person pushes black person; and
- white person pushes white person.

Subjects were asked to describe what they saw, using terms such as 'playing around' or 'violent behaviour'. Over 70 per cent used the term 'violent behaviour' when the protagonist was black!

When asked to explain the behaviour, they were more likely to ascribe the cause of the violence to personal characteristics in the black person, whereas when the protagonist was white, they were more likely to explain the behaviour in situational terms.

Role theory

Another factor that plays a part in our perception of another person is the role they play. We have expectations of how people should behave because in our heads we have a blueprint – *a cognitive prototype* – of roles that we use to categorize others (Cantor & Mischel, 1979). A role can be defined as a set of behaviours associated with a position in the social system (Harre & Lamb, 1986), and each of us will play many roles within the social system to which we belong.

Role behaviours have to be learned, and some roles are more prescriptive than others: in other words, expectations of certain behaviours are more rigidly defined. Compare our expectations of the behaviour of a doctor with the expectations of appropriate behaviour expected of a member of a friendship group. The latter may be interpreted in many different ways, but a doctor's role is more clearly defined. The other people with whom we interact in a particular social setting are called *the role set*. The role set is also responsible for defining the behaviours that are expected in a role.

Role conflict can occur when there is conflict within the individual about how to interpret the role; when two or more roles played by the same person place conflicting demands upon them; or conflict may arise between individuals playing different roles.

Intra-role conflict: the senior nurse on the unit has to discipline a junior nurse, but also understands that this nurse has personal problems, so wants to be supportive. How does the senior nurse manage this conflict of interest?

Inter-role conflict: the nurse whose child is sick has a duty both to her child and to her clients. Which role will win?

Conflict between different people's expectations of role behaviours: student nurses are often surrounded by differing expectations of them. The client may expect all nurses to be capable and not differentiate between qualified and unqualified staff, the senior nurse may expect all student nurses to be incompetent and ill-prepared for clinical work, the medical staff may expect unquestioning obedience. What effect will these differing expectations have on how the student nurse plays the role?

Roles tell us how to behave in given situations, and help us to predict the behaviour of other people based on our internal prototype schema. A role gives us certain rights (nurses can ask complete strangers to undress) and duties (the stranger expects the nurse to behave with respect and professionalism).

Talcott Parsons (1951) compared the rights and obligations conferred by the sick role with the rights and obligations of the medical profession. To be allowed to play *the sick role*, the individual must be genuinely ill, must seek professional help, and must recover as quickly as possible. In return, the sick person is excused from normal responsibilities and tasks, and is given sympathy and support. In contrast, the obligations or responsibilities of the medical profession are to be competent, to abide by the rules of professional practice, and to put patients' interests before their own. The privileges conferred by following these rules are that the doctor is given authority over patients and is allowed to touch them in intimate places, as well as having professional autonomy.

Groups and teams

So what exactly happens when a team first gets together? Teams can be defined as groups with complementary skills who work together to achieve a common purpose for which they hold themselves accountable (Schermerhorn et al, 2000). We work in groups or teams most of the time, and there are good reasons for this. Effective groups are better for problem-solving for three main reasons:

1 the old saying 'two heads are better then one' means that there are more people with expertise to draw on in a group;
2 tasks can be shared out among group members; and
3 creativity and enthusiasm is generated in a group (Schermerhorn et al, 2000).

All teams are groups, and therefore the peculiar dynamics that occur in groups will also occur in teams, and thus can affect how the team performs.

Think about experiences that you have had where the team worked well, and others where group members don't get on, and the job doesn't get done. Can you identify with any of the following? It has been suggested that all groups pass through a sequence of stages from initial setting-up to closing (Tuckman, 1965). Tuckman initially described four stages: later a fifth stage was added (Tuckman & Jensen, 1977).

Forming: This is the beginning of the group and is characterized by *Anxiety*. Group members are getting to know each other and testing relationships. There is much reliance on and questioning of the designated group leader. 'Why are we here?' 'What are we supposed to do?' 'What can the group offer me?' are common questions, and the group members are often preoccupied with the physical environment and 'creature comforts' ('Do we get a coffee break?'). Conversation is often irrelevant to the task at hand.

Storming: This second stage of the group's development is about *Conflict*. Rebellion and competition are fierce, and group members challenge the formal leader and 'test out' the boundaries. Roles are being established within the group, as well as the pecking order. Alliances and cliques form, and there is tension between those group members seen as silent (or 'passive') and those seen as 'active' within the group. Silent members are often attacked and their contributions disregarded by other group members.

Norming: This is the point in the group process when the group begins to develop an identity, and group members see themselves as belonging. Group norms or rules for behaviour are established, and *Cohesion* is the dominant theme. Members begin to trust each other and common goals and tasks are shared. Group roles are firmly established, and the group identifies reward and punishment systems for its members.

Performing: The group is now *Working* – energies are channelled into the group task, and members are motivated by group goals. The group structure is stable, and any disagreements between members are usually handled with greater flexibility. As the group matures, it should be able to respond appropriately to changes and challenges.

Adjourning: This final stage of the group's life is especially important for temporary working parties, project teams and committees, for instance, which are set up with a specific remit and time frame. If this stage is completed successfully, it should enable the group members to re-convene and work well together in the future, should the need arise (Adapted from Tuckman, 1965, Tuckman & Jensen, 1977).

There is no time scale over which these stages will occur, and some groups may become stuck at an early stage. For instance, where there is a high turnover of staff the group may constantly return to the forming and storming stages each time a new member joins the team, and never progress to the norming or performing stages. In this situation, the team's energies will be dissipated in conflict and little may be accomplished.

Within groups, individuals will play certain roles. A fundamental split that often occurs in groups is between the silent or passive members, and the more vocal, active members. The social psychologist Robert Bales (1950) suggested that people in groups were either 'task-oriented or maintenance oriented'.

Task-oriented group members are people whose behaviour is goal driven. They keep the group on target by constantly reminding them of the task, seek or provide information, and are good at clarifying problems and pushing for decisions. Task-oriented people do not tolerate confusion, and tend to limit debate in order to reach a solution. Too many task-oriented people in a group do not necessarily achieve the task quicker, as they may argue among themselves about what is the right answer and how to achieve the goal.

Maintenance-oriented group members are more interested in the social network in the group. They do not necessarily contribute directly to the task, but promote harmony and cohesion within the group, making the group experience more pleasant and increasing commitment to membership of the group. People who play a maintenance role support and encourage others, and reduce tension in the group by reconciliation and compromise. A group made up mainly of maintenance-oriented people may lack drive and the impetus to succeed.

Bales (1950) also identified a third type of behaviour sometimes seen in groups, which does not fall into either category.

Self-oriented behaviour is not aimed at doing the task or promoting group cohesion. Probably the most common example of this is withdrawal – we have all been in groups where one or more members make it quite clear they wish they weren't there by looking out of the window, physically distancing themselves, doodling, or refusing to co-operate with the group task. Other examples of self-oriented behaviour include:

- the *joker* is never serious;
- The *nitpicker* is always finding fault;
- The *hobby-horse* always has his or her own agenda; and
- The *red herring* always talks about irrelevancies (adapted from Douglas, 1978).

Think about groups of which you are a member – you can probably identify at least one of these roles, and there are others.

Most people will display self-oriented behaviour if they are attacked or feeling threatened; people who feel insecure in a group setting or are too concerned with meeting their own needs may also behave in this way. The group itself may be the problem – poor leadership, the wrong mix of members or simply a group that is too big can result in an increase in anxiety levels and therefore increase self-oriented behaviour in the group members.

This type of behaviour can be destructive and time wasting, so needs to be dealt with quickly. If most of the group is behaving in this way, it should be tackled as a group issue. If it is only one or two individuals, here are some ideas on how to deal with self-oriented behaviour:

- *Dont increase defensiveness* – here is someone who is already behaving defensively.
- *Include in a non-threatening way* – self-oriented behaviour often stems from feeling excluded.
- *Give the individual a job to do within the group* – this builds self-esteem, reduces anxiety and increases commitment.

Belbin (1981) identified eight team types characterized by certain personality characteristics that he felt were essential to a functioning team. He based his theory on observations of management training games, and used psychometric tests to relate team behaviour to psychological traits. Belbin came to the conclusion that most people have a 'preferred' team role, as well as a 'secondary' role that they could play in the absence of someone better able to take on that particular team behaviour.

Groups or teams that have been working well together for a long time can also have problems. One of these is called *'groupthink'*, and was first described by Janis (1982). Groupthink is characterized by extreme conformity within the group, and results in poor or downright disastrous decision-making (Janis cites a number of controversial US government decisions as examples of groupthink, such as the space shuttle 'Challenger' disaster). Groupthink can happen when members fail to question, individuals who rock the boat are censored or considered deviant, and outside opinions are not sought.

A second problem of long-standing groups is known as *'the risky shift'* – the group tends to make decisions that are more daring and controversial than those which might be made by an individual acting alone (Wallach et al, 1962). This seems to result from people feeling that they have no individual responsibility for the group's decision: if things turn out badly, the group members can say: 'It wasn't my decision, it was the group.'

Team types

Chairman – Not necessarily the appointed team leader, this person is able to control and co-ordinate the team in a facilitative way. Good at recognizing strengths and weaknesses in the team, and is able to bring out the best in others. The chairman is neither the most intelligent nor the most creative person in the team, but is practical and has a strong sense of objectives.

Shaper – Dynamic, assertive and impatient to get the job done, the shaper is charismatic, competitive and needs to be in charge! Can be intolerant and dislikes rules and regulations, but rarely holds a grudge and can be extremely effective at getting to the point. Inspiring when working well, but not always popular and works best in an informal setting.

Plant – So called because they act as the catalyst for new ideas within the team, the plant is usually highly intelligent and able to bring creative energy into the team. Not concerned with 'boring' detail or practicalities, some of their ideas are unworkable, while others are inspired. Can be sensitive and needs careful handling.

Monitor evaluator – The only other team member identified as being highly intelligent, the monitor evaluator is cool, objective and analytical the 'Mr Spock' of the team (with apologies to Star Trek)! Essential but irritating, the monitor evaluator is almost always right and can prevent the team from making costly mistakes. However, he or she can be seen as negative and may have a dampening effect on morale.

Company worker – The backbone of the team, the company worker is reliable and hardworking. He or she is able to translate ideas into practical action and gets the job done. Likes order and organization and is uncomfortable with change.

Resource investigator – Extrovert, enthusiastic and loves new ideas. The resource investigator has contacts everywhere – he or she is the team's liaison with the outside world and is able to bring new ideas back into the team. Usually to be found on the phone doing a bit of 'wheeling and dealing', this team member needs constant stimulation and variety, and will become de-motivated if socially isolated or bored.

Team worker – Person-oriented, the team worker can enhance morale and maintain harmony in the team. This is the person who will bring in the cream cakes when it's someone's birthday, and can sense when other team members are troubled. Often an unsung hero, this is the one member of the team who is missed when they are not there.

Completer-finisher – Obsessive and particular, the completer finisher ensures that the paperwork is done, jobs are completed on time, and even the smallest details are correct. Often perceived as a 'nagger' by colleagues but guards against slapdash work. (*Source*: Adapted from Belbin, 1981.)

Using interpersonal skills effectively

Working with other people is not always a harmonious experience. Conflict is part of human experience, and although we tend to think of conflict as a bad thing, without it new ideas would not always be tried, and change wouldn't happen. Nelson-Jones (1990) details the positive aspects of conflict as being greater trust and increased intimacy, arising from the sharing of honest feedback and being able to maintain a relationship in spite of differences in viewpoint; increased self-esteem resulting from managing conflicts well and creative solutions from successful problem solving.

How we deal with conflict in the workplace is what determines a successful outcome. It is suggested that there are three main styles when it comes to handling conflict (Nelson-Jones 1990).

The *competitive* style is a 'fight' response and the goal is to win. Competition is, therefore, seen as a win–lose situation, and the individual who views conflict in this way may be prepared to use any tactics in order to get what they want, including lying, denying mistakes and using aggressive verbal and non-verbal language.

In contrast, the *compliant* individual exhibits a 'flight' response, in which issues may be either avoided altogether, or the compliant individual will simply give in, even if they are in the right – anything for an easy life.

The ideal way of dealing with conflict is the *collaborative* approach, where people work together to maximize gains and minimize losses. Nelson-Jones (1990) describes this as the 'win–win' approach, but admits that it may not be so easy to put into practice when people have strong feelings about an issue and may not be prepared to compromise.

Confrontation is another way of dealing with conflict that can be helpful, although needs to be carefully considered first. Confrontation is about pointing out reality, encouraging people to look at themselves, their behaviour and its consequences. Burnard (1992a) offers this advice in relation to challenging and confronting.

- Be clear what you are confronting about.
- Only confront about one issue at a time.
- Don't moralize or blame.
- Say what you have to say clearly and calmly and repeat if necessary.

This is really about how we can use interpersonal skills to deal effectively with conflict in the workplace, and *Assertiveness* is the key to successful interpersonal relationships. Assertiveness enables us to deal with conflict, ask for what we want, and state what we think without intimidation or aggression. Kagan and Evans (1994) maintain that assertion is about demonstrating respect for others, not about power. Martin and Osborne (1989, p 150) describe assertion as *'exert[ing] one's rights as a human without subsequent offence'*.

Assertiveness needs to be differentiated from other less helpful ways of dealing with conflict situations. Three main approaches have been identified by a number of writers (see Table 27.1)

Assertiveness can be differentiated from non-assertiveness in a number of ways. For instance, assertive people make more requests, use fewer words to put their point across, and are more likely to make 'I' statements to express their feelings: that is, they are more likely to 'own' the feelings (Martin & Osborne, 1989). Non-verbal behaviours also differ, in that assertive people are more likely to maintain eye contact, stand straight, and have facial expressions congruent with what they are saying (Williams & Long, 1979).

Table 27.1 Approaches to dealing with conflict situations

Passive behaviour	Aggressive behaviour	Assertive behaviour	Alberti and Emmons (1986)
Compliant	Competitive	Collaborative	(Nelson-Jones, 1990)
The pussyfooting approach	The sledgehammer approach	The assertive approach	(Burnard, 1992)
A 'flight' response.	A 'fight' response.	A 'win/win' response.	
The person avoids issues or gives way	The person is determined to win and will use any methods. The situation is seen as a personal attack.	The person is calm, clear and communicates intentions with respect for the other person.	

We often find assertive behaviour difficult because of early messages we have picked up about being polite and respecting other people's feelings. Women in particular tend to find assertive behaviour difficult, which is more problematic in a male-dominated work environment (Martin & Osborne, 1989). The following list is a charter of assertive rights, adapted from Davis et al (1982), that might be helpful in dispelling some of the mistaken ideas we have about assertiveness.

Your assertive rights

- You have a right to put yourself first, sometimes.
- You have a right to make mistakes.
- You have the right to be the final judge of your feelings.
- You have a right to your own opinions and convictions.
- You have a right to change your mind or decide on a different course of action.
- You have a right to protest unfair treatment or criticism.
- You have a right to interrupt in order to request clarification.
- You have a right to negotiate for change.
- You have a right to ask for help or emotional support.
- You have a right to feel and express pain.
- You have a right to ignore the advice of others.
- You have a right to receive formal recognition for your work and achievements.
- You have a right to say NO.
- You have a right to be alone.
- You have a right to not have to justify yourself to others.
- You have a right to not take responsibility for someone else's problem.
- You have a right to not to have to anticipate the wishes and needs of others.

- You have a right to not always worry about the goodwill of others.
- You have a right to choose not to respond to a situation.

References

Alberti, R. E. & Emmons, M. L. (1986) *Your Perfect Right: A Guide to Assertive Living*, (5th edn), San Luis Obispo, CA: Impact Publishers.

Argyle, M. (1994) *Bodily Communication*, (2nd edn), London: Methuen.

Bales, R. F. (1950) *Interaction Process Analysis*,. Cambridge, MA: Addison-Wesley.

Baumgardner, A. H., Kaufman, C. M. & Levy, P. E. (1989) Regulating affect interpersonally; when low esteem leads to greater enhancement, *Journal of Personality and Social Psychology*, 56, 907–21.

Belbin, R. M. (1981) *Management Teams*, London: Heinemann.

Burnard, P. (1992a) *Know Yourself*, London: Scutari Press.

Burnard, P. (1992b) *Interpersonal Skills Training*, London: Kogan Page.

Cantor, N. & Mischel, W. (1979) Prototypes in person perception, in I. Berkowitz (ed.), *Advances in Experimental Social Psychology*, Vol. 2, New York: Academic Press.

Davis, M., Eshelman, E. R. & McKay, M. (1982) *The Relaxation and Stress Reduction Workbook*, Oakland, CA: New Harbinger Publications.

Department of Health and Home Office (1990) *National Health Service and Community Care Act*, London: HMSO

Douglas, T. (1978) *Basic Groupwork*, London: Tavistock Publications.

Duncan, S.L. (1976) Differential social perception and attribution of intergroup violence: testing the lower limits of stereotyping of blacks, *Journal of Personality and Social Psychology*, 34, 590–8.

Goffman, E. (1959) *The Presentation of Self in Everyday Life*, Garden City, NJ: Doubleday Anchor.

Griffiths, R. (1988) *Community Care: Agenda for Action*, London: HMSO.

Harre, R. & Lamb, R. (1986) *The Dictionary of Personality and Social Psychology*, Cambridge, MA: The MIT Press.

Heider, F. (1958) *The Psychology of Interpersonal Relations*, New York: Wiley.

Home Office (1988) *Childrens Act*, London: HMSO.

Janis, I. (1982) *Groupthink*, (2nd edn), Boston: Houghton Mifflin.

Johnson, T. (1993) *Professions and Power*, UK: Macmillan, now Palgrave Macmillan.

Jones, E. E. & Davis, K. E. (1965) From acts to dispositions: the attribution process in person perception, in I. Berkowitz (ed.), *Advances in Experimental Social Psychology*, Vol. 2, New York: Academic Press

Jones, E. E. & McGillis, D. (1976) Correspondent inferences and the attribution cube: a comparative peappraisal, in J. H. Harvey et al (eds), *New Directions in Attribution Research 1*, Hillsdale, NJ: Erlbaum.

Jones, E. E. (1964) *Ingratiation*, New York: Appleton-Century-Crofts.

Jones, E. E. & Pitman, T. S. (1982) Toward a general theory of strategic self-presentation. in J. Suls (ed.), (1995) *Psychological Perspectives on the Self*, Hillsdale, NJ: Erlbaum, 231–62.

Jones, R. V. H. (1986) *Working Together – Learning Together*, London: RGCP.

Kagan, C. & Evans, J. (1994) *Professional Interpersonal Skills for Nurses* Cheltenham: Nelson Thornes.

Leary, M. (1996) *Self-presentation*, Oxford: Westview Press Inc.

Mackay, L. (1995) *Conflicts in Care: Medicine and Nursing,* London: Chapman and Hall.

Martin, G. L. & Osborne, J. G. (1989) *Psychology, Adjustment and Everyday Living,* Englewood Cliffs, NJ: Prentice Hall.

Nelson-Jones, R. (1990) *Human Relationship Skills*, (2nd ed.), London: Cassell.

Parsons, T. (1951) *The Social System,* Glencoe, IL: Free Press.

Pietroni, P. C. (1992) Towards reflective practice – the languages of health and social care, *Journal of Interprofessional Case*, 6(1), 7–16.

Schermerhorn, J. R., Hunt, J. G. & Osborn, R. N. (2000) *Organizational Behaviour*, (7th edn), New York: John Wiley and Sons.

Spratley, J & Pietroni, M. (1996) Creative collaboration: inter-professional learning priorities in primary health and community care, in M. Pietroni & P. C. Pietroni (eds), *Innovation in Community Care and Primary Health,* London: Churchill Livingstone.

Obholzer & Roberts (eds) (1995) *The Unconscious at Work,* London: Routledege.

Tuckman, B. W. (1965) Developmental sequence in small groups, *Psychological Bulletin*, 63, 384–99.

Tuckman, B. W & Jensen M. A. C. (1977) Stages of small group development revisited, *Group and organizational Studies*, 2, 419–27.

Wallach, M. A., Kogan, N. & Bem, D. J. (1962) Group influence on individual risk taking, *Journal of Abnormal and Social Psychology*, 65, 75–86.

Williams, R. L. & Long, J. D. (1979) *Toward a Self-Managed Lifestyle*, (2nd edn), Boston: Houghton Mifflin.

CHAPTER 28

The Evidence Base

ANGELA MORGAN AND CHRIS STEVENSON

Indicative Benchmark Statements

▨ Participation in the provision of evidence-based family intervention programmes for service users with severe mental illness

▨ Retrieval and critical appraisal of mental health research and relevant evidence

▨ Utilization of appropriate research and relevant evidence to support decision-making relating to the selection and individualization of mental health nursing interventions

▨ A commitment to disseminating own evidence-based mental health research and practice development

---

Introduction

This chapter aims to facilitate an understanding of what evidence-based practice (EBP) is and its relevance to mental health nursing. This will be supported by exploring the nature of evidence and the methodologies that can be used to generate research-evidence. Also we will be examining the use of evidence to underpin day-to-day mental health nursing practice.

The suggestion that all nurses use evidence as a basis for practice has gained momentum over the past decade and a requirement to do so is now firmly embedded in the professional benchmark statements. However, EBP is not such a new concept and authors such as Hunt (1996), state that using evidence (as a basis for nursing care) has featured in the literature for the last 30 years. Hamer's (1999) analysis of factors that have contributed to a rise in the requirement for EBP generally, includes the following factors:

- economic factors – limited resources enhance the need to ensure value for money;
- technological advances – an increase in the availability of treatments and interventions has led to a need to ensure their effectiveness; and

- enhanced consumer awareness – this has resulted from increased availability of information, particularly via the World Wide Web and subsequently service users are more likely to question healthcare treatments and interventions.

In addition to this, the Department of Health's commitment to achieving effective practice is unquestionable and this is evident in documents such as the NHS Executive (1998) document *Achieving Effective Practice*. Colyer and Kamath (1999) propose that the EBP initiative stems from the dominant political ideology of the past 20 years. This liberal ideology, which promotes individual freedom and choice, resulted in the introduction of general management systems (Griffiths, 1983) and the free market in 1991. These two main factors, argue Colyer and Kamath (1999), have intensified the demand for service providers to improve the quality and effectiveness of healthcare and they have resulted in the emergence of the EBP initiative.

EBP undoubtedly has its roots in medicine (e.g., Rosenberg & Donald, 1995) but according to Regan (1998, p 245) its subsequent adoption by the nursing profession may have resulted from a move to increase the professionalism of nursing:

> To a profession that has struggled to establish itself as an equal partner and not handmaiden to the medical profession, the opportunity to prove the worth of nursing by measuring the effectiveness of its interventions could be seen as an exciting challenge and a real opportunity to raise the profile of nursing.

What is evidence-based practice?

A variety of terms are in existence including 'evidence-based medicine', 'evidence-based healthcare', 'evidence-based practice' and 'evidence-based nursing'. In addition, the NHS Executive (1998) uses the term 'clinical effectiveness', which incorporates the use of EBP. An attempt will be made here to clarify the meaning of some of these concepts but the reader is directed to French (2002), Bradshaw (2000) and Jennings and Loan (2001) for more in-depth reviews of definitions and concept analyses.

Evidence-based medicine is defined by Sackett et al (2000, p 246) as:

> the conscientious, explicit and judicious use of current best evidence in making decisions about the care of individual patients. The practice of evidence-based medicine means integrating individual clinical expertise with the best available external clinical evidence from systematic research.

Renfrew (1997) describes EBP as a culture based on enquiry and the use of research evidence to inform practice. This involves using the best possible information to help in making clinical decisions. The NHS Executive (1998) use the following, very complex definition of EBP from McKibbon et al (1995, p 737):

> evidence-based practice is the conscientious, explicit and judicious use of current best evidence, based on systematic review of all available evidence – including patient reported, clinician observed and research derived evidence – in making and carrying out decisions about the care of individual patients. The best available evidence, moderated by patient circumstances and preferences, is applied to improve the quality of clinical judgements.

This is a very complex definition, however it does recognize that there are other forms of evidence apart from research. We will discuss forms of evidence in more detail shortly.

The term EBP is frequently used in a nursing context and Jennings and Loan (2001) offer several definitions including the one from Ingersoll (2000, p 152): 'Evidence-based nursing practice is the conscientious, explicit and judicious use of theory-derived, research-based information in making decisions about care delivery to individuals or groups of patients and in consideration of individuals' needs and preferences.' Rosenberg and Donald (1995) describe four stages involved in EBP:

- Formulate a clear clinical question from the patient's problem.
- Search the literature for relevant clinical articles.
- Evaluate (critically appraise) the evidence for its validity and usefulness.
- Implement useful findings in clinical practice.

Case Study 28.1

As a mental health nurse, a relevant question might be 'what is the most effective method of working with an adolescent person with Anorexia Nervosa?'

A critical appraisal of available evidence would then be used to develop guidelines.

In the example given, research evidence suggests that *structural family therapy* (Minuchin, 1974) is the treatment of choice for cases where the person is a young adolescent and living at home and being seen on an out-patient basis (Eisler et al, 1997; Robin et al, 1995; Russell et al, 1987). However, as McKibbon et al's (1995) and Ingersoll's (2000) definitions indicate, the implementation of such guidelines may need to be moderated to take into account individual circumstances.

A pervasive staff view on people who eat differently is that it has been impossible for them to move on with life and they are 'stuck' at a developmental life stage that is not congruent with their chronological age. Staff members sometimes talk about 'the missing years'. In this circumstance, it is possible for family meetings to be effective with adult patients despite the lack of congruence with research evidence that indicates the treatment is effective with adolescents. The need to judge the specific clinical situation is even more convincing in the light of *lack* of convincing evidence about what *is* the most effective treatment option for adults in anorexia (Dare et al, 2001).

Implicit in the earlier discussion, was an assumption that EBP is related to clinical effectiveness. The NHS Executive (1998, Section 1, p 6) defines clinical effectiveness as: 'the extent to which specific clinical interventions, when deployed in the field for a particular patient or population, do what they are intended to do. That is, maintain or improve health and secure the greatest possible health gain from the resources available'.

EBP implies that health professionals should use evidence *of some form* in their decision-making. McKenna et al (2000) identify that this concerns the *process* of decision-making and definitions rarely make explicit reference to the outcomes of those decisions. Clinical effectiveness, McKenna et al (2000) propose, relates to both the *process* and the *outcomes* of decision-making.

Clinical effectiveness, therefore, introduces the notion that we should utilise interventions that promote the greatest health gain for the lowest cost.

Case Study 28.2

So, if our review of the evidence relating to Anorexia Nervosa (disregarding age factor) reveals two equally effective interventions in terms of health gain, family therapy and psychoanalytic psychotherapy (Dare et al, 2001), to comply with clinical effectiveness, the least expensive option should be selected.

The Government has set up the National Institute for Clinical Excellence (NICE) to develop guidelines around particular aspects of service delivery to assist practitioners. An example of clinical guidelines of relevance to mental health nurses is the guidelines on 'Schizophrenia; Core Interventions in the Treatment and Management of Schizophrenia in Primary and Secondary Care (available from http://www.nice.org.uk).

However, such a view regarding the way in which decisions about the treatment of choice are made may be naïve. Returning to our example, family therapy is, superficially, more resource hungry, as it requires a team of practitioners. Psychoanalytic psychotherapy does not. Yet, any cost benefit analysis needs to take into account the whole system. For example, Proctor et al (2000) suggest that the assessment of service utilization may be a simplistic measure on which to base treatment decisions. A more comprehensive model is to take account of indirect costs, e.g., the cost of informal caring offered by family members, which may be offset by an *apparently* more expensive intervention.

The NHS Executive (1998) states that the key activities needed to support clinically effective practice include:

- selecting a particular aspect of practice to question or examine;
- finding out from the literature and professional networks and other sources what is current best practice and critically appraising the available literature and sources;
- implementing and/or learning how to provide best known practice;
- confirming that you're providing best practice on a day-to-day basis; and
- changing practice to make improvements if necessary.

This clinical effectiveness process seems to incorporate the stages of EBP. However, it goes further in that it uses clinical audit to monitor whether or not EBP is being achieved and implementing changes in practice if necessary. The NHS Executive (1998, Section 5, p 3) define clinical audit as: 'a clinically led initiative which seeks to improve the quality and outcome of patient care through structured peer review whereby clinicians examine their practices and results against agreed explicit standards and modify their practice where indicated'.

So, to summarize, Evidence Based Practice is about systematically finding, appraising and using evidence as a basis for clinical decisions; clinical effectiveness is about ensuring care is effective by applying EBP and clinical audit and implementing change where appropriate. Clinical audit encourages professionals to examine their practices and results against agreed explicit standards (developed using appropriate evidence) and modify their practice where indicated. All of these processes are integral strands of the government's agenda for quality. This is implemented via clinical governance, the framework by which NHS organizations demonstrate accountability for continuously improving the quality of their services (NHS Executive, 1999).

What constitutes evidence?

Central to an understanding of EBP is an analysis of what constitutes appropriate evidence. Sackett et al's (2000) definition does not identify types of evidence. Ingersoll's (2000) definition suggests that evidence includes theory-derived and research-based information and McKibbon et al (1995) add in clinician-observed and patient-reported data. However, even within this pluralistic approach, it seems that much more weighting is given to research-derived evidence. McKenna et al (2000) report on the following commonly used hierarchy of evidence:

- Level 1 – meta-analysis of a series of randomized controlled trials;
- Level 2 – at least one well-designed randomized controlled trial;
- Level 3 – at least one controlled study without randomization;
- Level 4 – non-experimental descriptive studies; and
- Level 5 – reports or opinions from respected authorities.

However, EBP is constantly evolving and Harbour and Miller (2001) as part of the Scottish Intercollegiate Guidelines Network Grading Review Group (SIGN) have further refined the hierarchy and have developed a grading system for levels of evidence.

Implicit within hierarchies of evidence is the assumption that Level 1 offers the strongest form of evidence while Level 5 is the weakest. Only level 5 utilizes a source of evidence that is not research-based, which adds some weight to the assumption that EBP is synonymous with research-based practice.

While patient-reported and clinician-observed data are included in some definitions of EBP, they rarely appear explicitly in evidence hierarchies. Jennings and Loan (2001) offer three examples of evidence hierarchies and all of them mainly focus around the use of experimental research studies. The Cochrane library which commissions and reports systematic reviews of the literature limits inclusion to experimental studies and sees the randomized controlled trial as the gold standard. Bury (1998) highlights that this is generally appropriate for questions relating to the effectiveness of interventions and this is usually the focus of Cochrane reviews. They also advocate that the hierarchy of evidence should be tailored to the type of question being posed and suggest that questions of 'appropriateness' should include qualitative research much higher up the hierarchy.

Humphris (1999) offers the following hierarchy of research evidence, which again places more emphasis on quantitative research methods:

- Randomised controlled trial;
- Case-controlled study (participants are recruited who have the condition or diagnosis under study and a control group is recruited with participants who are free of the condition but matched on important variables);
- Cohort study (studies a group of participants over time);
- Survey;
- Qualitative studies; and
- Professional consensus.

While it is beyond the remit of this chapter to discuss research designs in detail, an attempt will be made to explore some of the key features of those research designs identified in the above hierarchy of evidence. Research is a systematic process that involves the collection of primary data with the intention of generating knowledge. In a simplistic overview, research designs are underpinned by one of two philosophical traditions. Quantitative research collects data that can be manipulated numerically and it is based on the belief that there is an objective world that exists independently of our existence that can be measured objectively. This is often referred to as *positivism*.

Positivists believe that laws and mechanisms determine events, as they do in the natural sciences. They also believe that these laws can be discovered via research and such discoveries can be used to predict events and behaviours. There is an interest in linking cause and effect and generalizing findings from the study situation to other situations.

Broadly speaking, there are two types of study that fit within the positivist tradition; experiments and surveys. While both of these collect numerical data, there is a distinction. Surveys collect naturally occurring data, generally using structured questions i.e.: the researcher does not administer an intervention of any kind. Surveys are considered to be a weak form of evidence in the hierarchy. In contrast, an experiment such as *a randomized controlled trial (RCT)* is a type of research that introduces an intervention to one group of people (e.g., a community team approach) and measures the effect that it has on particular outcomes. In order to be confident that any changes in outcomes wouldn't have occurred anyway, the intervention group are compared with a control group who didn't receive the intervention. The allocation of the subjects to the intervention or control group is performed randomly (i.e., every member has an equal chance of being allocated to the intervention group) to reduce bias and ensure that the intervention (experimental) and control groups are similar in all respects except for the intervention. Any difference observed in the outcomes can then be attributed to the intervention and a cause and effect relationship can be established. In addition to being similar in all respects, the two groups must also be treated in an identical way in order to achieve experimental control. If they are not, then differences in outcomes cannot be attributed to the intervention, they may be due to the groups being treated differently in other ways. Healthcare experiments are often difficult to control because human subjects are autonomous and strict control (e.g., ensuring that participants adhere to the prescribed intervention) is often difficult to maintain. In addition, attempts to exert such control result in an artificial situation that often doesn't represent real life. Generalizing such findings to more natural situations is then problematic.

Occasionally, for practical or ethical reasons, random allocation and strict control cannot be achieved. The researcher may then choose to study a naturally occurring group of people experiencing an intervention (e.g., a particular form of nursing care or therapy) and compare them to a similar group of people who haven't. This is called a *case-controlled study* (Humphris, 1999) or a quasi-experiment. Such studies are considered as weaker in the hierarchy because differences in outcomes may result from inherent differences between the groups rather than being directly attributable to the intervention.

The hierarchy, therefore, places great emphasis on RCT's, particularly when assessing the effectiveness of interventions. How useful then is it for mental health nursing interventions? Repper and Brooker (1998) remind us that in order to evaluate healthcare interventions, it is necessary to measure the health of those receiving it before and after the intervention. In relation to physical health, outcome measures may include physiological measurements, but when considering mental health, outcome measures are problematic. Repper and Brooker (1998) report that often, proxy outcome measures are used such as service use and mortality, although there is widespread recognition that as indicators, they are unreliable. Such outcome measures also generally fail to consider the service users' perspectives and these are often different from those of the mental health service provider. Repper and Brooker (1998) also argue that outcome studies usually focus on single, rather than multiple interventions, whereas in reality, usually a range of interventions and services are offered. For example, a recent paper by Stevenson et al (2002), which reported the development of a model to evaluate the Tidal Model for Psychiatric Nursing, was criticized for not being RCT based (Gamble and Wellman, 2002). Barker and Stevenson (2002) point out in reply that it is naïve to think that all variables apart from the intervention can be controlled in clinical settings, and that outcome measures can be taken that accurately reflect the effect of an intervention. Rather they advocate looking at what happens within a system when a new practice is introduced. Such qualitative research offers a deeper more individualized picture regarding clients' experiences of an intervention and their feelings regarding it.

In contrast to the positivist view that sets out to measure phenomena objectively, qualitative researchers believe that there is no one objective reality. They also believe that human behaviour is inextricably linked to the context in which it occurs and that human behaviour can only be understood when the context in which it takes place is studied. This philosophical approach is sometimes called naturalism or *interpretivism*. Qualitative research methods are often used in order to gain a holistic understanding of the meaning that healthcare situations have for the users of mental health services. Qualitative data cannot be manipulated numerically and it is collected using in-depth data collection methods such as unstructured interviews and observation. It is inductive (theory generating) as opposed to deductive (theory testing) and the findings are not generalizable to the population under study because they are inextricably linked to the context in which they were generated. Such findings can provide the mental health nurse with a meaningful insight into the patient's world or experience. For example, a study reported by Aldridge and Stevenson (2001) used in depth interviewing in order to elicit the meaning for one client of being diagnosed as schizophrenic. The focus was on her personal feelings and adaptations, but also on how the psychiatric system (composing both professionals and other service users) responded, and how that in turn was important in constructing her experience. In addition to utilizing qualitative research methods to gain an insight into practice, Morse et al (2000) propose that they can be used to rigorously evaluate nursing interventions. This deviates from the accepted view that it is only the RCT that can do this. They discuss a process they label Qualitative Outcome Analysis (QOA) which takes into account the dynamic nature of nursing interventions and includes two stages. The initial project collects qualitative data to illuminate the patients' experiences, while the second QOA phase identifies strategies and evaluates their efficacy. However, whether this approach becomes accepted as a legitimate form of evidence by the 'scientific community' remains to be seen, although, we would argue, it seems eminently suitable for developing and evaluating mental health nursing interventions.

Instead of becoming embroiled in the quantitative/qualitative debate, McKenna et al (2000) offer an alternative typology that focuses on the quality of evidence-based nursing. They refer to this as an 'evidence-egg' that contains four areas:

- Area one contains those nursing interventions that are informed by good research evidence (what is meant by good evidence is not explained). These interventions tend to do more good than harm. An example given is the use of cognitive behavioural therapies in reducing the frequency and intensity of medically unexplained physical symptoms (Speckens et al, 1995).

- Area two contains interventions that are not based on sound research but are supported by the opinions of experts. These interventions tend to do more good than harm. The use of models of nursing and psychoanalysis are cited as examples of interventions in this area.

- Area three contains those nursing interventions that are not based on research evidence or expert opinion, but on tradition as identified by Walsh and Ford (1989). It is not known whether or not such interventions cause more harm than good. The cited example here is the continued use of the therapeutic community method of treatment for patients with borderline personality disorder that Cornah et al (2000) believe has uncertain results.

- Area four contains those nursing interventions that actually do more harm than good such as the use of 'tilt chairs' for older patients.

McKenna et al (2000) argue that the nursing profession should strive to increase areas one and two and eradicate area four. In relation to area three, such interventions should be evaluated and if found to be beneficial, they will be subsumed within area one. They also propose that the idea of achieving an ideal of 100 per cent of nursing interventions being research-based is unrealistic and naïve. In fact, extensive analysis of the types of knowledge that nurses use to underpin their practice identifies that scientifically derived knowledge is only one type of knowledge used by nurses in their every day practice. Carper's (1978) analysis of nursing knowledge is widely accepted and identified four types of knowledge used by nurses:

- *Empirics* – this knowledge originates from theory and empirical research. This is sometimes referred to as propositional knowledge.

- *Aesthetics* – this is referred to as the art of nursing. According to Rolfe (2001) this is essentially tacit or unspoken and is expressed in practice rather than language. McKenna et al (2000) explain that aesthetic knowledge is individual and unique and includes intuition.

- *Personal knowledge* – this includes knowledge about the patient/client and knowledge about oneself. This includes how the nurse relates to others and it seems to incorporate the interpersonal aspects of knowledge.

- *Ethical knowledge* – this involves an evaluation of what is right and wrong and according to McKenna et al (2000) this type of knowing is expressed through moral codes and ethical decision-making (Adapted from McKenna et al, 2000).

McKenna et al (2000) propose that there are four types of evidence in EBP, based on Carper's (1978) four ways of knowing. The first is *'empirical evidence'*, based on rigorous and systematic research. McKenna et al (2000) argue that the practitioner can use the other three types of evidence to reject empirical evidence. The second type of evidence is *'ethical evidence'*. For example, a patient may refuse a particular treatment or intervention and acting as the patient's advocate, the nurse would reject the empirical evidence and accept the right of the patient to refuse. Likewise, empirical evidence may be rejected for *'aesthetic evidence'* (e.g., intuitive expertise) and *'personal evidence'* (that emerges from the interpersonal relationship that the nurse has with the patient/client). McKenna et al (2000) liken this to the use of patient-reported and clinician-observed evidence cited in EBP definitions.

So, how are we to make sense of these debates around what constitutes evidence in EBP? Colyer and Kamath (1999) summarize by stating that the medical profession and to a certain extent the nursing profession espouse randomized controlled trials (RCTs) as the gold standard in EBP. In addition to RCTs the NHS Executive (1998) identifies other types of research studies and expert opinion as legitimate forms of evidence, although who should be awarded the status of 'expert' is not clarified. Colyer and Kamath (2000, p. 189) suggest that:

'good practitioners synthesise their clinical expertise and best available external evidence, recognising that neither is sufficient alone. Without clinical expertise, practice may become tyrannised by evidence that is inapplicable or inappropriate for an individual patient. Without best evidence, practice runs the risk of becoming both ineffective and inefficient. Either way, the inherent subjective aspects of unique practitioner–patient interactions are prominent.'

So far, we have discussed what EBP is and what constitutes evidence. We identified that the first stage of the process, according to Rosenberg and Donald (1995) was to identify a clear clinical problem or question. The next stage is to search the literature for relevant studies or evidence. Where can such evidence be found?

Sources of evidence

Locating appropriate evidence can be a daunting task for professionals working in healthcare. Because of the increase in online information in healthcare, it is now acknowledged that information literacy (including electronic information retrieval skills) is essential for all healthcare professionals (DoH, 1998). However, it is beyond the remit of this chapter to assist in the development of information retrieval skills and critical appraisal skills and the reader is directed to Palmer and Brice (1999) and the Critical Skills Appraisal Programme (http://www.phru.org.uk/~casp/casp.htm) for further details.

Books are potential sources of evidence but as Palmer and Brice (1999) acknowledge, they become out of date very quickly. Journals are more up to date sources of primary research evidence, although there are still delays in publication. However, manually searching journals is very time consuming. More effective literature searches can be carried out using electronic databases such as CINAHL and MEDLINE. Relevant health related databases can be searched via the OVID interface if the institution subscribes to the service. There are also specific information gateways to healthcare related websites such as OMNI (the UK's gateway to high quality Internet resources for health and medicine – found at http://omni.ac.uk/) and NMAP a specific gateway for nurses, midwives and health visitors (http://nmap.ac.uk).

Information gateways offer access to high quality web-based resources that have been evaluated and their use is preferable to using general search engines, which may identify websites of questionable quality. However, probably the most important resource currently available is NELH, the National Electronic Library for Health (www.nelh.nhs.uk). This gives access to many of the other sources of evidence such as the Cochrane Library, NICE guidelines and other virtual libraries such as the National Electronic Library for Mental Health Nurses, which includes gateways to information on depression, schizophrenia and suicide (see http://www.psychiatry.ox.ac.uk/cebmh/elmh/nelmh/index.html).

Systematic reviews of evidence are now commonplace. If undertaken properly, systematic reviews are extremely useful, because they reduce the need for individual health professionals to appraise a large body of complex research evidence. Taylor (2000) explains that a systematic review is a review and synthesis of the research literature on a particular topic. It will attempt to locate all published and unpublished literature and studies are only included if they meet predetermined criteria of research quality. They differ from other types of review in that they attempt to minimize bias by adhering to a strict scientific design and so ensuring their reliability. Rather than reflecting the views of the authors or being based on only a (possibly biased) selection of the literature, they contain a comprehensive summary of the available evidence and may include a conclusion regarding the effectiveness of a specific intervention.

Examples of centres that undertake systematic reviews are NHS Centre for Reviews and Dissemination (http://www.york.ac.uk/inst/crd/) based at the University of York and the UK Cochrane Centre (http://www.nelh.nhs.uk/cochrane.asp). As mentioned earlier, the National Institute for Clinical Effectiveness also review and publish evidence-based guidelines following systematic reviews of the literature. There are also journals such as *Evidence Based Nursing* and *Effective Healthcare Bulletins* that report on systematic reviews of evidence.

Some systematic reviews (e.g., those undertaken by the Cochrane Library) apply a statistical technique called meta analysis to the studies included in a systematic review. Taylor (2000) informs us that meta analysis is a statistical technique that is used to assemble the results of several studies into a single numerical estimate. For example, Pharoah et al concluded in their meta analysis that family intervention may decrease the frequency of relapse for schizophrenia. The odds ratio for this was 0.57 (CI 0.4–0.8). Generally speaking, an odds ratio (and accompanying confidence intervals) of less than 1 indicates a better outcome in the intervention group, which provides evidence for the efficacy of the intervention (family therapy). However, overall the reviewers concluded that they couldn't be confident of the effects of family intervention from the findings of the review and recommended that further trials should be undertaken.

While meta analysis is a useful tool, we do have some reservations about its use and we suggest that results should be interpreted in light of these. Meta analyses combine data from disparate studies that have used different variations on an intervention (e.g., a family intervention in one study may be different from an intervention in another study) and different outcome measures and combine them into one measure of efficacy. While the rationale for doing so is generally sound, in that it answers the criticism that many studies are underpowered (i.e., on their own, they do not have sufficient subjects to detect differences between groups), the logic of trying to compare 'apples and pears' may be flawed.

In parallel with quantitative systematic reviews and meta analyses, it is possible for a research team to take a systematic overview of qualitative studies. Paterson et al (2001) describe how the theory, methods and findings of primary qualitative studies can be re-examined. She suggests that there are distinct processes within a meta study. In the first instance, the researcher must formulate tentative questions, e.g., how do nurses and patients inter-relate, and choose a theoretical framework, e.g., interpersonal relations theory (Peplau, 1952), as the lens through which to view the primary studies. Evaluation criteria are set against which the studies are assessed, inclusion/exclusion criteria are specified and systems are put in place for retrieving and storing data. Once retrieved, the data reported in the studies are (re)categorized and a critical interpretation is made of the strengths and weaknesses of the various research studies' contributions to understanding in the field.

How can EBP be incorporated into mental health nursing?

So, how do Mental Health Nurses make sense of all of this in their day-to-day practice? At the point of registration, mental health nurses are required to 'use evidence-based knowledge from nursing and related disciplines to select and individualize nursing interventions' (Exit Profile Competency 2.8). This chapter has attempted to explore issues relating to the development of an evidence base for mental health nursing. We have suggested that some of what mental health nurses do can be underpinned by empirical evidence that is generated using both quantitative and qualitative research methods. However, much of what nurses do rests within the aesthetic, personal and ethical domain and nurses may use evidence from these domains to reject research evidence if this is in the best interest of individual service users.

The Tidal Model of Psychiatric and Mental Health Nursing (Barker, 2000) epitomizes such an approach. It was developed from theory (Peplau, 1952), research (Jackson and Stevenson, 2000), and the expert opinion of patients, nurses, and other disciplinary colleagues. In its enactment, the Tidal Model requires an aesthetic appreciation of the context of assessment and treatment, for example, in working out how to be with someone who is distressed, using intuition in relation to finding creative solutions to the immediate concern. The Tidal Model places the person central to her/his own care and looks at the person in context. The person's own interpretation of their problems *in her/his own words* directly influences the care negotiated, within ethical boundaries. The model requires the nurse to prioritize and reflect on the interpersonal relationship within which all care is offered. This holistic approach to evidence-based practice, we argue, is more appropriate for mental health nursing than adopting a more medically focused philosophy of evidence-based practice.

References

Aldridge, D. & Stevenson, C. (2001) Social poetics as research and practice: living in and learning from the process of research, *Nursing Inquiry*, 8, 19–27.

Barker, P. J. (2000) The Tidal Model of Mental Health: person centred caring within the chaos paradigm, *Mental Health Care*, 4(2), 59–63.

Barker, P. J. & Stevenson, C. (2002) A reply to Gamble and Wellman, *Journal of Psychiatric and Mental Health Nursing*, 7, 743–5.

Bradshaw, P. L. (2002) Evidence-based practice in nursing: the current state of play in Britain, *Journal of Nursing Management*, 8(6), 313–16.

Bury, T. (1998) Evidence-based healthcare explained, in T. Bury & J. Mead (eds), *Evidence-Based Healthcare: A Practical Guide for Therapists*, Oxford: Butterworth Heinnemann.

Carper, B. H. (1978) Fundamental patterns of knowing in nursing, *Advances in Nursing Science*, 1(1), 13–23.

Colyer, H. & Kamath, P. (1999) Evidence-based practice. A philosophical and political analysis: some matters for consideration by professional practitioners, *Journal of Advanced Nursing*, 29(1), 188–93.

Cornah, D. et al (2000) The therapeutic community method of treatment for borderline personality disorder, bristol: R&D Directorate, NHS Executive South and West, cited in McKenna, H., Cutcliffe, J. & McKenna, P. (2000) Evidence-based practice: demolishing some myths, *Nursing Standard*, 14(16), 39–42.

Dare, C., Eisler, I., Russell, G., Treasure, J. & Dodge, L. (2001) Psychological therapies for adults with anorexia nervosa: randomised control trial of out-patient treatments, *British Journal of Psychiatry*, 178, 216–21.

Department of Health (1998) *Working Together with Health Information. A Partnership Strategy for Education, Training and Development*, London: HMSO.

Eisler, I., Dare, C. & Russell, G. F. M. (1997) Family and individual therapy in anorexia nervosa, *Archives of General Psychiatry*, 54, 1025–30.

French, P. (2002) What is the evidence on evidence-based nursing? An epistemological concern, *Journal of Advanced Nursing*, 37(3), 250–7.

Gamble, C. & Wellman, N. (2002) Judgement impossible, *Journal of Psychiatric and Mental Health Nursing*, 9, 741–3.

Griffiths, R. (1983) *The NHS Management Inquiry*, London: DHSS.

Hamer, S. (1999) Evidence-based practice, in S. Hamer & G. Collinson (eds), *Achieving Evidence-Based Practice. A Handbook for Practitioners*, Edinburgh: Balliere Tindall, ch 1.

Harbour, R. & Miller, J. (2001) A new system for grading recommendations in evidence based guidelines, *British Medical Journal*, 323, 334–6.

Humphris, D. (1999) Types of evidence, in S. Hamer & G. Collinson (1999) (eds), *Achieving Evidence-Based Practice. A Handbook for Practitioners*, Edinburgh: Balliere Tindall, ch 2.

Hunt, J. (1996) Barriers to research utilisation, *Journal of Advanced Nursing*, 23(3), 423–5.

Ingersoll, G. L. (2000) Evidence-based nursing: what it is and what it isn't, *Nursing Outlook*, 48(4), 151–2, cited in Jennings, B. M. & Loan, L. (2001) Misconceptions among nurses about evidence-based practice, *Journal of Nursing Scholarship*, 33(2), 121–7.

Jackson, S. & Stevenson, C. (2000) What do people need psychiatric and mental health nurses for? *Journal of Advanced Nursing*, 31, 378–88.

Jennings, B. M. & Loan, L. (2001) Misconceptions among nurses about evidence-based practice, *Journal of Nursing Scholarship*, 33(2), 121–7.

McKenna, H., Cutcliffe, J. & McKenna, P. (2000) Evidence-based practice: demolishing some myths, *Nursing* Standard, 14(16), 39–42.

McKibbon, K. A., Wilczynski, N., Hayward, R. S., Walker-Dilkes, C. J. & Haynes, R. B. (1995) The medical literature as a resource for healthcare practice, *Journal of American Society for Information Science*, 46, 737–42, cited in NHS Executive (1998) *Achieving Effective Practice. A Clinical Effectiveness and Resource Information Pack for Nurses, Midwives and Health Visitors*, London: HMSO.

Minuchin, S. (1974) *Families and Family Therapy*, London: Tavistock.

Morse, J. M., Penrod, J. & Hupcey, J. E. (2000) Qualitative outcome analysis: evaluating nursing interventions for complex clinical phenomena, *Journal of Nursing Scholarship*, 32(2), 125–30.

NHS Executive (1996) *Promoting Clinical Effectiveness: A Framework for Action in and Through the NHS*, London: HMSO.

NHS Executive (1998) *Achieving Effective Practice. A Clinical Effectiveness and Research Information Pack for Nurses, Midwives and Health Visitors, Number 1, Clinical effectiveness – What its all about*, London: HMSO.

NHS Executive (1999) *A First Class Service. Quality in the New NHS*, London: HMSO.

Nursing and Midwifery Council (2001) *Requirements for Pre-registration Nursing Programmes*, London: HMSO.

Palmer, J. & Brice, A. (1999) Information Sourcing, in S. Hamer & G. Collinson (eds), *Achieving Evidence-Based practice. A handbook for practitioners*. Edinburgh: Balliere Tindall, ch 4.

Paterson, B. L., Thorne, S., Canam, C. & Jillings, C. (2001) *Meta-Study of Qualitative Health Research*, London: Sage.

Peplau, H. (1952) *Interpersonal Relations in Nursing*, New York: Putnam.

Pharoah, F. M., Mari, J. J. & Streiner, D. (2003) Family intervention for schizophrenia (Cochrane Review), Oxford: *The Cochrane Library, Issue 1,* Update Software Ltd. (accessed online via www.nelh.nhs.uk/cochrane.asp).

Proctor, S., Watson. B., Byrne, C., Bremner, J., van Zwanenberg, T., Browne, G., Roberts, J. & Gafni, A. (2000) The development of an applied whole-systems research methodology in health and social research: a Canadian and UK collaboration, *Critical Public Health,* 10(3), 331–42.

Regan, J. (1998) Will current clinical effectiveness initiatives encourage and facilitate practitioners to use evidence-based practice for the benefit of their clients? *Journal of Clinical Nursing,* 7(3), 244–50.

Renfrew, M. J. (1997) The development of evidence-based practice, *British Journal of Midwifery,* 5(2), 100–4.

Repper, J. & Brooker, C. (1998) Difficulties in the measurement of outcome in people who have serious mental health problems, *Journal of Advanced Nursing,* 27(1), 75–82.

Robin, L., Siegel, P. T. & Moye, A. (1995) Family versus individual therapy for anorexia: impact on family conflict. Topical section: treatment and therapeutic processes, *International Journal of Eating Disorders,* 17, 313–22.

Rolfe, G. (2001) *Knowledge and Practice,* London: Distance Learning Centre.

Rosenberg, W. & Donald, A. (1995) Evidence-based medicine: an approach to clinical problem solving, *British Medical Journal,* 310, 1122–6.

Russell, G. F. M., Szmukler, G., Dare, C. & Eisler, I. (1987) An evaluation of family therapy in anorexia and bulimia nervosa, *Archives of General Psychiatry,* 44, 1047–56.

Sackett, D. L., Straus, S. E., Richardson, W. S., Rosenberg, W. & Haynes, R. B. (2000) *Evidence-Based Medicine. How to Practice and Teach EBM,* Edinburgh: Churchill Livingstone.

Speckens, A. E., van Hemert, A. M., Spinhoven, P., Hawton, K. E., Bolk, J. H. & Rooijmans, G. M. (1995) Cognitive behavioural therapy for medically unexplained physical symptoms: a randomised controlled trial, *British Medical Journal,* 311, 1328–32, cited in McKenna, H., Cutcliffe, J. & McKenna, P. (2000) Evidence-based practice: demolishing some myths, *Nursing Standard,* 14(16), 39–42.

Stevenson, C., Barker, P. J. & Fletcher, E. (2002) Judgement days: developing an evaluation of an innovative nursing model of mental health care, *Journal of Psychiatric and Mental Health Nursing,* 9, 271–6.

Taylor, M. C. (2000) *Evidence-Based Practice for Occupational Therapists,* Oxford: Blackwell Science.

Walsh, M. & Ford, P. (1989) *Nursing Rituals: Research and Rational Actions,* London: Heinemann.

CHAPTER 29

Learning: from Self-development to Competency

STEPHAN D. KIRBY AND DENIS A. HART

> You cannot be wise without some basis of knowledge; but you may easily acquire knowledge and remain bare of wisdom. (Whitehead, 1967)

Introduction

Between 1990 and 1996 pre-registration nurse education converted from apprentice-type training located in hospitals to tertiary training conducted by the higher education institutions and resulted in the 'Project 2000' (UKCC, 1986) diploma courses. When polytechnics were given university status in 1992 the remaining colleges of nursing were incorporated into the expanding universities.

This move into the higher education institutions was driven by the nursing profession itself in the early 1980s following concern being expressed for the future of nurse education. It was felt that the status and effectiveness of the apprenticeship style nurse training was out of date, thus badly equipping nurse trainees for the demands of rapidly changing and expanding health care systems, and consequently lowering the morale of nurse trainees due to the conflicting educational and service demands being placed upon them. This training was seen to provide lower professional status in comparison to other non-medical health care professions (whose training was conducted in the university), and to be contributing to student recruitment and retention problems (RCN, 1985; UKCC, 1986).

The Judge Report (RCN, 1985) linked wastage levels among student nurses during training to their exploitation as a vital component of the nursing workforce and argued that student nurses should be freed from the obligations of work in order to concentrate on learning. The obvious solution was seen by the professional bodies to be the recommendation of the termination of hospital-based training, and the transfer of nurse education into the higher education sector.

These (and other) recommendations (e.g. ENB, 1985, UKCC, 1986) were symptomatic of the growing concern regarding the ability of nurse education to produce a sufficient number of qualified nurses with the increasingly sophisticated skills that were necessary to operate in the growing health service (Humphreys, 1996). Certainly there was concern throughout the nursing profession, regarding the future direction for nurse education in light of the changing nursing environment. The consensus from these three reports stated that educational standards could best be enhanced by breaking the traditional apprenticeship model, and placing nurse education under the control of educationalists. Thus the relationship between the student and clinical workplace would be greatly altered, with the onus now being on theoretical education rather than meeting workforce needs. The reports agreed further that the nurse education award should take place in higher education institutions. Thus the changing and challenging demands of the future NHS would be met by a highly qualified and more flexible nurse; her/his role extending beyond traditional areas to cover health education, sophisticated clinical practice, and community care.

These changes to nurse education obviously stood to benefit the nursing profession as a whole, as well as creating a more effective system of nurse training. It has long been agreed that two of the key aspects of professionalization of occupations are those actions that improve the group's status, and maintain or enhance its control over entry to the profession (Johnson, 1972). The move of nurse training to higher education has achieved these aims. It has brought nurse education more into line with the training for comparable non-medical health professions (e.g. occupational therapy, physiotherapy, etc) and hence has improved the status of nursing as a career.

This 'revolution' is taking place, not only in the planning of the curriculum for pre-registration nurse education, but also how this is delivered in the most effective manner reflecting the principles of adult learning. It is a revolution that deals with:

- the philosophy of how students learn and how academics teach;
- the relationship between teacher and student;
- the way in which a classroom is structured; and
- the nature of curriculum (Norman & Spohrer, www).

At the heart of this philosophy is a powerful constructivist (Marsh, www) learning theory and strategy, one that embraces social issues, the culture of the classroom, lifelong learning concerns, technology and places the student firmly at the centre of the learning process. Central to this is the idea that people learn best when engrossed or immersed in the topic, motivated to seek out new knowledge and skills because they need them in order to solve the problems at hand. The goal is active exploration, construction and learning rather than the passivity of lecture attendance and text book reading.

Learning

A fairly standard definition of learning is: 'a relatively permanent change in behaviour that results from practice or experience' (Atkinson et al, 1993). Learning, therefore, can be thought of as a process whereby a person acquires the ability to carry out a task or procedure of some sort in a natural – and relatively effortless – way, as if it were an innate part of his or her behaviour pattern. However, we are reminded by Smith (2001) that the term '*learning*' does not mean – *learning* – the lifeless, sterile, futile, quickly forgotten stuff that is crammed in to the mind of the poor helpless individual tied into his seat, but – LEARNING – the insatiable curiosity that drives the student to explore and absorb everything they see or hear (Ellington et al, 1997).

There are several schools of thought relating to theoretical models of how people learn. One of the most useful for adult learning has, according to Smith (2001), proved to be that developed by David Kolb, where learning is presented as a cycle see Figure 29.1.

Honey and Mumford (1982) subsequently adapted Kolb's original cycle to that shown in Figure 29.2.

While it is proposed that a learner would consciously move through *every* stage in the cycle in *every* learning situation, the practicalities are that not all learners are equally at home at all stages of the cycle. Many show marked preferences for one or more of the stages and sometimes positive dislike of one of the others. Honey and Mumford (1982) identified four different preferences, or ways in which people prefer to learn, each relate to a different stage

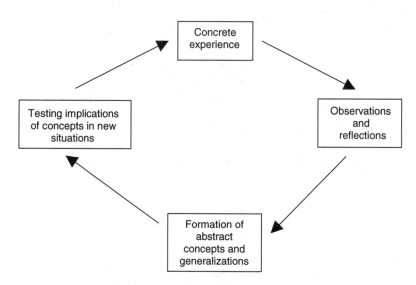

Figure 29.1 A Kolb-type learning cycle
Source: Adapted from Anon, http://www.ic.polyu.edu.hk

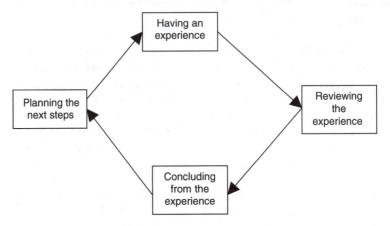

Figure 29.2   Revised learning cycle
Source: Anon, http://www.ic.polyu.edu.hk

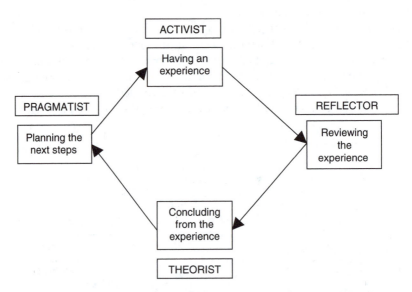

Figure 29.3   Honey and Mumford's four learning styles
Source: Adapted from Anon, http://www.ic.polyu.edu.hk

of the learning cycle. These preferred 'learning styles' they call 'Activist', 'Reflector', 'Theorist' and 'Pragmatist' (see Figure 29.3).

While there have been various additions and variations to these themes in the literature it is the work of Kolb (1976, 1981, 1984) and with Fry (Kolb & Fry, 1975) that still provides the central reference point for discussion.

Self-assessment

Self-assessment is an appraisal of the following questions:

- Where am I now? and
- What do I need to acquire to enable me to develop, improve and move forward?

It is thus the recognition of your strengths and of your needs self-assessment needs to address the following questions:

- What do I know (underpinning knowledge)?
- What can I do (skills/competences)? and
- How do I do it (values requirements)?

Self-development

Self-development is made up of two components that frequently become blended together:

- personal development; and
- professional development.

Figure 29.4 shows two different routes to self-development. Route 1 follows a purely personal development approach, while Route 2 follows a predominantly professional development approach – but does not exclude personal development.

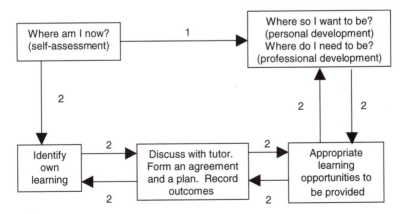

Figure 29.4 Two routes to self-development

Route 1

When we seek to change a part of ourselves, say for example, to lose weight, we begin by making a baseline assessment (we weigh ourselves) and then set a target (calculate our ideal weight). We follow Route 1 in the diagram as no other party is directly involved and the target is one chosen by us and for us.

Route 2

Professional training is much more complex. You are not learning for your own sake, but in order to work effectively and appropriately with service users. Your target is to meet the requirements set down by the NMC and delivered through the Competence-based Exit Profile for Pre-registration Mental Health Nursing.

Unlike losing weight, you cannot do this by yourself. To make the journey you need:

● to identify the route to be taken;
● to work out where you are (your baseline);
● to meet your personal and modular tutor(s) to agree a strategy for profes-sional and personal development; and
● to keep a learning journal to monitor your progress on your journey.

Competence and the portfolio

> Competence is a successful amalgamation of knowledge, values and skills together with a process of understanding one's own self and what effects that process has on others as well as on the outcomes of supervision, intervention and interpersonal relations with colleagues, users and other agencies (Vass, 1996, p 195).

Dominelli (1997, p 62) says: 'What is taught, how it is taught, what is assessed, how it is assessed and by whom are matters which must be openly discussed and resolved'. Competence is essentially 'knowledge' plus 'skill' conducted within an 'appropriate values' framework (see Figure 29.5).

Within this Mental Health Nurse Training Programme Competence involves: '. . . demonstrating skills, knowledge and understanding performed to a specified standard and carried out with the attitude, values and ethical principles consistent with professional nursing practice' (University of Teesside, 2003, p 7). The Core Competencies for the programme are detailed throughout this text and are illustrated in depth in the Appendix but they include (by way of an example):

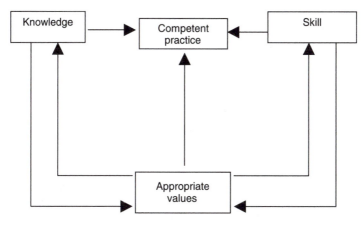

Figure 29.5 Competence

- Practice in accordance with an ethical and legal framework which ensures the primacy of patient and client interest and well-being and respects confidentiality.
- Practice in a fair and anti-discriminatory way, acknowledging the difference in beliefs and cultural practices of individuals or groups.
- Engage in, develop and disengage from therapeutic relationships through the use of appropriate communication and interpersonal skills.
- Enhance the professional development and safe practice of others through peer support, leadership, supervision and teaching.

(Adapted from University of Teesside, 2003)

Kolb (1993) produced a cycle of competence to encourage both reflective learning and reflective practice (see Figure 29.6).

Identifying learning needs is very much an individual activity. There are likely to be a number of needs that have implications for the way the learning experience is organized. Perhaps you recognized the need to receive some new and relevant knowledge before taking up your next practice placement. If so you may have thought about a need to make stronger links between theory and practice.

As such, new knowledge allows a deeper understanding of practice and facilitates reflection as to how the ideas can be incorporated into good practice. Hearn (1982, p 7) elaborates: 'theory has to be understood in terms wider than "what is learned" at college.' By examining the gap in your knowledge, experience and values, the activity moves you behind self-assessment. You have now reached the stage of conscious incompetence and are thus embarked in the first stage of self-development.

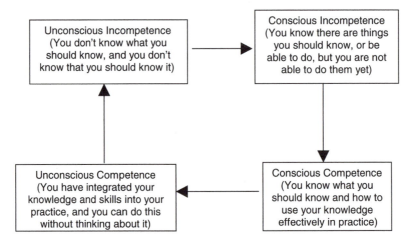

Figure 29.6   Kolb's cycle of competence
Source: Adapted from Kolb (1993)

The exit profile portfolio

Your mental health nurse training has programmes outcomes, which are drawn from the competencies identified within the framework of four practice domains (UKCC, 2000). These provide a framework for meeting statutory requirements and competencies in accordance with the Amendment Rules (Training) changes to the Nurses, Midwives and Health Visitors Act (2000). They are adapted to emphasize the integration of theory and practice which is combined to encourage an integrated approach to knowledge acquisition and skills development. Reflection, together with the four domains of practice as identified by the UKCC (UKCC, 2000) are considered to be the major influences in these programmes. The four domains are (University of Teesside, 2000, p 24):

- Professional and ethical practice;
- Care delivery;
- Care management; and
- Personal/professional development.

Professional and ethical practice

Students will exit the programme with a sound knowledge of the *Code of Professional Conduct* (UKCC, 1992), the concepts and principles that underpin it, and realize the importance of adhering to it. This requires students to consider the primacy of patient interests, well being and confidentiality as well as practising in a fair and anti-discriminatory manner, which acknowledges differences in the beliefs and cultural practices of individuals and groups.

Care delivery

Students exiting the programme will demonstrate competence when carrying out essential nursing skills, which include maintaining dignity and privacy, effective observation and communication skills, safety and health, essential first aid and emergency procedures, administration of medicines and emotional, physical and personal carer. Their care delivery will be informed by best available evidence in order to assess effectively and safely, plan, implement and evaluate care.

Care management

The student will exit the programme with a range of key skills that support and create a safe working environment. In doing so they will contribute to public protection through the use of quality assurance and risk management strategies. Through effective inter-professional working practices the student will demonstrate the value of collaboration with all members of the health and social care team.

Personal/professional development

The student will exit the programme recognizing the importance of life-long learning in order to continue personal and professional development. Through peer support, supervision and teaching they will also promote the professional development and safe practices of others within the health and social care team.

The learning outcomes for your mental health nurse training are clearly laid down within the Programme Portfolio. The overall aim of this approach to training is to prepare mental health nurses who are fit for practice, purpose and award upon registration.

There are two elements to the Exit Profile Portfolio:

- It is a cumulative record of your personal and professional development.
- It is the means by which your achievement of the practice module benchmarks will be assessed.

The portfolio, therefore, should include documentary evidence, which demonstrates progress towards, and acquisition of, the pre-requisite knowledge, skills, attitudes and competencies. In order to demonstrate achievement of portfolio benchmarks, students are required to keep a practice portfolio. This must provide a documentary record illustrating practice, the nature of the learning, and the evidence collected to demonstrate achievement of the benchmarks and the NMC competencies for entry to the professional register.

The portfolio keeping process includes:

- reflection upon existing knowledge and skills;
- exploration of the NMC competencies and practice module benchmarks;
- identification of learning needs;
- identification of learning opportunities in the current placement area;
- matching learning opportunities to learning needs;
- development of a plan or learning contract to meet learning needs;
- identification of essential evidence to support achievement of learning needs, and benchmarks for practice;
- implementation of the plan/learning contract and collection of supporting evidence;
- reflection upon learning and achievement of practice module benchmarks; and
- presentation of the portfolio within the tripartite meeting.

Table 29.1 provide a key to essential evidence.

Reflection and reflective practice

In the past number of years, the terms 'reflection', 'critical reflection' and 'reflective practice' have increasingly appeared in descriptions of approaches to higher (and especially nursing) education. It is clear however that the terms are often ill-defined, and have been used rather loosely to embrace a wide range of concepts and strategies.

Arguably, Dewey has made the most significant contribution to the development of educational thinking in the twentieth century. He considered it to be a special form of problem-solving thinking to resolve an issue, which involves active chaining, a careful ordering of ideas linking each with its predecessors. Within this process, consideration is to be given to any form of knowledge or belief involved and the grounds for its support (Adler, 1991; Calderhead, 1989; Cutler et al, 1989; Farrah, 1988; Gilson, 1989). His basic ideas indicate that reflection may be seen as an active and deliberative cognitive process, involving sequences of interconnected ideas, which take account of underlying beliefs and knowledge. Reflective thinking generally addresses practical problems, allowing for doubt and perplexity before possible solutions are reached.

Four key issues with regard to reflection emerge from Dewey's original work and its subsequent interpretation:

Table 29.1 Key to essential evidence

	Essential evidence
AV: Audio / Visual Presentation	During your time in clinical practice you will be expected to work educationally with patients and other health professionals the material used within this role could be used as evidence. For example the use of relaxation tapes you devised as part of an anxiety management programme. Skills demonstrated in the laboratory setting can also be audio or video tapes to provide evidence of achievement
CD: Completed Documentation (with written critique, including a rationale for actions / decisions)	
D: Dialogue / discussion in 'Tripartite Meeting'	This invites discussion within the final tripartite meeting which demonstrates understanding of issues. Oral dialogue evidence will be graded the same way as written evidence
LC: Learning Contract	This should include identification of student's personal learning needs, these should be related to the specific learning environment, negotiated with the Practice and Academic Mentor during the first tripartite meeting
O: Observed Practice (by Practice Assessor)	This involves direct observation of your practice skills, abilities, attitudes and conduct by your Practice Mentor. Evidence that your practice is safe (year 1) safe and effective (year 2) and safe, effective and efficient (year 3 will be provided by the Practice Mentor who will assess the student and determine their ability to meet the practice module competencies. This will be based upon the student demonstrating appropriate knowledge, skills, professional attitude and behaviour in practice.
S: Simulation in Skills Laboratory	This includes simulated learning experiences within the skills laboratory. In order to use that as evidence to demonstrate achievement of a specific benchmark it must be authenticated and signed by the person running the workshop.
T: Testimony of others (i.e.: written materials, letters, consumer feedback)	The testimony must be relevant and specific to the student's experience. Such testimony provides further supporting evidence of their achievement of benchmarks. Testimony may be obtained from the Practice Mentor and other health and social care professionals
PJ (PW): Project Work (i.e.: poster displays, scrapbooks, group presentations, teaching packs)	During your time in practice you could be asked to do presentations to the multi-disciplinary team or to your peers and/or complete teaching packs for junior members of staff or patients, therefore the material used could be added as evidence. You should evaluate this process and this could form the basis of written reflection (WR)
WR: Written Reflection	Written reflection should identify the reflective model used and the associated stages of the model and can be separate pieces of work or integrated within the Care Study. Where appropriate one piece of reflection can be offered as evidence for more than one competency. The level of reflection expected varies i.e. year 1 – descriptive; year 2 – analytical; year 3 – critical reflection.

Table 29.1   *(Cont'd)*

Essential evidence	
GS/WB: Guided Studies/Workbooks	These are used to facilitate the application of the concepts underpinning the art and science of nursing practice to holistic patient care. Specified guided studies/workbooks are identified for each year of the practice module.
CS: Care Study	The care study should demonstrate the relationship between the patient's health status, care provision and evidence-based practice. It should be focused upon the relevant benchmarks that the student is providing evidence for rather than a descriptive/anecdotal account of care. Consent must be sought from the patient and the appropriate Informed Consent Form must be signed by the Practice Mentor.

Source: Adapted from University of Teesside (2003, p 10)

1 The first is whether reflection is limited to thought processes about action, or is more inextricably bound up in action (Grant & Zeichner, 1984; Noffke & Brennan, 1988).
2 The second relates to the time frames within which reflection takes place, and whether it is relatively immediate and short term, or rather more extended and systematic (Farrah, 1988; Schön, 1983).
3 The third has to do with whether reflection is by its very nature problem-centred or not (Adler, 1991; Calderhead, 1989; Schön, 1987).
4 Finally, the fourth is concerned with how consciously the one reflecting takes account of wider historic, cultural and political values or beliefs in framing and reframing practical problems to which solutions are being sought, a process which has been identified as 'critical reflection' (Gore & Zeichner, 1991; Noordhoff & Kleinfeld, 1988; Smyth, 1989).

The notion of 'reflective practice' offers a highly challenging paradigm of learning (Evans, 1997). There is considerable evidence from learning style research (Kolb, 1984), from consumer research into the education for such caring professions as social work (Coulshed, 1986; Davies, 1984; Walker et al, 1995), nursing (Clark et al, 1996; Davies et al, 1996) and teaching (Back & Booth, 1992) and from adult learning theory, which suggests that a large proportion of caring profession students prefer to learn inductively. The challenge, therefore, is how to develop inductive learning strategies throughout education for the professions, particularly in higher education institutions, and also how to assess whether that learning is taking place.

Inductive learning – central to the learning process is a specific practice event, experienced uniquely and differentially by a small number of people, from which a number of more abstract generalizations will hopefully be derived.

Deductive learning – abstract generalizations, often available to many people through the printed word, are understood and then possibly, but only possibly, applied to specific concrete situations. (Adapted from Evans, 1997)

Schön (1987) differentiated between reflection-in-action (practice) and reflection-on-action (practice). The former occurs during (nursing) practice when the attentive practitioner watches, interacts and adjusts reactions and approaches through thinking in a focused way while working. There is some debate as to whether reflection-in-action (practice) is really possible, given the need to act quickly in complex situations (Clinton, 1998). Reflection-on-action (practice) occurs after the action when details are recalled through rich description and analysed through careful unpicking and reconstructing of all aspects of the situation, to gain fresh insights and make amendments if necessary (Taylor, 2000). Schön emphasized the idea that reflection is a way in which professionals (nurses) can bridge the theory-practice gap, based on the potential of reflection to uncover knowledge in and on action (practice) (Schön, 1983).

The processes of reflection as outlined particularly by Schön (1987), Boud et al, (1985), Mezirow (1981) and Kolb (1984) can be summarized as: *analysis, synthesis, evaluation* and *feeling*. Evans (1997) includes under *'synthesis'* such processes as 'transfer of learning' and 'relating theory and practice' and under *'evaluation'* the critical evaluation of practice contexts (Brookfield, 1987) as well as of practice processes and outcomes (Evans, 1991). A crucial facet of reflective practice is its participants. Some, theorists (e.g, Kolb, 1984), seem to concentrate on the practitioner as the principal if not sole participant in the reflective process. Others (e.g, Schön, 1987) include a second key contributor: the coach, mentor, supervisor, consultant, teacher. A proposed (Evans, 1997) final facet is time.

Schön's framework is able to incorporate all levels or kinds, including critical reflection. His reflection-in-action/practice and reflection-on-action/practice involve a structure of professional (nursing) practice based upon knowing-in-action/practice and knowledge-in-action/practice (Altrichter & Posch, 1989; Munby & Russell, 1989). Reflection-in-action, an element of knowing-in-action occurs while an action is being undertaken. It is therefore seen to be one means for distinguishing professional from non-professional practice, (Feiman-Nemser, 1990; Schön, 1983, 1987). It may be characterized as part of the artistry or intuitive knowledge derived from professional experience (Gilson, 1989) and includes engaging in a reflective conversation with oneself, shaping the situation in terms of the reflector's frame of reference, while consistently leaving open the possibility of reframing by employing techniques of holistic appraisal (Altrichter & Posch, 1989).

Learning opportunities and practice skills

Opportunities to address your practice skills must be provided at all times and in all practice settings. To this end, and in line with *Making a Difference*

(DoH, 1999) and *Fitness for Practice* (UKCC, 1999) the 'Common Foundation' element of the programme was reduced from 18 months to 12, but the practice component of was increased to 50 per cent. The importance of placements and the practice mentor(s) in your learning experience cannot be overstated: '[Practice Mentors] hold critical positions in facilitating students to negotiate a valid and rigorous route to demonstrate competence' (Walker et al, 1995, p 15). The role of the Practice Mentor is to provide you with a patient-centred approach to caring in the clinical setting in which your individual learning can be negotiated and facilitated. The Practice Mentor will be supported in their role by a clinical mentor.

Within this clinical placement, your role as student, is to become progressively (as the training programme progresses) more involved in negotiating your own learning with both the Academic Mentor and as well as the Practice Mentor, in order to develop an increasing level of self-reliance in practice and academic competence.

Together this 'Tripartite Relationship' (Academic Mentor; Practice Mentor and Student) facilitates student-centred learning and reflective practice focused upon the programme practice outcomes.

Programme practice outcomes

- Provide a rationale for care delivery across a range of differing professional and care delivery contexts.
- Under supervision, select and employ appropriate communication methods when interacting with patients, clients and health care professionals.
- Work in a collaborative fashion with clients, carers and significant others in health care delivery.
- Plan and implement health promotion activities for patients/clients.
- Contribute to team or group activities within a range of learning situations.
- Under supervision, plan appropriate nursing care and interventions for a small group of clients.
- Choose appropriate approaches, models of framework of care to support client centred care.
  (Adapted from University of Teesside, 2003, p 16)

Learning opportunities and the learning experience

So far we have looked at prior learning and experience, we will now look at the central role that the provision of appropriate opportunities plays in the learning experience (see Figure 29.7).

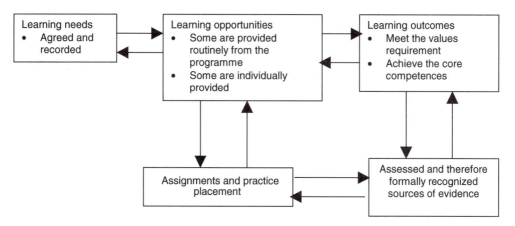

Figure 29.7   The role of opportunities in the learning experience

Learning opportunities and values

There is an interesting debate as to whether or not values can be taught. We believe the answer is 'probably not' – but you will need learning opportunities on your programme to:

- give you a greater understanding of the needs of people who are oppressed, discriminated against and/or vulnerable – the person with the mental health problem;
- enable you to develop greater insight as to how such people feel; and
- consider your own values in terms of their appropriateness.

Pearce (1996) provides a helpful framework when focusing upon the value base of practice. While this is directly related to social work, it is also useful for mental health nurses to consider and possibly adopt. She identifies a number of aspects of values which can be taught:

- The right to freedom from harm or abuse – This includes an understanding of power dynamics within families and their impact on individual members. It includes the right to protection for children and women but also recognizes the potential for all family members to act as carers.
- The need for appropriate practice which includes participation, accountability and accessibility. This is about the rights of the individual.
- Valuing differences and diversity – This is about the need to avoid stereotypical assumptions in the decision-making process on behalf of mental health service users and the need to work in partnership and enable these users to set their own agenda for help, support or change.

- Commitment to social justice and social welfare – The practitioner has the responsibility to communicate clearly with mental health service users, informing them of their rights and choices and, where welcomed and appropriate, taking up issues on their behalf.

Learning opportunities and anti-discriminatory practice

All staff involved in health care must do so without any form of prejudice. The programme has been designed to ensure that students are exposed, from the earliest point, to the concept of practice without discrimination. Two distinct strategic approaches are taken in the application of the programme with practice competencies relating specifically to anti-discriminatory care incorporated within the programme and a specific programme module designed to allow students to explore issues of culture, beliefs and their influences upon healthcare.

Practice competencies ensure that a student's behaviour towards colleagues and patients must always be in line with current NHS directives insisting on equality of access to treatment and care without prejudice for all. In order for students to practice without discrimination, they need to understand and debate issues raised by differing personal behaviours and attitudes.

Conclusion

Nursing has fought hard for many years to ensure that it has a place in higher education alongside the other health professionals. In many universities nurses are the largest single student group and the money paid to the universities from the NHS forms a substantial part of the income of the institution (Hale, 2001). It is now important to ensure that nursing continues to have its presence felt within the higher education sector and that nursing academics have the opportunity to contribute to the governance of the universities and thereby ensure that the funding that the Government provides for the education of nurses is used for that purpose.

One of the challenges for nursing education is to further apply adult educational theories and principles to a unique educational environment. The nursing learning process does not take place in the isolation of a formal educational system and is not a solo or individual affair. Rather, the learning takes place in a complexity of the clinical environment where people interact collectively in a social context. The nurse is part of a multi-disciplinary and multi-faceted team that involves relationships with peers, the organization, allied health professionals and of course the recipient of that care – the patient. However, we are aware that there is still a considerable amount to be learnt about developing effective teaching and learning strategies for such a dynamic environment where individuals' educational needs are not necessarily nor traditionally a priority.

References

Adler, S. (1991) The reflective practitioner and the curriculum of teacher education, *Journal of Education for Teaching*, 17(2), 139–50.

Altrichter, H. & Posch, P. (1989) Does the 'grounded theory' approach offer a guiding paradigm for teacher research? *Cambridge Journal of Education*, 19(1), 21–31.

Anon *Learning to Learn* online at: http://www.ic.polyu.edu.hk/posh97/student/Learn/Learning_to_learn.htm

Atkinson, R. L., Atkinson, R. C., Smith, E. E. & Bem, D. J. (1993) *Introduction to Psychology*, (11th edn), Fort Worth: Harcourt Brace Jovanovich.

Back, D. & Booth, M. (1992) Commitment to mentoring, in M. Wilkin (ed.), *Mentoring in Schools*, London: Kogan Page.

Boud, D., Keogh, R. & Walker, D. (1985) Promoting reflection in learning: a model, in D. Boud, R. Keogh & D. Walker (eds), *Reflection: Turning Experience into Learning*, London: Kogan Page.

Brookfield, S. D. (1987) *Understanding and Facilitating Adult Learning*, San Francisco: Jossey Bass.

Calderhead, J. (1989) Reflective teaching and teacher education, *Teaching and Teacher Education*, 5(1), 43–51.

Clark, J. M., Maben, J. & Jones, K. (1996) *Project 2000, Perceptions of the Philosophy and Practice of Nursing*, London: English National Board for England and Wales.

Clinton, M. (1998) On reflection-in-action: un-addressed issues in re-focusing the debate on reflective practice, *International Journal of Nursing Practice*, 4(3), 197–202.

Coulshed, V. (1986) What do social work students give to training? A survey, *Issues in Social Work Education*, 6, 119–28.

Cutler, B., Cook, P. & Young, J. (1989) *The Empowerment of Preservice Teachers Through Reflective Teaching*, paper presented at the Annual Meeting of the Association of Teacher Educators, St Louis.

Davies, M. (1984) Training: what we think of it now, *Social Work Today*, 24/1/84, 12–17.

Davies, S., White, E., Riley, E. & Twinn, S. (1996) How can nurse teachers be more effective in practice settings? *Nurse Education Today*, 16, 19–27.

Department of Health (1999) *Making A Difference: Strengthening the Nursing, Midwifery and Health Visiting Contribution to Health and Healthcare*, London: HMSO.

Dominelli, L. (1997) *The Blackwell Companion to Social Work*, (2nd edn), Oxford: Blackwell.

Ellington, H., Earl, S., McConnell, M. & Middleton, I. (1997) *How Students Learn: A Course Booklet for the Postgraduate Certificate in Tertiary Level Teaching*, Aberdeen: Robert Gordon University, online at: http://www.rgu.ac.uk/subj/eds/pgcert/how/how.htm

English National Board for England and Wales (1985) *Professional Education/Training Courses: Consultation Paper*, London: ENB.

Evans, D. (1991) *Assessing Students' Competence to Practise*, London: Central Council for the Education and Training of Social Workers.

Evans, D. (1997) *Reflective Learning Through Practice-Based Assignments*, paper presented at the British Educational Research Association Annual Conference 11–14 September: University of York.

Farrah, H. (1988) The reflective thought process: John Dewey re-visited, *Journal of Creative Behaviour*, 22(1), 1–8.

Feiman-Nemser, S. (1990) Teacher preparation: structural and conceptual alternatives, in W. T. Houston (ed.), *Handbook of Research on Teacher Education*, New York: Macmillan, now Palgrave Macmicllan.

Gilson, J. (1989) Reconstructive reflective teaching: a review of the literature, ED, 327 481.

Gore, J. & Zeichner, K. (1991) Action research and reflective teaching in preservice teacher education: a case study from the United States, *Teaching and Teacher Education*, 7(2),119–36.

Grant, C. & Zeichner, K. (1984) On becoming a reflective teacher, in C. Grant (ed.), *Preparing for Reflective Teaching*, Boston: Allyn & Bacon.

Hale, C. (2001) Nursing education in the UK, *Nyhedsbrev fra Udviklingsinitiativet for Sygeplejerskeuddannelsen i Århus Amt*, online at: http://www.aaa.dk/ufs/dec2001.pdf

Hearn, J. (1982) The problem(s) of theory and practice in social work and social work education, *Issues in Social Work Education*, 2(2), 95–118.

Honey, P. & Mumford, A. (1982) *Manual of Learning Styles*, London: P Honey.

Humphreys, J. (1996) English nurse education and reform in the National Health Service, *Journal of Education Policy*, 11, 655–79.

Johnson, T. (1972), *Professions and Power,* Bostingstoke: Macmillan, now Palgrave Macmillan.

Kolb, D. A. (1976) *The Learning Style Inventory: Technical Manual*, Boston: McBer.

Kolb, D. A. (1981) Learning styles and disciplinary differences, in A. W. Chickering (ed.), *The Modern American College*, San Francisco: Jossey-Bass.

Kolb, D. A. (1984) *Experiential Learning*, Englewood Cliffs, NJ: Prentice Hall.

Kolb, D. A. (1993) The processes of experiential learning, in M. Thorpe, G. Edwards & A. Hanson (eds), *Culture and Process of Adult Learners*, London: Routledge.

Kolb. D. A. & Fry, R. (1975) Toward an applied theory of experiential learning, in C. Cooper (ed.), *Theories of Group Process*, London: John Wiley.

Marsh, G. E. Constructivism, online at: http://www.bamaed.ua.edu/ail601/const.htm

Mezirow, J. (1981) A critical theory of adult learning and education, *Adult Education*, 32, 1.

Munby, H. & Russell, T. (1989) Educating the reflective teacher: an essay review of two books by Donald Schön, *Journal of Curriculum Studies*, 21(1), 71–80.

Noffke, S. & Brennan, M. (1988) *The Dimensions of Reflection: A Conceptual and Contextual Analysis*, paper presented at the Annual Meeting of the AERA, New Orleans: April.

Noordhoff, K. & Kleinfeld, J. (1988) Rethinking the rhetoric of 'reflective inquiry' in teacher education programs, in H. Waxman et al (eds), *Images of Reflection in Teacher Education*, Virginia: ATE.

Norman, D. & Spohrer, J. C. *Learner Centered Education*, online at:

http://it.coe.uga.edu/itforum/paper12/paper12.html

Pearce, J. (1996) The value of social work, in A. Vass (ed.), *Social Work Competences*, London: Sage.

RCN (1985) *The Education of Nurses: A New Dispensation (The Judge Report)*, London: Royal College of Nursing.

Schön, D. (1983) *The Reflective Practitioner: How Professionals Think in Action*, New York: Basic Books.

Schön, D. (1987) *Educating the Reflective Practitioner*, San Francisco: Jossey Bass.

Smith, M. K. (2001) Learning, T*he Encyclopaedia of Informal Education*, online at: http://www.infed.org/b-learne.htm

Smyth, J. (1989) Developing and sustaining critical reflection in teacher education. *Journal of Teacher Education*, March–April, 2–9.

Taylor, B. J. (2000) *Reflective Practice: A Guide for Nurses and Midwives*, Buckingham: Open University Press.

United Kingdom Central Council for Nursing, Midwifery and Health Visiting (1986) *Project 2000: A New Preparation For Practice*, London: UKCC.

United Kingdom Central Council for Nursing, Midwifery and Health Visiting (1992) *Code of Professinal Conduct*, London: UKCC.

United Kingdom Central Council for Nursing, Midwifery and Health Visiting (1999) *Fitness For Practice: The UKCC Commission for Nursing and Midwifery Education (The Peach Report)*, London: UKCC.

United Kingdom Central Council for Nursing, Midwifery and Health Visiting (2000) *Supporting Nurses, Midwives and Health Visitors Through Lifelong Learning*, London: UKCC.

University of Teesside (2000) *Pre-registration Nursing Framework for BSc (Hons) in Nursing Studies Programme and Diploma/Advanced Diploma in Nursing Studies: Framework Document*, Cleveland: University of Teesside.

University of Teesside (2003) *Pre-registration Nursing: BSc (Hons) Mental Health: Student Portfolio*, Cleveland: University of Teesside.

Walker, J., McCarthy, P., Morgan, W. & Timms, N. (1995) *In Pursuit of Quality: Improving Practice Teaching in Social Work*, Newcastle-Upon-Tyne: Relate Centre for Family Studies.

Whitehead, A. N. (1967) *The Aims of Education and Other Essays*, New York: Free Press.

Vass, A. (1996) *Social Work Competences*, London: Sage.

CHAPTER 30

A Framework for Success:
A Student's Perspective

COLIN ROWLEY

This is a personal account of the applicability, appropriateness and usefulness of the competency framework, inherent within the Exit Profile for Pre-registration Mental Health Nurses (Northern Centre for Mental Health, 2000) when delivered as a 3-year mental health student nurse portfolio.

This chapter is based on the experience of being among the first cohort of 'Making a Difference' students to complete the original version of this portfolio that was designed in 2000 (the first stage being completed at the end of the first year of training in 2001) and its subsequent updated and revised versions in 2001 (completed at the end of the second year of training in 2002) and 2002 (to be completed at the end of the programme in late 2003).

As the portfolio has evolved and developed since its original conception many of its earlier 'teething troubles' have been ironed out. Originally it presented as complex, unclear in its definition of what was expected, and overly academic rather than practical in its usage. This contemporary version, while still retaining a degree of complexity, is a much more streamlined affair and clearly defines what is necessary for completion. However, the competency framework remains much the same, advancing each year, guided by the national *Making a Difference* programme (DoH, 1999), which is at the core of the portfolio and is designed to develop practice and prepare students to become qualified mental health nurses. This chapter aims to present the user perspective (that of the student nurse) and demonstrate how useful the competency framework was in developing practice, its relevance, and how achievable the competencies actually were in practice.

In the student nurses' first year the competency framework centres on the basic tenets of nursing practice, such as generic physical care skills and appropriate personal and interpersonal attitudes. You are required to provide evidence that shows your ability to grasp these. Competencies here include 'demonstrating a positive approach to learning'; 'a professional approach to practice'; 'showing an ethical attitude'; 'maintaining confidentiality' and other similar aspects of character. The first impression here is that rather than develop practice the aim of the competencies is to ascertain whether you have the personal qualities to be a nurse. The focus in many ways seems to be on *what you have done* and *what you are* rather than *what you need to do* to develop in practice in order to achieve your ultimate goal.

This appears quite daunting at first but when viewed from an alternative perspective it can be seen to give you the opportunity to evidence skills that are already present (or at least should be), and to recognize these skills. When the individual competencies and the larger domains are examined in further detail by viewing their component benchmarks it is then possible to see how small elements of practice combine in order to produce significant knowledge bases and complex skills. You may consider that you fulfil the criteria for a selected competency but by breaking it down (to the level of the benchmarks) you are able to identify areas of weakness that can be improved upon. For example, being able to maintain confidentiality of information is not just about only telling those who are required to know, it is about accurate communication skills, being consistent with legislation and policy and storing and recording information correctly. It is knowledge of these constituent parts of a competency (and the wider domain) that promotes development in practice. Viewing the competency framework in this way aids greater understanding of your actions.

Each domain and competency is effectively broken down into benchmarks detailing what is required to achieve each one. This is where the problems begin. Differing types of evidence are quoted to show the achievement of each competency. This can be in the form of a case study, written reflection, completed documentation, testimonies and such like. Where the difficulty lies is in matching the evidence to a number of competencies at once. The portfolio has a word limit, for example the limit for case studies may be set at 4,000 words. This may have to include a specific number of competencies and benchmarks and the difficulty here is paying sufficient homage to each of these to be able to demonstrate that they are effectively and thoroughly evidenced.

A significant factor here is that not all the specified competencies may actually be achievable within the case study. Nursing and mental health in particular is not an exact science and to work on the pretext that a defined number of factors will occur within the scope of a case study (that can be used to provide evidence) is optimistic at the very least. Whether they occur in the case study or not you are still required to provide evidence in order to have that competency 'signed off'. What is needed here is a more creative and flexible approach.

The competencies themselves are theoretically related to practice and therefore should be achievable more globally. If for example a specific benchmark is unachievable in the scope of the case study then this is not to suggest it cannot be achieved elsewhere and then attributed or 'cross referenced' to the case study. While this removes a degree of genuineness in the case study this is only in the academic sense. In practical terms the competency has still been achieved and practice has been developed. Surely this is a much more beneficial and realistic approach than trying to incorporate interventions into the care of an individual purely for academic reasons.

While the framework itself is quite rigid and prescriptive, particularly in the first year where clear and specific physical skills have to be developed and evidenced, it is still possible to approach it flexibly. Partly due to inexperience there is an urge to evidence work descriptively and to highlight every accomplishment by identifying it in the literature. With the benefit of hindsight this is not the way forward. Many of the techniques and skills required by the competency framework are things you are already doing. Rather than set out to tackle each one individually and 'tick it off' once it is completed, you need to recognize that many of these skills are already present and that they can be recognized and applied to the competency framework. With this comes the knowledge that skills are not individual, in fact they are complementary to each other. The achievement of one competency often leads to the achievement of another.

A simple format is to choose an area such as 'written reflection' then list all the competencies and benchmarks requiring this. Grouping them in such a way makes it easier to identify which ones can be achieved at the same time. Doing this with each required area of evidence enables you to see exactly what is required to complete the written work for that particular area. As can be seen by doing this a lot of competencies (and therefore benchmarks) are very similar and it is a noticeable weakness of the framework that it over complicates such areas by differentiating matters when it may not be necessary.

Upon completion of the first year framework competencies and the experience thus gained it is now possible to gauge their benefits. Rather than directly influencing practice I am of the opinion that these provided the foundations and the belief from which growth was encouraged. The competencies promote the realization of an existing skill base and oblige and require the student to identify what is necessary to move forward. Once they were simplified into a workable concept and the expanse of 'explanatory' literature that served as a dressing to the portfolio was recognized as just that, the competencies did actually serve their purpose. Adversely the teething problems that were experienced actually served to develop confidence through the simple fact that they had to be, and were, overcome with considerably little guidance available.

The second year of the portfolio showed obvious developments from the first, however it still remained academic rather than practical in its usage. A degree of user (student) input in the development stages may have improved its ease of use here. The competency framework focuses on intervention and interaction and is much more client centred than the original portfolio. Rather than question character and attitude it questions practice directly and promotes development by asking for the student to be much more proactive in achieving their outcomes. This is the point where expectations are increased and the protective atmosphere of the first year dissipates.

You are expected to be efficient as well as competent in practice and take on a considerable degree of responsibility regarding the care of clients. Evidence has to be provided within the portfolio for all of this.

The number of competencies increases accordingly and initially this can be quite overwhelming. These can however be combined to make them more achievable. Many are focused around assessment issues that are entirely relevant to the placement and concurrent teaching. The problem here was their achievability. Some of the issues highlighted by the competency framework (such as some of the psychotherapies), were so contemporary that practice in the placement areas had not yet caught up. In the case of some of the more advanced psychosocial interventions there were hardly any professionals with sufficient knowledge to learn from and to be honest very few had an advanced knowledge of traditional interventions. This leaves students in the position of having to introduce little known concepts into practice areas with a distinct lack of supervision. From a personal point of view, I acknowledge and applaud the need to introduce new ideas and the benefits this has on existing practice, but complex ideas that impact upon client care need to be learned first, preferably with adequate supervision. Books alone cannot be expected to produce competency in practice.

The way forward for myself was to use and develop brief interventions through client interaction and then expand upon these using theoretical knowledge in order that this could be presented as evidence. It is unrealistic to expect to be fully competent in all aspects of chosen care upon qualifying, or even close. Competence will come with experience and this is what the competency framework seeks for the student to understand. A simplistic approach to wording the competencies may be beneficial here. Particular competencies appear unclear in their meanings and are easily misinterpreted. The student and the practice assessor must work together to decipher these if they are to be successfully achieved. Considering that the competency framework also guides the assessor who in turn is expected to guide the student, very few if any speak in the form of language it is presented in.

To make this process more clear and understandable each portfolio has assessment guidelines that highlight indicative content, areas of skill development, and what problem-based learning should concentrate upon. These are relevant to the placement areas and can be effectively broken down into two or three defining areas that incorporate all of the learning needs. For example, the area of risk will incorporate team supervision as a means of support and concern for the safety of others, this in turn covers effective communication skills and so on. This devolves the portfolio into manageable sections and as can be seen here, integrates achievement of the benchmark competencies. This brings the competency framework much more into focus and does not make each competency seem so insular and complex.

On a more positive note, once the framework can be comprehended its relevance to practice becomes apparent. It is extremely closely linked with the *Code of Professional Conduct* (Nursing and Midwifery Council, 2002) and serves to instil these codes into everyday practice. This helps to develop a secure understanding of the rights and wrongs and ethical underpinnings in nursing. Rather than portray the codes as unbreakable and inflexible rules that you must abide by no matter what, the competency framework encourages and cajoles you into questioning the moral and ethical reasons for these codes and therefore your practice. Forcing you to examine your practice at such a micro-level increases your self-awareness and allows weaknesses and strengths to be recognized. I personally feel that this process of critical evaluation is the key to moving practice on to a higher level. Being able to identify limitations and areas of strength promoted confidence that my practice could be developed yet remain safe, supposedly attributes of a qualified and competent staff nurse.

While it can be seen that the competency framework strongly advocates the critical evaluation of practice, it appears overly concise in how it asks for it to be evidenced. To evaluate your practice you must reflect as an individual, therefore making this an autonomous process. You can be given guidance on how to reflect or asked to reflect upon a chosen area, but for the reflection to be worthwhile it must have specific meaning to you. This is where the competency framework fails somewhat in the manner of evidence it requests. The wordage for reflection is extremely limited, which in itself is not a problem as writing is expected to be concise. What is a problem is the amount of significantly different competencies you are expected to cover within these limitations. The written reflection is guided so much by the competencies that it ceases to be true personalized reflection and merely pays tribute to the competency framework. This makes it extremely difficult to discuss any issue in depth and provides an unrealistic account of what was really felt.

When the contemporary focus on being reflective practitioners is considered, it would seem a logical suggestion that this is encouraged rather than turned into an unsatisfactory experience due to the rigidity of the structure. The approach used to overcome this was to incorporate evaluation that was reflective in its essence in the completion of items such as 'case studies' and 'critique of completed documentation'. While this was not evidenced in the manner the portfolio asked for it nevertheless gave the reader an overall impression that the stipulated competencies had been reflected upon. In terms of practice it is acknowledged that reflection is an everyday component of the nurse's thinking but the process of writing this down allows for a more in-depth examination of feelings that can be referred to rather than forgotten.

The competency framework in the second year portfolio, in hindsight is pivotal in changing the way you look at things. The first year is viewed from the standpoint of a student, recognizing existing skills and indicating developmental areas. The second year encourages you to take the standpoint of a qualified nurse, taking responsibility and becoming accountable. This is necessary for expectations are constantly increasing in preparation for qualification. This is very much a framework that looks at the development of skills with the implication being that the third year is about the implementation of these skills.

The third year portfolio itself is a much more streamlined and user-friendly effort than its predecessors. While academically more advanced as would be expected at this stage, there is less repetitive work involved and it clearly states what is required to progress. The competency framework is very similar in style and admittedly is more comfortable to work with due to the previous two years experience. The differences that do exist pertain to the management of care issues rather than assessing and evaluating. My own feelings are that previously the competency framework had guided practice by basically letting you know what you should be doing and achieving. With practice now at an advanced level this is not the case. Clinical placements tend to be in specialist services that require adaptable approaches. Operating at this higher level of practice essentially incorporates the achievement of most of the benchmarks. At this stage the competency framework is extremely relevant to practice. You do not have to attempt each competency, it is simply the case of acknowledging what part each plays in your overall practice.

This seems easier in essence and indeed it is for many of the simpler competencies. However, some of them are quite specific in what they ask for. For example, issues such as violence and community interventions are expected to be experienced at some point. Dependent upon the placement area you choose these may not be easily achieved. This can be quite frustrating and lead to the evidence that is presented being tenuous to say the least. What is required here is a versatile approach, viewing the competency in a different light. To illustrate this point, family work is required to be evidenced in the case study. In a secure environment there may be no contact with the family, however, if viewed from a different angle it can be seen that the nursing team and fellow clients actually represent the role of the family and it is this that needs referring to. The competency framework needs to be interpreted creatively for it to be fully achievable. With experience and a flexible approach this becomes entirely possible.

Even the most difficult of competencies should be achievable, helped significantly by considerable placement length. The time span enables you to create opportunities and prompt situations that allow for the correct skill development. What can be limited in the placement area (as mentioned earlier) is the lack of availability of professionals with specialist skills that are able to give you the time to learn. Specialist areas as can be expected are busy the majority of the time and assessor observation of the student's practice or vice versa may be limited due to the sensitivity of situations restricting the number of people present. It is possible and invariably helpful that within the placement time structured tutoring in specialist areas such as the range of possible therapies can be arranged. Even if client participation is not possible you can still use the knowledge gained by discussing its possibilities in relation to a client as evidence for the competency framework.

What is evident and particularly relevant in the third year is the amount of dialogue and discussion required with the placement mentor in order to assess competency and achievement levels. While the majority of assessors seem only to have a rudimentary knowledge of the portfolio and its benchmarks, at this stage you should have developed a reasonable level of knowledge and possess the ability to describe the competency framework as you interpret it. It is possible that the assessor may have entirely different interpretations and, rather than view this as a difficulty, in reality it is an opportunity to impart your knowledge and assert your views on what you believe and why. This can promote healthy debate on issues that allows the assessor to gain an understanding of your knowledge base and what stage of development you are at. The relevance this has to practice is that as a qualified nurse you will be expected to have knowledge that you can defend but also have the ability to take the views of others on board.

Returning to the competency framework, it is feasible that you can provide written evidence that shows knowledge and understanding but that you actually have difficulty achieving this in practice. Alternatively you may be able to achieve this in practice but lack the ability to evidence it appropriately. The fact that this can now be evidenced through discussion and dialogue removes such dilemmas. It is a fundamental aspect of nursing and one of the primary benchmarks in the portfolio that you are able to be an effective communicator. Through observation and interaction your assessor should be aware of your capabilities and skills and can question your underpinning knowledge of these. The process of discussion allows for simple and uncomplicated achievement of competencies without increasing academic workload. This provides a clinical representation of your competence as opposed to an academic one. It is highly relevant to practice due to the fact this is how the majority of information is passed. If you are unable to communicate as a qualified nurse, the obvious conclusion is you will have major difficulties in practice.

The strength of the competency framework becomes much more apparent in the final year. As has been mentioned previously, placements are more advanced, as are the interventions you are expected to deliver. It is easy to get carried away and overly focus upon such areas as this in the belief that this is what really is behind personal advancement. What the framework does here however, is pull you back and make you concentrate on the basics of nursing also. It never allows you to forget the importance of issues such as ethical consideration, confidentiality, safe practice and the recognition of limitations. These and similar competencies are what underpins real development in my opinion. They provide the foundation for you to build your skills to the levels to which you aspire. Without incorporating these into practice, life may seem easier but decisions are uninformed and risky. Practice cannot be justified and the purpose of your nursing will be called into question. As a student you are supported in much of your decision making until you are fully able to digest what the competency framework is trying to introduce to your practice. It has to be recognized that this is not just a paper exercise it is a crucial part of the developing process that will turn us into effective nurses.

An overall impression of the competency framework is that it is highly relevant to practice. Undeniably it may be possible to simplify it and still achieve the same results. An interesting point is that the finished portfolio is marked highly on accessibility and conciseness of information contained within. These are areas of considerable weakness in the document itself but admittedly they appear to be improving with time. This may sound slightly pedantic but bearing in mind the length of time it initially takes to come to grips with the competency framework this does not help. This is time that could be better spent concentrating on clinical practice. However this issue is not as prominent in the third year where it is possible to return to previous formats and incorporate existing knowledge of the competency framework. This degree of comfort allows you to delve deeper into the meaning of the competencies and hopefully demonstrate understanding and meaning in practice.

As the three annual portfolios develop they turn out to be more satisfying in their achievement as they become more personal in their content. Writing is more reflective of actual practice than it is of theory. The achievement of the competency framework fits more naturally into practice without requiring sustained effort. Minor difficulties can be overcome by ensuring a creative approach is developed over time. The experience is more enjoyable because the subsequent lessening of the academic workload means it no longer encroaches into practice time and allows for placements to be more fulfilling and therefore more beneficial. This is not to deny that at first this is a daunting task that creates apprehension but if it makes it any easier it is a process that serves its purpose and provides us with the necessary skills and foundations to be competent practitioners.

Acknowledgements and thanks to my fellow students Chris Lawton, Jill Luke and Vicky Moir for their input, inspiration and support throughout the writing of this chapter.

References

Department of Health (1999) *Making a Difference*, London: HMSO.

Northern Centre for Mental Health (2000) *A Competence-based Exit Profile For Pre-Registration Mental Health Nursing*, Durham: Northern Centre for Mental Health.

Nursing and Midwifery Council (2002) *Code of Professional Conduct*, London: Nursing and Midwifery Council.

Suggested reading

Boud, D., Keogh, R. & Walker, D. (eds) (1985) *Reflection: Turning Experience Into Learning*, London: Kogan Page.

Brooker, C. & Repper, J. (1998) *Serious Mental Health Problems in the Community Policy, Practice & Research*, London: Harcourt Publishers.

Chaloner, C. & Coffey, M. (eds) (2000) *Forensic Mental Health Nursing: Current Approaches*, Oxford: Blackwell Science.

Dexter, G. & Wash, M. (1997) *Psychiatric Nursing Skills: A Patient-Centred Approach*, (2nd edn), Cheltenham: Stanley Thornes Ltd.

Fortinash, K. M. & Holoday-Worrat, P. A. (1999) *Psychiatric Nursing Care Plans*, (3rd edn), Missouri: Mosby.

Fowler, D., Garety, P. & Kuipers, E. (1995) *Cognitive Behaviour Therapy for Psychosis, Theory and Practice*, Chichester: John Wiley & Sons.

Gamble, C. & Brennan, G. (2000) *Working with Serious Mental Illness: A Manual for Clinical Practice*, London: Harcourt Publishers.

Healy, D. (2002) *Psychiatric Drugs Explained*, (3rd edn), Edinburgh: Harcourt Publishers.

Kettles, A., Woods, P. & Collins, M. (eds) (2002) Therapeutic Interventions for Forensic Mental Health Nurses, London: Jessica Kingsley.

Newell, R. & Gournay, K. (2000) *Mental Health Nursing: An Evidence Based Approach*, London: Harcourt Publishers.

Palmer, A., Burns, S & Bowman, C. (eds) (1994) *Reflective Practice in Nursing: The Growth of the Professional Practitioner*, Oxford: Blackwell Science.

Schultz, J. & Videbeck, R. (2000) *Lippincotts Manual of Psychiatric Nursing Care Plans, Edition 6*, Philadelphia: Lippincott, Williams & Wilkins.

Thomas, B., Hardy, S. & Cutting, P. (eds) (1997) *Stuart and Sundeen's Mental Health Nursing Principles and Practice (UK Version)*, London: Mosby.

CHAPTER 31

A Day in the Life of . . .

MIKE FIRN, STEVE HARRISON AND PETER MELIA

Editors' Note:

This chapter is intentionally different from the ones that you have just read. As the preceding chapters are underpinned by the Benchmarks derived from the 'Exit Profile for Pre-registration Mental Health Nursing', they then have hopefully allowed you to gain an insight into, as well as an understanding of, the theories and rationale(s) behind what and why mental health nurses do in practice.

This chapter is the opportunity for Senior Clinicians to share with you valuable day-to-day experiences that are encountered as well as highlighting issues relating to working in a selection of diverse clinical areas. These contributors write straight from the heart and 'tell it like it is' drawing on their considerable experience within their chosen areas to give you an insight into 'A Day in the Life of . . .'

Working in Assertive Outreach

MIKE FIRN

Introduction

Assertive Outreach teams form one of the specialist services comprising the modern framework set out by the Department of Health to meet the needs of those patients living in the community with more severe and enduring mental health problems (DoH, 1999, 2001). The skills and competencies required to work in this field derive from the global problems faced by the type of patients who require this model of working.

As a community service, outreach teams embrace integrated psychiatric and social care delivery from the resources of one team. This recognizes that services have in the past been fragmented into functional areas, governed by separate professions or agencies, which were not easily negotiated by patients with the most severe psychotic illness.

A patient with many years of regular hospital admissions due to schizophrenia is very concerned about benefit payments not arriving and the rent not having been paid by housing benefit. At the same time he is prescribed depot anti-psychotic medication but is hard to engage in services, somewhat chaotic and regularly avoids or misses appointments. The Care Co-ordinator identifies concerns about missed treatment for his persistent psychotic symptoms, the risk of losing his flat due to arrears, a lack of money to provide for food, gas and electric, poor coping strategies and high levels of distress.

This is not an extreme example but a common situation faced by people living with psychosis. Often the degree of organization and motivation required to fill in benefit forms, negotiate with the benefit agency or housing department and seek medical treatment is lacking. These procedures themselves can be complex and stressful. Small caseload sizes enable workers in Assertive Outreach to take high levels of responsibility for delivering care across these functional areas and for co-ordinating across agencies to ensure that the patient can survive outside hospital. Assertive Outreach is labour intensive and a long-term commitment. It involves working closely and frequently with patients to sustain support and gradually move towards greater self-sufficiency.

Generic working

There is a commitment in the model to workers from different professional groups blurring traditional boundaries to deliver patient care according to client need. The work is intensive, with extended hours and extended roles. This is a step towards generic roles and requires confidence and experience to feel comfortable stepping out of the safety of the role envisaged and prepared for by basic training and professional bodies. A working knowledge is needed which spans psychiatric and psychological interventions for psychosis and social interventions to protect the essentials of community living. This remit is not the preserve of one profession or agency. Indeed some necessary tasks are not generally regarded as the work of trained professionals. Helping a patient clean up their flat to prevent them being evicted or getting them some food in may be the most pressing intervention for some patients.

Assertive Outreach person specification

Perhaps one way of looking at the skills required for assertive outreach is to look at an actual person specification used to recruit staff for our team (see Table 31.1)

Table 31.1   Assertive Outreach person specification

	Essential	Desirable
Qualifications and experience	• Trained mental health professional. • Minimum of two years qualified mental health experience. • Experience of assessing and managing crisis in the severely mentally ill.	• Experience in community-based work • Certificate or diploma in psychosocial interventions or similar • Experience of assertive outreach work.
Skills	• Can demonstrate a flexible approach to care. • Can demonstrate an ability to work independently, yet function as part of a team. • Can demonstrate an ability / experience / willingness to work in a creative manner that is not constrained by disciplinary boundaries. • Can understand and meet the particular needs of the black and ethnic minority client group. • Can demonstrate experience of creating a total package of care for a client that may require access to more local resources. • Can demonstrate an ability to work with the client and their carers / family (as appropriate) in an educational / therapeutic way.	
Attitude and personal qualities	• Can demonstrate a willingness to cope with the particular problems of working with a client group that is difficult to engage in services. • Can demonstrate a flexible approach to care and patient need. • Possess good communication skills both written and verbal. • Can demonstrate the use of initiative when dealing with clients.	• Is enthusiastic about the prospect of working in a new role
Other	• Are able to undertake evening and weekend work. • Can adopt a flexible working schedule. • Is a car driver.	

This brief specification is for a Clinical Case Manager who would act as Care Co-ordinator with a caseload of team patients. It refers to a trained mental health professional rather than specifying which training or profession. The team as a whole needs a skills mix of staff in order to maintain multi-disciplinary input and a healthy debate. Although training and experience in Assertive Outreach provides an overview of generic skills, there are often team members who can provide a lead or give supervision in specific interventions. Traditionally psychologists may have greater knowledge and practice in schizophrenia family work or occupational therapists have more in-depth knowledge for the assessment of daily living skills compared to other professions. Nurses, of course, may have greater knowledge about the effects and side effects of medicine.

In Assertive Outreach, Care Co-ordinators have an identified caseload but routinely see many other team patients to provide interventions. This is especially the case where patients are seen seven days a week, since no individual Care Co-ordinator could sustain this frequency, but also as a deliberate attempt to manage challenging behaviour or the risk of over-dependency on one Care Co-ordinator.

Communication and structuring the work

The routine practice of sharing contact with patients throughout the team, and the high levels of patient contact required, demand good co-ordination and communication. This is achieved by morning handover meetings where every patient is mentioned by name, and visits and interventions planned. Most teams meet first thing and plan visits using a white board, allocating visits according to available staff. Rarely would visits be allocated according to the intervention needed since all professions work to a generic model. The culture of staff from all professions helping patients manage their medication, or structure their day is engrained in theory and practice.

Boxes 31.1 and 31.2 from Burns and Firn (2002) outline the format and purpose of these meetings.

Similarly the level of responsibility for helping patients manage all aspects of their life is a heavy responsibility to be carried by one case manager. The facility of daily group support and multi-disciplinary problem solving maintains a healthy team.

Engagement

You will notice that the word flexible is used several times throughout the person specification. No patients' needs fit into neat boxes along diagnostic or service unit demarcations. Nor should they. Assertive Outreach is a collaborative enterprise and the process of effectively engaging with a patient

---

Box 31.1   Format for handover/briefing

- Takes place first thing in the morning. (Some teams meet at the beginning and the end of the day when using a shift system).
- 15–30 minutes depending on caseload size.
- Chairperson to mention each client by name (alphabetical order or by Care Co-ordinator).
- Discussion only occurs if there has been a change, development, concern or advice needed for that client or where visit allocation or cover needed.
- Chairperson to curtail lengthy discussion or refer to clinical supervision or weekly review meeting.
- Junior Doctor present.
- Monday handover may be more involved in allocating tasks for the week throughout the team e.g. Clients on daily visits, support worker tasks allocation.
- Friday handover may include time for planning support over the weekend if cover is limited

Source: Burns & Firn (2002)

Box 31.2   Functions of handover/briefing

- Structured information exchange on every patient in a time efficient forum.
- Allocation of tasks and visits.
- Organization of cross cover for staff on leave, training or sick.
- Organization of joint visits either for safety or specific input
- Group support and multidisciplinary problem solving.
- Prioritization of resources for the day.
- Regular access to a doctor for advice, prescription, medicine titration or changes.
- Reinforces 'teamness' through face-to-face planning and discussion.

Source: Burns & Firn (2002)

---

means listening to their agenda, and working towards mutual goals not attempting to control the patient's life for them.

Paul was referred to the team because he had many admissions and was labelled hard to engage. He was ambivalent at best to the involvement of mental health services and often refused access to staff on home visits telling them to leave him alone. The team continued to attempt home visits as a way of monitoring risk as he had a history of severe self-neglect and withdrawal, and would be picked up by the police after arguments with his neighbours precipitated by persecutory delusions.

On one of the few occasions that Paul allowed us in we offered to give him some practical help by using our car to take his television to be repaired. After this Paul started to allow us access and gradually a rapport built up enough to discuss issues of symptoms, treatment and social needs.

Patients will disengage from services repeatedly and present moral and ethical dilemmas to the team and individual worker about how assertively we should attempt contact, when to intervene, and when to use the statutory powers of the Mental Health Act (DoH, 1983). Engagement related activity could be classified into three approaches (Burns & Firn, 2002). The ideal is to work collaboratively with the patient to foster a positive attitude towards the service. This 'constructive approach' would include advocacy, empower-ment, befriending and a non-judgemental attitude. Helping with financial problems, housing and support with employment are often the first items on the patient's agenda.

If the therapeutic alliance breaks down the care co-ordinator may be required to maintain frequent contact because of history of rapid relapse or risk. An 'indirect approach' may be one option where the patient refuses access to their home. This involves communicating with the patient's family, carers and third parties such as housing or the benefits agency. Have complaints been made by neighbours about the patient's behaviour, is the patient claiming their benefits, have they seen their GP recently? Where the family is involved they will know if the usual behaviour of the patient has changed. Should this indi-rect information indicate risk then the team must decide when to intervene.

Statutory powers available in the UK include compulsory admission, and aftercare under supervision (Section 25 of the Mental Health Act 1983). The latter is often referred to as 'Supervised Discharge'. It is in effect a contract with the patient to allow access to their home, reside at a specified place or to attend appointments for the purpose of medical treatment, occupation edu-cation or training.

In summary 'the foundation for effective Assertive Outreach services will be engagement and persistence with a constructive rather than restrictive approach to keeping track of people' (Sainsbury Centre for Mental Health, 1998).

Symptom management

No one has ever got better from simply being engaged in mental health ser-vices or just being a patient with an Assertive Outreach team. We see our patients frequently and intensively in order to appraise their clinical and social condition, which in turn serves to guide effective treatment and rehabilitation. It is the latter that produces changes in the outcomes, whether these are reduced hospitalization, better quality of life, or a reduction in distressing psychotic symptoms.

The evidence supports several interventions. Regular prescription, monitoring and supervision of medication are core features of helping patients manage with psychotic illness. Medication is used for both acute treatment and maintenance of schizophrenia and bipolar affective disorder. Care Coordinators require the skills to explain these potential benefits to patients in a way that is relevant to their circumstances. They require the knowledge and the rapport of trust to work through the patient's ambivalence to medication and their concerns about side effects. More sophisticated approaches to this educational, prompting and supporting approach are described as 'Compliance Therapy' (Kemp et al, 1997). This is a structured programme based on collaboration, motivational interviewing (Rollinick et al, 1992) and cognitive behavioural techniques (Kingdon & Turkington, 1994). Patients unable to enter into formal and demanding programmes can benefit from daily visits to supervise the taking of medication, and the small caseloads in Assertive Outreach facilitate this option.

Cognitive Behavioural Therapy is beginning to be used for psychosis to restructure patients' beliefs about delusions and hallucinations. Patients can also be taught simple strategies for coping with persistent symptoms (Tarrier et al, 1998) and early intervention plans to deal with relapse. Helping patients recognize their individual early warning signs can ensure that they participate in heading off relapse.

Formal programmes of schizophrenia family work are well established and effective in reducing rates of relapse albeit to a lesser extent than maintenance medication (Pharoah et al, 1999). Involving and supporting carers at all times is a vital part of community work and does not involve the level of training necessary for formal schizophrenia family work.

Conclusion

Assertive Outreach calls for an expansion of the traditional role of the mental health nurse. 'It does not detract from nursing's professional identity and core values which are focused on acting in the best interests of the patient' (Gough, 1998, p 23).

An expansion of roles beyond that envisaged in core training requires both experience on the part of the nurse and a system of providing additional training, clinical supervision and assessing competence within the organization. The level of patient need calls for intensive work, which can only come from a highly organized team. Daily meetings and co-ordination structure the delivery of interventions and provide multi-disciplinary support and problem solving for team members in a challenging job.

Nursing Young People With Mental Health Problems

Steve Harrison

Introduction

Professionally I'm selfish. I want children who are trying to deal with mental health problems to be helped by the most able nurses. This is not only because I think a civilized society should put its children first, but also because I think the earlier we can tackle mental health problems the greater our chances of progress.

So what should a newly qualified nurse working in the Child and Adolescent Mental Health (CAMH) arena be thinking about and doing? Space is limited so I will focus on some key ideas which will, I hope, make readers curious to discover more about this fascinating area of nursing.

Initial reflections

My early experience as a newly qualified Staff Nurse working with adolescents on an inpatient unit, was characterized by confusion. Was I there to befriend these children? Was I a surrogate father or brother? Was I a teacher? I didn't know, and what is more the young people knew that I didn't know! They duly had a good deal of fun at my expense and I learned experientially, or 'the hard way' as it was known then.

I recognize that the confusing and challenging part of working with children, is actually the part I find most enjoyable. In fact if I wasn't constantly asking myself questions I'd be worried. I think a nurse who works with children needs not only to acknowledge this fact but to embrace it. A fair question to ask at this point is 'Why?'

First of all, theory and practice don't always fit neatly. Schön (1987) holds the view that knowledge, developed out of context in academic settings, struggles to take root in the clinical world. Croom et al (2000) note that in the Child and Adolescent Mental Health arena, as much as any other, the relationship between academia and clinical action is not only difficult in the sense of the problems of transferring dry theory into complex interpersonal practice. There is also the issue of 'perpetuating custom and practice'. That is to say, the tendency for professionals to confer the status of 'knowledge' on practice that has developed idiosyncratically. This then is a challenge for the newly qualified nurse getting to grips with taking theoretical maps and applying them to an unfamiliar terrain.

In terms of the CAMH arena there is an extra puzzle to contend with. That is, in terms of child mental health even the maps are unclear and badly drawn. To illustrate this let us consider basic principles.

Basic principles

A simple fundamental question to start with is 'What is a Child?' On 7 September 2000, after some procrastination, the United Kingdom became signatories to the United Nations Convention on the Rights of the Child. At least we were ahead of the United States, which is still to get round to this task. This protected rights of children in law and helpfully defined a child as being a person under 18 years of age. Because of its merit as a current and clear definition it is this meaning we use here, however in practice, things aren't so clearly defined. Other laws say adulthood starts at 16 and even before in some instances.

It is not the aim of this chapter to tackle this issue in detail, merely to illustrate that, the laws that nurses must work within are 'unclear and extremely contentious' (NHS Health Advisory Service, 1995).

If childhood is not a sharply defined area then what of the notoriously slippery concept 'mental health'? Graham et al (1999) suggest that this concept is more difficult to define in a child and mental health context than in most other areas. This is, in their view, due to the number of factors that will influence a child's mental health. The child's development, family influences and the wider environment all have a part to play. The Audit Commission (*Children in Mind*, 1999) suggest that there is a broad agreement in recent research that at any one time one-fifth of children will be suffering from mental health problems. The term 'mental health problems' in this case covers a broad range of psychological difficulties experienced by young people. This could arguably mean anything from pre-GCSE anxiety to psychosis. The 'milder' end of this continuum could be viewed as essential elements of a person's defences.

At what point should we judge which situations are best dealt with by supportive parents and friends and which require professional help? Pearce (1993) is helpful in suggesting the following criteria in tracking the change from problem to disorder. He suggests that a mental health disorder is a change in the usual behaviours, thoughts or feelings. Difficulties should persist for more than two weeks. They should be pervasive and intense enough to disrupt day-to-day functioning.

What is clear is that the fundamentals are not easy to grasp. Perhaps it should be like that. Childhood is about growth, change and uncertainty. That is the exciting challenge of nursing in the child mental health arena. Because problem situations are new and part of a developing process, important changes can often be made more easily. Which brings us to an interesting question. If the picture is a complex and uncertain one where should we target our efforts? I would suggest nurses think about two key ideas. The child's development and the child as part of a family 'system'.

The developmental context

Although we are all changing all of the time, our childhood is a period of the most intense developmental activity. Bee (2000) sees this period not only as a time where frantic change and consolidation takes place but also as a time where developmental changes have dramatic effects upon each other. For example, our success at developing our language will impact upon our social development, which will in turn influence our sense of self and our personality. Such an enormous topic as this can barely be touched upon here but in Bee's (2000) work we can find a number of helpful frameworks to shape our thoughts.

One such schema which seems useful not only in its original context of infancy, but in a holistic sense is the idea of four developmental processes that play key roles in our overall maturation. Physical maturation is a process that is at its most active in our first 18 years. Why should we be so interested in this from a mental health perspective? Because factors like our size, shape, appearance, strength and so on help us construct our identity, our sense of self. People respond to these characteristics giving us reassuring or discouraging messages to which we, in turn, can react in a multitude of ways. A complex multi-layered interaction develops, between the child, other people and the groups around them.

A second developmental process to be aware of is the child's explorations. We are born with a bias to enquire. We carry out increasingly complex experiments to understand our world and how we fit within it. In a mental health context, many of a child's painful and self-limiting conclusions may arise from these explorations. They may feel worthless because they've been bullied. They may experience a sense of guilt or being 'dirty' because they've been sexually abused by a grown up. These are extreme illustrations and not all of these explorations are that pronounced and fundamental. I can clearly recollect warnings given to me in my first working week saying that the youngsters would 'test me out'. The connotation at the time was that I would be 'confronted'. Another way to view it was that they were naturally 'testing' me, tackling their developmental tasks of understanding who I was, how I responded to them, what my arrival meant to the group and a multitude of other questions.

A third key developmental idea is that of attachment. The pioneer of this notion John Bowlby, (1969) holds the view that as infants we are driven to form a key attachment to a caregiver. The quality of this relationship is considered to be enormously influential in other developmental processes. There is strong evidence that even in the midst of adolescence, though peer relationships are becoming increasingly important, the quality of attachment between teenagers and parents is critically important. Levitt et al (1993) hold the view that in adolescence as much as childhood, this relationship is generally more important to a sense of well being than those with friends, teachers and so on. The value of this concept to a mental health nurse is self-evident. We need to be attuned to the quality of this relationship in practice if the evidence available to us indicates that it is at the heart of a person's well being.

The fourth key developmental process to consider at this stage is linked to those mentioned so far. That is the results of these processes of enquiry or as Bee (2000) terms it, 'internal working models'. It is suggested here that from our earliest days we develop our theory of reality around us based on our explorations. Epstein (1991) feels that we focus on four key themes. We decide how much the world is a place of pain or pleasure. We develop a belief about how chaotic or meaningful the world is. We develop a view about to what extent people are friendly or threatening, and finally we gain an estimation of our self-worth. Challenges to Epstein's idea could be made in terms of how universal a process it is, and whether his view is suspiciously simplistic, failing to take into account the complexities of human development. Nevertheless, a nurse who is able to safely and meaningfully explore these questions with a youngster is engaged in critical and potentially fruitful nursing practice.

There are broad implications for nursing practice arising from the area of development. But before we turn to them we must think more about children in their most important context, that of their family.

The family context

As we have discovered, any child is experiencing immense change, commonly termed 'development'. Carr (1999) sees these forces as primarily social factors and cites the family as the main place where we try to deal with these processes. A key question constantly posed in the CAMH arena is 'To what degree has the family facilitated the child's development?' The most commonly used model for understanding family complexities is to think of it as a system. That is to say, an interconnected structure that has an identity beyond the sum of its parts. (Graham et al, 1999) For example, this book is comprised of a series of words and pages but as a whole it forms an organized set of ideas and concepts. A second important characteristic of a system is its ability to interact with its surroundings, constantly giving and receiving messages, and required to change as a result of this.

In families complex change must be dealt with. I have three children – two are teenagers and the other a toddler. My commitment to them all is equal.

However, to be effective, my approach to them has to be different and constantly open to change. One needs constant attention and to be fed, changed and kept safe from risks on nearly all occasions. The others need to practice problem solving and to have a greater degree of freedom within certain limits.

Having briefly touched upon this central idea of the family system, how do we address this question of a family's ability to nurture development? Wilkinson (1998) gives us some clues. Here five dimensions are considered as helpful themes to think about.

First of all closeness and distance. Emotionally, how 'near' are family members to each other? Are they stifling each other's growth or are they so distant as to be barely connected? Is there a combination of these two extremes? Are these patterns of proximity changing, and importantly, what are the net gains and losses for the child who is suffering in mental health terms?

Second, how is power managed in the family? Are the 'grown ups' in the family discharging their legal and moral responsibilities clearly and effectively? Are responsibilities distributed in a way that matches people's developmental needs and abilities?

Third, what emotional climate exists in this family? Regardless of theoretical background, there is much support for the notion that the emotional culture of a family is key in fostering or undermining mental health. Pettit et al (1997) established that children given warm supportive parenting are less likely to display aggression or delinquency despite being raised in impoverished conditions.

A fourth aspect is the degree of stress placed upon the family. It is impossible to conceive of a family that is not experiencing stress to some degree, the key questions are how much, how intense is the pressure and how well are the family equipped to cope?

Finally there is the question of the family's own developmental journey. Is it a new system discovering its own identity? Are older children starting to establish their own independence and preparing to 'fly the nest'. Has these been a merger of two previous families which forces this new family to address issues of structure, power, emotional climate and proximity?

These are clearly complex issues, however, we must be aware of such important forces and develop our capacity to understand a child's mental health problems from a developmental and family perspective as well as crucially, developing a working relationship with them. Even in this brief overview of some key ideas the task seems daunting. So to be effective CAMH nurses where do we begin?

Implications for practice

What do we know for certain? It is clear that the formative nature of childhood presents us with challenges and chances to have a major beneficial impact upon the mental health of young people. It is also clear that we need to be able to see a child's situation from a number of complex standpoints and carry in our heads several explanatory models to organize our thinking. My view is that it would be unrealistic to expect a newly qualified nurse to have mature skills, knowledge, and experience in all these aspects of nursing. These can be developed with time, organizational commitment and a healthy team ethos. What a nurse must bring with them are some active values, principles that they are prepared not just to describe but to act upon. Egan (1998) views this 'bias toward action' as a 'cardinal value'. Nowhere is this more true than working with children. There must be a willingness to learn about these ideas and actively implement the principles in practice, even at the risk of seeming foolish or confused. This is how skills and knowledge, consolidated by experience and driven by an ethical attitude, add up to a high level of competence.

There must be a value of respecting children and their families, and recognition of the fact that as a nurse you are in a privileged position of power. You are developmentally more mature with often a greater command of language, more education, and more sophisticated thinking. From an NHS perspective you are part of an enormous organization. You will often be in familiar surroundings instead of in a place which is new and daunting to you. You will often have greater physical strength, and in certain rare and extreme circumstances you may have the power to detain young people in hospital against their will, albeit briefly, under the Mental Health Act (DoH, 1983). It is paramount therefore that this considerable array of powers is used with respect to address the needs of the child you are nursing. An extension of this is a willingness to relate to children on their terms and seek a medium that they can use to find a voice. This may be using play materials or creative media such as clay, paint and so forth. Structured games, diaries, magazines, group activities; the list is endless.

Perhaps the easiest value to have but the hardest to keep is to maintain genuineness in the way that you listen and respond to young people. As we acquire knowledge, skills and experience it is easy to adopt attitudes of peers so that you conform to your own peer group pressure, or to replicate newly acquired knowledge and skills. These are understandable affectations but the fact of the matter is we are paid to go beyond them and attempt to give the best nursing care that we can. That means being authentic in our interactions with young people and their families. The most effective nurses that I have worked with have not necessarily been the most knowledgeable, but those who have been able to combine enthusiasm, a calm demeanour and the above values. Even the most ill young people have recognized this and have been prepared to work at daunting problem situations as a result.

If we are able to take these values and back them with an ongoing learning of key academic and clinical concepts and the emerging evidence base the results will be rewarding for ourselves, illuminating for our colleagues and, most importantly, therapeutic for children and their families.

Reflections of a Forensic Mental Health Nurse

PETER MELIA

Walking into the forensic mental health environment you can't help but be struck by the fact that much of its frippery and regalia is more akin to a prison than a hospital. I suppose you do get used to that. All the same, it still feels funny having to go into work through double electronic doors with a 'sterile' airlock and then 'arm' yourself with keys, personal alarms and in some cases two-way radios before you even get near the ward to start your job.

Having to go through what feels like endless numbers of doors, continually unlocking and locking them can be a bit of a pain, and having to count and check things like cutlery, snooker equipment, lighters, scissors, needles and even batteries is a positive nuisance. But those things are just time consuming, it's having to rub-down search your clients and search their rooms and private possessions that feels really intrusive and untrusting. This more than anything makes you wonder whether you can really develop a positive and therapeutic relationship with your clients.

I remember reading a paper by Tom Mason and Dave Mercer (1990) describing psychiatric patients detained under the provisions of the Mental Health Act (DoH, 1983) as being like 'medical hostages'. It's easy to see why they would argue such a point and it makes you really think about the legal and political framework in which we work. Of course compulsion in the treatment of psychiatric patients per se is fairly common but we get taught never to let what is common or usual simply become routine. Broadly you have to remember that compelling a patient to some part of treatment must be essential and not simply tradition and that you must always have a clear and demonstrable decision making process based on sound ethical principles to edify this.

It can be complicated because we always think of compulsory treatments as things like formally admitting someone to a hospital under the provisions of the Mental Health Act (DoH, 1983) or administering medication against the expressed wishes of the patient after obtaining a second opinion. These are obviously very important decisions where compulsion is necessary but there are many more basic things we do on an almost daily basis that are equally as important to the life of the patient and require sound ethical consideration before being carried out. A good example would be encouraging a patient with depression or high negative symptoms to get out of bed to engage in therapeutic activities. The patient may express the wish to remain in bed but should we compel him or her otherwise?

The guidelines outlined in *Who Decides?* (Lord Chancellors Department, 1997) state there are three conditions that must be met before employing compulsion in the care and treatment of mental health patients, viz capacity, best interest of the patient and necessity.

- Capacity – relates to the individual's ability to make a choice on the basis of (a) being able to understand and retain information relating to that choice and (b) to use that information in arriving at their decision.
- Best interest of the patient – necessitates that the health practitioner and those responsible for care are satisfied that the treatment to be compulsorily administered is entirely and directly beneficial to the patient and not simply to the benefit of, or to make life easier for, others.
- Necessity – requires the health care practitioner to consider all options and only compel an individual to a treatment intervention where absolutely necessary and where no alternatives more suitable to the patient are apparent or available.

Only when all three criteria are met can we safely argue that compulsion is ethically appropriate and/or justifiable and that we are consequently acting in a professional manner and upholding the terms of our professional code of conduct. Even then it can feel uncomfortable and intrusive to encourage your patient out of bed when they so obviously don't want to get up.

You just have to keep reminding yourself that the need for compulsion as part of mental health law is not only necessary but actually helps keep many of our patients out of prison and gets them the help they need. Melia et al (1999) remind us that mental health law in this country is fairly unique as it is prophetic rather than historic. They point out that the Mental Health Act (DoH, 1983) is the only piece of peace-time legislation that allows an individual to be detained against their will, for long periods of time, on the grounds of what we (the clinicians) think they might do rather than what they have already done.

I know in prisons people get a fixed sentence for some misdemeanour for which they have been found guilty and sentenced to a period of imprisonment as punishment. In fact the Criminal Justice and Public Order Act (Home Office, 1994) actually dictates that individuals found guilty will be detained 'on pain of punishment'. Clearly then, the criminal justice system is punitive and based on past behaviours deemed by a court to be criminal. There is no issue of assessment of risk or dangerousness because an individual will be released at the EDR (earliest date of release), irrespective of whether the authorities believe that individual may commit some further criminal act or not. This then would be the history part of the argument.

The Mental Health Act (DoH, 1983) conversely accepts that even though an individual may have been found guilty of committing a criminal act their culpability or responsibility is diminished because of some mental disorder and therefore detention is for treatment, not punishment. Detention here though works differently to criminal justice because we aren't detaining an individual for a fixed period of time 'on pain of punishment' but for treatment. That detention can continue until it is the opinion of the clinical team that the individual's mental disorder has been treated and consequently the risk of further offending reduced. This then is prophecy, what we think might happen if that individual was at liberty. From this then, it's clearly a main priority that we treat both the individual's mental disorder and associated psychological pathology, as obviously the sooner we can reduce an individual's risk of further offending, the sooner we can give that individual back his or her liberty. Crucial to this is establishing a good therapeutic relationship with your clients, despite the complexities of the system and those components of mental health legislation, which seem to conspire to confound our best efforts. This is obviously not easy or automatic and has to be worked at.

It is important to remember the forensic mental health nurse's role is to help the individual recover from mental disorder or, where that's not entirely possible, to reduce the disabling components of their disorder to help the client live with their disability. In essence our role is to minimize functional impairment and associated subjective distress. This can be made more difficult as many of our clients use a language which portrays us as a sort of psychiatric prison and will talk about 'doing time' and will attend therapy only as a means to help them have a chance of 'getting out'. It can be tempting to actually invest in this language as an important part of the recovery process is giving the client the opportunity to formulate their own story of mental ill health and to outline their personal journey. This helps in understanding the nature of the disorder and helps them identify and recognize symptoms or relapse triggers for the future. As Said (1993) pointed out however, people create their own realities through story telling so you have to be careful not to invest in prison type language or the 'reality' of forensic mental health care services could really become psychiatric prisons.

It can seem a bit of a contradiction but as part of the relationship-building process it is necessary to maintain a strict professional detachment and not get too emotionally involved with your clients. This is partly because working in forensic mental health services you have a dual role, both to care for those clients receiving treatment and to protect the public. But more importantly it's imperative to the treatment process that clinical integrity is maintained.

We know from numerous public inquiries that there is a significant risk of staff colluding consciously or unconsciously with clients due to the long-term nature of care afforded to forensic mental health patients and the ongoing contact with individual nurses. It seems in most instances where there has been a serious breach of security staff collusion has been a factor. But when you think about it no staff would knowingly and wantonly risk their professional qualification and status by deliberately acting in a way that compromised either security or professional integrity, so how do these things come about?

The Ashworth Inquiry (Fallon et al, 1999) highlighted that in the Personality Disorder Unit at Ashworth Hospital clinicians had attempted to engender trusting and open relationships with their clients as they would in any area of mental health practice. The pitfall in the process seemed to be, however, that in their eagerness to establish trust and trying to prove themselves trustworthy they were doing or telling things to the clients that they should strictly not. The current received wisdom is that in fact the issue of 'trust' should be avoided at all costs and that the focus of the nurse should rather be on maintaining absolute professional integrity. The rationale for this is that if we always act with absolute integrity then trust will follow as a natural consequence.

I can remember that when I first came to work in forensic mental health services I was quite afraid because I thought the clients would be really different. In fact the clients are no different to those I've nursed in the adult mental health services and for the most part just appear to be regular guys who've had a few problems. There probably are more clients with recognizable personality problems in the forensic mental health services and we do have clients who have never suffered any psychotic type mental illness but have personality disorders. This is not unusual as a lot of research (see for example, Dolan & Coid, 1993) indicates that individuals who commit serious offences against other people often have a lot of narcissistic traits. Sometimes these traits are so pronounced they warrant a diagnosis of Narcissistic Personality Disorder.

Of course it's predicated by the nature of the unit that nearly all the clients have been convicted of some sort of offence. In some cases these can be really serious offences including rape and murder and you have to be continually aware of how that knowledge affects your demeanour towards individual clients. Supervision is really important here because if your judgement becomes influenced by feelings that stem from your own fears and fantasies, rather than facts, you risk doing your clients (and yourself) a great disservice. A really important part of our role, then, is offence analysis as we have to advise the courts on disposal (be it prison or hospital). To do that you have to be able to understand the nature of the individual's mental disorder (if any) and the relationship between the disorder and their history of offending behaviours. This is not always easy or obvious and sometimes you have to really separate things out. For example you might have an individual who has a diagnosable personality disorder who also has a history of sexual offences against children. We know there is no causal relationship between psychopathy and paedophilia and so it seems reasonable to conclude that being a psychopath would not in itself cause an individual to offend against children.

This is really important when you're looking at what is mostly referred to as 'dangerousness' but is actually better described as risk. Psychopathy or personality disorders on their own do not in any way make individuals dangerous, nor does mental illness. It's a question of whether the nature of the disorder precludes the individual's capacity to limit his or her behaviour to the confines of those moral and social codes of what is acceptable or not. Most important is that to realize the potential for serious offences to take place there also has to be some additional motivation. So someone who has aberrant sexual predilections (e.g. rape, masochism, paedophilia) may fantasize about their own predilections but never actually act on them. But if that individual also has a narcissistic or antisocial personality disorder then they will be less constrained by social proprieties and more ready to act to satiate those aberrant sexual desires.

In instances like the above where an individual has both sexual urges towards children and a diagnosable personality disorder then we would have to look at the facets of the individual's disorder and explore contributory aspects. Perhaps, for example, the individual lacks empathy and consequently acts on his own sexual predilections with impunity or perhaps the individual lacks the emotional and cognitive processes to understand what he was doing was wrong. Whatever the case may be, however, it is still imperative that on the basis of our assessment we come to some opinion as to whether this individual would be likely to benefit from treatment or not.

In considering the issue of disposal the court will require clear advice on this issue because if the individual is likely to benefit from treatment they will probably be given a hospital order (for treatment), if not, they will almost certainly receive a custodial sentence and be sent to prison. So to really examine the risks presented by any individual client then we need to give close attention to previous offending behaviours and associated thinking. We get taught to look at such issues on the basis of four broad questions which need to be asked and answered, thus:

1. Why was the offence committed? (MOTIVE);
2. Why that date, time, place, person (victim)? (GROOMING);
3. Can we do anything to prevent it happening again? (TREATABILITY); and
4. How do we minimize the chances of re-offending in a similar way? (RELAPSE PREVENTION).

Obviously each of these questions demands considerable attention as each area can be hugely complex and convoluted but it's really important we get it right. The nursing contribution is particularly valuable because it is our best chance of observing patterns of behaviour that could lead to high risk situations (or further offences) in the future. It also offers our best chance to test the clients self-reporting and awareness of relapse indicators against actual interactions so if there are tensions or conflicts we can pick them up and do something before further offences occur. This process of exploration is really begun before the individual comes into the unit. Part of our assessment (a significant part in terms of the advice we will offer the court) is that if the individual does need to come into hospital for treatment then what level of security will he or she require to enable safe treatment to take place? This is more complex than you might imagine, for if we advise less security than is required the risk to the individual and others is considerable, if we advise too high we infringe the right of the individual to receive care in a place that offers a level of security no greater than is absolutely necessary.

There is no magic formula for assessing this issue but broadly we follow the process of coming to an opinion on the four 'D's, these being Diagnosis, Dangerousness, Detainability and Discharge.

Diagnosis. This is partly a legal requirement under the Mental Health Act (DoH, 1983) and this is of course essential if we are to detain an individual for treatment under mental health legislation. Equally important, however, is that the process of diagnosis also facilitates a comprehensive description and classification of the main components or symptoms of that individual's disorder and how they impact on the client's life and his or her human environment.

Dangerousness. This is really a bit of a misnomer because the term 'dangerous' implies a state of being permanently dangerous and of course no one is dangerous 24 hours a day – 7 days a week. In practice we tend to talk about 'risk' rather than dangerousness. The major difference here is that risk is contextual so you have to try to isolate in what circumstances is an individual most likely to realize their own risk potential to commit some offence or cause serious harm to others. In many ways it's similar to grooming as mentioned above as it asks that on the basis of what we know about their previous behaviours in what circumstance(s) may this individual offend again, what will be his/her motive, what will be his/her victim type (man, woman, child, policeman, sexual partner etc)?

Detainability. This is to some extent predicated by the first two 'D's as if someone continues to exhibit symptoms of a mental disorder and as a result is considered to present a risk to others then obviously that individual needs to be detained for treatment. What needs to be given more thorough consideration here, however, is the issue of what level of security is required to safely manage the individual and this can be more complex.

Discharge. The real value in thinking this through at such an early stage is that you're really asking what do we need to do to get our patient from where they are now (usually charged with some serious offence and in need of psychiatric treatment) to the point where they can be safely given back their liberty. Or put another way what are the treatment needs? To adequately answer this question demands a clear understanding of mental health needs and risk with additional attention to the susceptibility to treatment (treatability) in the case of individuals with personality disorder or learning disability.

There needs to be continuous attention to these issues and the nursing role is really important as we need to try and identify patterns of interpersonal functioning that have previously contributed to offending behaviour and look for how these might replicate themselves in the individual's current demeanour. For example individuals who have a history of rape and still objectify women or maintain those sort of Victorian attitudes towards women (Mother, Madonna, Whore) or individuals who have history of paedophilia and still spend a lot of time watching children's TV or amass pictures of children from catalogues; or even people who have a history of violent offences and still exhibit problems with anger control or have difficulty in seeing other people's point of view on a specific issue. Basically the rough and ready formula for looking at dangerousness or risk is to comparatively give regard to an individual's history of offending behaviours and his or her current attitude to the object or objects of those behaviours.

All-in-all it's not the sort of work most of us thought we would be doing when we make the decision to train as a mental health nurse but it is an essential role and one that demands all your traditional psychiatric nursing skills and then a few more. You just have to look at the history of forensic psychiatry to see why the role is so important and why we need to have people who are clear thinking and with unwavering commitment. You also have to remember that without our services most of our clients would be in and out of prison and there would be a lot more victims out there, wanting to have their accounts heard by a sympathetic public.

Still, it's nice to hand in your keys and alarms at the end of the day, though!

References

Audit Commission (1999) *Children in Mind*, Abingdon: Audit Commission Publications.

Bee, H. (2000) *The Developing Child*, (9th edn), London: Allyn & Bacon.

Bowlby, J. (1969) *Attachment and Loss: Volume 1 – Attachment*, New York: Basic Books.

Burns, T. & Firn, M. (2002) *Assertive Outreach in Mental Health; A Practitioners Manual*, Oxford: Oxford University Press.

Carr, A. (1999) *Child and Adolescent Clinical Psychology: A Contextual Approach*, London: Routledge.

Croom, S., Procter, S. & Le Couter, A. (2000) Developing a concept analysis of control for use in child and adolescent mental health nursing, *Journal of Advanced Nursing*, 31(6), 1324–32.

Department of Health (1983) *Mental Health Act 1983*, London: HMSO.

Department of Health (1999) *Modern Standards and Service Models: National Service Framework For Mental Health*, London: HMSO.

Department of Health (2001) *The Mental Health Policy Implementation Guide*, London: HMSO.

Dolan, B. & Coid, J. (1993) *Psychopathic and Antisocial Personality Disorders: Treatment and Research Issues*, London: Gaskell.

Egan, G. (1998) *The Skilled Helper* (5th edn), California: Brookes Cole.

Epstein, S. (1991) *Cognitive-Experiential Self Theory: Implications for Developmental Psychology*, London: Allyn & Bacon.

Fallon, P., Bluglass, R., Edwards, B. & Daniels, G. (1999) *Report of the Committee of Inquiry into the Personality Disorder Unit, Ashworth Special Hospital*, London: HMSO.

Gough, P. (1998) Multiskilling: here to stay, *Nursing Standard*, 12(31), 22–4.

Graham, P., Turk, J. & Verhulst, F. (1999) *Child Psychiatry, A Developmental Approach* (3rd edn), Oxford: Oxford University Press.

Home Office (1994) *Criminal Justice and Public Order Act*, London: HMSO.

Kemp, R., Hayward, P. & David, A. (1997) *Compliance Therapy Manual*, London: King's College School of Medicine and Dentistry and Institute of Psychiatry.

Kingdon, D. G. & Turkington, D. (1994) *Cognitive-Behavioural Therapy for Schizophrenia*, New York: Guilford Press.

Levitt, M. J., Guacci-Franco, N. & Levitt, J. L. (1993) Convoys of social support in childhood and early adolescence: structure and function, *Developmental Psychology*, 29, 811–18.

Lord Chancellor's Department (1997) *Who Decides?* London: HMSO.

Mason, T. & Mercer, D. (1990) Forensic psychiatric nursing: visions of social control, *Australian New Zealand Journal of Mental Health Nursing*, 5(4), 153–62.

Melia, P., Moran, A. & Mason, T. (1999) Triumvirate nursing for personality disordered patients: crossing the boundaries safely, *Journal of Psychiatric & Mental Health Nursing*, 6, 15–20.

NHS Health Advisory Service (1995) *Together We Stand*, London: HMSO.

Pearce, J. (1993) Child health surveillance for psychiatric disorders: practical guidelines, *Archives of Disease in Childhood*, 69, 394–8.

Pettit, G. S., Bates, J. E. & Dodge, K. A. (1997) Supportive parenting, ecological context, and children's adjustment: a seven-year longitudinal study, *Child Development*, 68(5), 908–23.

Pharoah, F. X. I., Mari, J. J. & Steiner, D. (1999) *Family Interventions for Schizophrenia*, Oxford: Cochrane Library Database.

Rollinick, S., Heather, N. & Bell, A. (1992) Negotiating behaviour change in medical settings: the development of brief motivational interviewing, *Journal of Mental Health*, 1, 25–37.

Said, E. (1993) *Culture and Imperialism*, London: Chatto & Windus.

Sainsbury Centre for Mental Health (1998) *Keys to Engagement: A Review of Care for People with Serious Mental Illness Who are Hard to Engage with Services*, London: Sainsbury Centre for Mental Health.

Schön, D. A. (1987) *Educating the Reflective Practitioner*, New York: Jossey-Bass.

Tarrier, N., Yusupoff, L., Kinney, C., McCarthy, E., Gledhill, A., Haddock, G. et al (1998) Randomised controlled trial of intensive cognitive behavioural therapy for patients with chronic schizophrenia, *British Medical Journal*, 17(7), 154, 303–7.

Wilkinson, I. (1998) *Child and Family Assessment: Clinical Guidelines for Practitioners* (2nd edn), London: Routledge.

Overview

STEPHAN D. KIRBY, DENIS A. HART, DENNIS CROSS AND
GORDON MITCHELL

The text we have presented has addressed a wide range of issues that mental health nurses will need to be aware of and address in their practice. The text has been written around the competency-based approach and has consistently attempted to address the benchmark criteria. As editors we became very aware of the need to present you with breadth rather than depth and we now take this opportunity to suggest aspects which you may need to consider further as you integrate your enhanced awareness once you qualify (or for your personal and professional development if you are already a qualified mental health nurse).

Perhaps, most importantly we have emphasized the need to keep abreast of new and emerging issues, this should dovetail appropriately to the critically reflective, and evidence-based approaches that have permeated your training and have been reflected in your portfolio and learning log.

The pace of change is, if anything, likely to accelerate yet further. There is no time to sit and become entrenched; rather the clarion call is to adapt and respond and to see challenges as potential opportunities.

Keeping up means maintaining a sharp eye to revised Government practice and the latest reports produced by the Department of Health and other professional bodies, it also entails being aware of new treatment modalities, best practice and effective strategies for delivering services in a world ever constrained by limited resources. Long hours, and high expectations create pressure. It is easy for this to become overwhelming. We hope you will consult key texts to help you avoid burn out and that you will find the supervision experience in the workplace supportive and energizing rather than oppressive and debilitating.

As has been demonstrated in the text, values cannot be taught – we either do or do not believe in a sensitive and anti-discriminatory approach to practice. Of course, there are minimum requirements placed upon us by virtue of the values framework required to be evidenced prior to qualification and registration. That said, an open mind, a preparedness to try out things new, underpinned by a belief as to what constitutes acceptable and unacceptable behaviour is the way forward in this difficult territory.

We are acutely aware that this text has been limited to the extent that it can discuss and apply specific concepts about gender, race culture and sexuality, and integrate them as thoroughly into main stream theory and practice as we would have liked. These issues should be exploited further and we hope you will find the list of additional reading texts, specifically related to these issues of value.

Finally, we hope that this text has provided you with the necessary foundation knowledge and a variety of different perspectives stimulating original thought as well as providing a helpful source of theoretical perspectives.

We thank you for reading this text

Stephan D. Kirby, Denis A. Hart, Dennis Cross and Gordon Mitchell

University of Teesside, 2003

A Competence-based 'Exit Profile' For Pre-registration Mental Health Nursing

Domain	UKCC Competencies for entry to the Register	Benchmarks for the Mental Health Nursing Branch	Essential Evidence	NSF Link Standard
1. Professional/ Ethical Practice	1.1 Manage oneself, one's practice, and that of others, in accordance with the UKCCs *Code of professional conduct*, recognizing one's own abilities and limitations. • Practice in accordance with the UKCC Code of Professional Conduct; • Use professional standards of practice to self-assess performance; • Consult with a registered nurse when nursing care requires expertise beyond one's own current scope of competence; • Consult other health care professionals when individual or group needs fall outside the scope of nursing practice; • Identify unsafe practice and respond appropriately to ensure a safe outcome; • Manage the delivery of care services within sphere of own accountability.	Be able to demonstrate: • A positive approach and optimism when working with mental health and social care users' of services; • Consideration to the needs of mental health and social care service users who may be particularly vulnerable to attacks or abuse; • Consideration of the power differential between users of services, carers and mental health and social care workers; • Skills in reflecting on the impact of own attitudes to mental health and social care; • Non-judgmental, non-blaming and non-punitive attitudes to users of mental health services and their carers; • Consideration of the different perspectives and needs of mental health clients, their carers and mental health care professionals to manage situations of conflict;	 O, WR T, WR D, WR O, WR T, WR, S D, WR	 All 1 7 All 1 4
1. Professional/ Ethical Practice	1.2 Practice in accordance with an ethical and legal framework which ensures the primacy of patient and client interest and well-being and respects confidentiality.	Be able to demonstrate: • Application of the mental health policies and frameworks for service delivery; • Identification of the scope and range of comprehensive,	 O WR	 All 3

Domain	UKCC Competencies for entry to the Register	Benchmarks for the Mental Health Nursing Branch	Essential Evidence	NSF Link Standard
	• Demonstrate knowledge of legislation and health and social policy relevant to nursing practice;	integrated mental health and social care services; • Contribution to the current systems of care e.g. Care Co-ordination;	CD, O	4
	• Ensure confidentiality and security of written and verbal information acquired in a professional capacity;	• Participation in the application of mental health law and related legislation;	O, S	3
	• Demonstrate knowledge of contemporary ethical issues and their impact on nursing and healthcare;	• An appreciation of mental health service users and carers civil rights, consent to treatment and the utilization of powers of compulsion and detention;	WR, T	All
	• Manage the complexities arising from ethical and legal dilemmas; • Act appropriately when seeking access to caring for patients and clients in their own homes.	• Ability to act for mental health services users who lack capacity to make decisions for themselves.	S, O, WR	4, 5
1. Professional/ Ethical Practice	1.3 Practice in a fair and anti-discriminatory way, acknowledging the difference in beliefs and cultural practices of individuals or groups.	Be able to demonstrate: • Ability to assess the impact of culture, race, gender and lifestyle on the needs of mental health service users and their carers;	T, WR, CS	1
		• Contribute to the development of culturally sensitive packages of mental health and social care;	CD, WR	4
	• Maintain, support and acknowledge the rights of individuals or groups in the health care setting;	• Identification of the impact of stigma on mental health service users, their families and carers, and the motivational basis of prejudice;	WR	1
	• Act to ensure that rights of individuals and groups are not compromised; • Respect values, customs and beliefs of individuals and groups;	• Ability to assist mental health service users and their carers in making informed choices about their care through the provision of culturally appropriate forms of communication;	O, WR	4
	• Provide care that demonstrates sensitivity to the diversity of patients and clients.	• Ability to work in mental health and social care settings in a non-discriminatory way.	O, D	1
2. Care Delivery	2.1 Engage in, develop and disengage from therapeutic relationships through the use of appropriate communication and interpersonal skills.	Be able to demonstrate: • The application of helping relationships as the cornerstone of their mental health nursing practice;	O, WR, AV	All
	• Utilize a range of effective and appropriate communication and engagement skills;	• Identification of the main characteristics and needs of the mental health and social care users and their carers;	CS	4

Continued

Domain	UKCC Competencies for entry to the Register	Benchmarks for the Mental Health Nursing Branch	Essential Evidence	NSF Link Standard
	• Maintain and, where appropriate, disengage from professional caring relationships which focus on meeting the patient's or client's needs within professional therapeutic boundaries.	• Facilitation of therapeutic co-operation with mental health service users and their carers, taking account of those who nurses find difficult to engage;	S, O, WR	4, 5
		• Maintenance of therapeutic alliances with users of mental health and social care services through partnership, intimacy and reciprocity;	CS, O	4, 5
		• A caring and empathetic attitude to users of mental health and social care services and their carers;	O, T, AV	All
		• Participation in negotiation, formulation and communication of therapeutic interventions with users of mental health and social care services and their carers;	WR, O, S	4
		• Appropriate disengagement from mental service users and their carers.	WR, O	4, 7
2. Care Delivery	2.2 Create and utilize opportunities to promote health and well being of patients, clients and groups.	Be able to demonstrate:		
		• A commitment to health promotion for users and carers of mental health and social care services in accordance with the 'Public Health Strategy' and Health Improvement Programmes;	WR, PW	1
	• Consult with patients, clients and groups to identify their need and desire for health promotion advice;	• Awareness of the relationship between NHS Direct, Primary Health Care Groups and Specialist Mental Health Services;	D, PW	3
	• Provide relevant and current health information to patients, clients and groups in a form which facilitates their understanding and acknowledges choice/ individual preference;	• Recognition of the prodromal signs of mental illness;	WR, O	4
		• Awareness of the effectiveness of early interventions in mental health and social care;	WR, D	4
	• Provide support and education in the development and/or maintenance of independent living skills;	• Recognition of relapse signatures in users of mental health and social care services;	O, D, CS	4
	• Seek specialist/expert advice as appropriate.	• Education of users of mental health and social care services and their carers about their condition, care and treatment;	O, WR, PW	1
		• Education of users of mental health and social care services and their carers about preventative medicine and health promotion;	O, CS, PW	1

Domain	UKCC Competencies for entry to the Register	Benchmarks for the Mental Health Nursing Branch	Essential Evidence	NSF Link Standard
		• Participation in mental health user and carer groups to problem solve health and personal problems.	O, WR, T	2, 4
		• Promotion of the understanding and acceptance of people with mental health problems in the wider community.	AV, PW	1
		• A commitment to promote mental health and well being in local communities.	S, PW	1
		• Participation in developing appropriate housing and vocational opportunities with users of mental health services and their carers;	O, T	4
		• Participation in activities to aid financial management with users of mental health services and their carers.	O, T	4
2. Care Delivery	2.3 Undertake and document a comprehensive, systematic and accurate nursing assessment of the physical, psychological, social and spiritual needs of patients, clients and communities.	Be able to demonstrate:		
		• Ability to undertake comprehensive, needs-led mental health nursing assessment;	CD, O	2, 4
		• Contribution to a family and social systems mental health assessment;	O, T, CD	2, 4
	• Select valid and reliable assessment tools for the required purpose;	• Participation in the assessment and management of factors of co-morbidity and precursors to mental illness;	O, WR	2, 4
	• Systematically collect data regarding the health and functional status of individuals, clients and communities through appropriate interaction, observation and measurement;	• Participation in the systematic assessment of the physical, psychological and social, spiritual needs of mental health carers;	CD, CS	6
	• Analyse and interpret data accurately to inform nursing care and take appropriate action.	• Identification of the needs, characteristics and key principles of care for a range of subgroups of people with severe mental illness across the age and setting continua.	WR, D	4
2. Care Delivery	2.4 Formulate and document a plan of nursing care, where possible in partnership with patients, clients, their carers and family and friends, within a framework of informed consent.	Be able to demonstrate:		
		• Enablement of users, their families and carers in establishing their own meaningful goals in the formulation of their care plans;	CD, O, T	4
	• Establish priorities for care based on individual or group needs;	• Contribution to the planning of mental health nursing care that facilitates communication among disciplines and across care setting and agencies;	O, WR	2, 4

Continued

Domain	UKCC Competencies for entry to the Register	Benchmarks for the Mental Health Nursing Branch	Essential Evidence	NSF Link Standard
	• Develop and document a plan of care to achieve optimal health, habilitation, rehabilitation based on assessment and current nursing knowledge; • Identify expected outcomes, including a time frame for achievement and/or review in consultation with patients, clients, their carers and family and friends and with members of the health and social care team.	• Involvement of users, their families and carers in planning and evaluating mental health and social care services.	WR, T	All
2. Care Delivery	2.5 Based on the best available evidence, apply knowledge and an appropriate repertoire of skills indicative of safe nursing practice.	Be able to demonstrate:		
		• Awareness of the importance of the integration of effective practice development into routine mental health nursing care;	WR	All
	• Ensure that current research findings and other evidence are incorporated in practice;	• Application of basic principles from the psychodynamic, behavioural, social and humanistic conceptual models of mental health interventions;	CS, AV	2, 4
	• Identify relevant changes in practice or new information and disseminate it to colleagues;	• Contribution to the care and treatment of service users with severe mental illness which is underpinned by the stress-vulnerability model and a bio-psycho-social approach;	O, CS	4
	• Contribute to the application of a range of interventions to support patients and clients and which optimize their health and well-being;	• Application of the basic principles of cognitive behavioural interventions;	O, CS	2, 4
	• Demonstrate the safe application of the skills required to meet the needs of patients and clients within the current sphere of practice;	• Participation in the provision of evidence-based family intervention programmes for service users with severe mental illness;	O, CS	4
	• Identify and respond to patients and clients' continuing learning and care needs;	• Application of the basic principles of person-centred counselling interventions	S, O, T	2, 4
	• Engage with, and evaluate, the evidence base which underpins safe nursing practice.	• Application of the fundamental knowledge of psychopharmacology;	O, WR, CD	2, 4
		• Contribution to the management of mental health medication, including prevention, detection and alleviation of side effects;	O, D	2, 4
		• Participation in techniques useful in increasing adherence to appropriately prescribed mental health medication and other treatments.	O, WR	2, 4

Domain	UKCC Competencies for entry to the Register	Benchmarks for the Mental Health Nursing Branch	Essential Evidence	NSF Link Standard
2. Care Delivery	2.6 Provide a rationale for the nursing care delivered which takes account of social, cultural, spiritual, legal, political and economic influences.	Be able to demonstrate:		
		• Participation in the identification and access of the range of supports needed to optimize the quality of life of mental health and social care service users and carers;	O, D	3
	• Identify, collect and evaluate information to justify the effective utilization of resources to achieve planned outcomes of nursing care.	• Participation in the practice of psycho-social rehabilitation;	O, CS	4, 5
		• Identification of the complexities of mental health and social care within acute settings;	WR	4, 5
		• A commitment to the guidance from the National Institute for Clinical Excellence to ensure efficiency and cost effectiveness of services.	WR, D	All
2. Care Delivery	2.7 Evaluate and document the outcomes of nursing and other interventions.	Be able to demonstrate:		
		• Contribution to the range of administrative duties, which are essential to effective case management;	O, D, T	4, 5
	• Collaborate with patients and clients and, when appropriate, additional carers to review and monitor the progress of individuals or groups towards planned outcomes;	• Maintenance of comprehensive mental health nursing records;	CD, O	2, 4, 5
		• Involvement of mental health service users, their families and carers in the evaluation of nursing care;	O, WR	2, 4, 5
	• Analyse and revise expected outcomes, nursing interventions and priorities in accordance with changes in individual's condition, needs or circumstances.	• Participate in the evaluation of mental health care and social care packages in collaboration with the care co-ordinator;	D, T	4, 5
		• Participation in the application of standardized measures for the purpose of monitoring mental health service user outcomes e.g. HONOS, BPRS, LUNSERS.	CD, S	2, 4, 5
2. Care Delivery	2.8 Demonstrate sound clinical judgement across a range of differing professional and care delivery contexts.	Be able to demonstrate:		
		• Retrieval and critical appraisal of mental health research and relevant evidence;	PW, CD	All
	• Use evidence based knowledge from nursing and related disciplines to select and individualize nursing interventions;	• Utilization of appropriate research and relevant evidence to support decision-making relating to the selection and individualization of mental health nursing interventions;	O, WR	All
	• Demonstrate the ability to transfer skills and knowledge to a variety of circumstances and settings; • Recognize the need for adaptation and adapt nursing	• Flexibility in the care of mental health service users, their families and carers to meet their changing needs and circumstances;	WR, T	2, 4, 5, 7

Continued

Domain	UKCC Competencies for entry to the Register	Benchmarks for the Mental Health Nursing Branch	Essential Evidence	NSF Link Standard
	practice to meet varying and unpredictable circumstances; • Ensure that practice does not compromise the nurse's duty of care to individuals or the safety of the public.	• Participation in therapeutic risk-taking in mental health and social care contexts;	S, WR	2, 4, 5, 7
		• Awareness of the need to share mental health nursing information with other agencies involved in maintaining public safety.	D, O	All
3. Care Management	3.1 Contribute to public protection by creating and maintaining a safe environment of care through the use of quality assurance and risk management strategies.	Be able to demonstrate: • Assessment and management of risk in mental health and social care settings;	O, CD, S	4, 7
		• Contribution to the audit processes used to monitor the quality of mental health nursing care in all settings;	O, CD	All
	• Apply relevant principles to ensure the safe administration of therapeutic substances; • Use appropriate risk assessment tools to identify actual and potential risks; • Identify environmental hazards and eliminate and/or prevent where possible; • Communicate safety concerns to a relevant authority; • Manage risk to provide care that best meets the needs and interests of patients, clients and the public.	• Participation in mental health nursing practice development initiatives;	O, T	All
		• Observation skills to maintain a safe environment within mental health and social care settings;	O, D	7
		• Participation in the management of violent and aggressive behaviour;	S, O, T	3, 4, 5, 7
		• Recognition of the importance of identifying and removing environmental dangers within mental health and social care settings;	S, WR	7
		• A critical awareness of the need to build healthier communities to ensure the safety of mental health service users, their families and carers.	WR	1
3. Care Management	3.2 Demonstrate knowledge of effective interprofessional working practices which respect and utilize the contributions of members of the health and social care team.	Be able to demonstrate: • Identification of specialist and non-specialist resources and the roles and responsibilities of local agencies;	WR, PW	3
		• Identification of the main roles and tasks of the mental health and social care multidisciplinary team;	D	3
	• Establish and maintain collaborative working relationships with members of the health and social care team and others; • Participate with members of the health and social care team in decision making concerning patients and clients;	• Participation in mental health multidisciplinary team working;	O, WR	2, 4, 5, 7
		• Identification of the range of settings within which mental health and social care take place;	WR	3
		• identification of the key tasks and functions of the following services: Assertive Outreach, Liaison Psychiatry, Mental Health	WR, PW	3, 4, 5

Domain	UKCC Competencies for entry to the Register	Benchmarks for the Mental Health Nursing Branch	Essential Evidence	NSF Link Standard
	• Review and evaluate care with members of the health and social care team and others.	Crisis Intervention Teams, CAMHS, Older People, Primary Care, Forensic, Drug and Alcohol , CMHT's, Day Care and Voluntary Sector, Helplines, Specialist Psychological Therapy Services;		
		• Ability to contribute to multidisciplinary Care Co-ordination meetings.	O, T	4, 5
3. Care Management	3.3 Delegate duties to others, as appropriate, ensuring that they are supervised and monitored.	Be able to demonstrate:		
		• Identification of the role and contribution to mental health and social care of non-specialist and support staff;	WR, D	3, 4, 5
	• Take into account the role and competence of staff when delegating work;	• Ability to provide support and supervision to mental health and social care non-specialist and support staff;	O, T	1
	• Maintain one's own accountability and responsibility when delegating aspects of care to others; • Demonstrate the ability to co-ordinate the delivery of nursing and health care.	• Assertiveness, conflict management and problem-solving skills within the multidisciplinary mental health and social care team.	O, T, S	1, 4, 5
3. Care Management	3.4 Demonstrate key skills	Be able to demonstrate:		
	• Literacy – interpret and present information in a comprehensible manner; • Numeracy – accurately interpret numerical data and their significance for safe delivery of care;	• Critical awareness of information systems which are needed to support mental health and social care services and improve the management of resources;	WR, PW	All
	• Information technology and management – interpret and utilize data and technology, taking account of legal, ethical and safety considerations, in the delivery and enhancement of care;	• Interpretation of mental health and social care data and its significance for care delivery; • Report writing in multidisciplinary and multi-agency mental health and social care context.	CD, PW

CD | All

4, 5, 7 |
| | • Problem solving – demonstrate sound clinical decision making which can be justified even when made on the basis of a limited information. | | | |

Continued

Domain	UKCC Competencies for entry to the Register	Benchmarks for the Mental Health Nursing Branch	Essential Evidence	NSF Link Standard
4. Personal/ Professional Development	4.1 Demonstrate a commitment to the need for continuing professional development and personal supervision activities in order to enhance knowledge, skill, values, and attitudes needed for safe and effective nursing practice	Be able to demonstrate:		
		• Identification of the need for lifelong learning within the modernized functions and organizations of the mental health and social care sector;	WR, D	All
		• Critical awareness of own competence and needs for future mental health nursing professional development;	WR, D	All
	• Identify one's own professional development needs by engaging in activities such as reflection in, and on, practice and lifelong learning;	• A commitment to continuing professional development and educational opportunities within the speciality of mental health nursing;	LC, WR	All
	• Develop a personal development plan which takes into account personal, professional and organizational needs;	• Support peers and others with special needs when working in mental health and social care settings.	O, T	1
	• Share experiences with colleagues and patients and clients in order to identify the additional knowledge and skills needed to manage unfamiliar or professionally challenging situations;			
	• Take action to meet any identified knowledge and skills deficit likely to affect the delivery of care within the current sphere of practice.			
4. Personal/ Professional Development	4.2 Enhance the professional development and safe practice of others through peer support, leadership, supervision and teaching.	Be able to demonstrate:		
		• Identification of strategies to enhance staff preservation and prevent individual and team burnout;	WR, D	1
	• Contribute to creating a climate conducive to learning;	• Participation in multi-disciplinary team clinical supervision;	WR, T	All
	• Contribute to the learning experiences and development of others by facilitating the mutual sharing of knowledge and experience;	• Participation in peer supervision strategies and learning sets;	WR, T	All
		• Teaching skills required to address the special challenges across mental health and social care settings;	S, O, WR	1

Domain	UKCC Competencies for entry to the Register	Benchmarks for the Mental Health Nursing Branch	Essential Evidence	NSF Link Standard
	• Demonstrate effective leadership in the establishment and maintenance of safe nursing practice.	• Application of the fundamentals of mental health nursing leadership by positive attitudes towards power and influence, clarifying the essential qualities and functions of leadership, identifying own strengths and weaknesses, developing 'action points' to improve personal leadership skills;	S, WR, D	All
		• A commitment to disseminating own evidence-based mental health research and practice development.	AV, PW	All

Key to essential evidence:

AV:	Audio/Visual Presentation
CD:	Completed Documentation (with written critique, including a rationale for actions/decisions)
CS:	Case/Care Study
D:	Dialogue/discussion in 'Tripartite Meeting'
LC:	Learning Contract
O:	Observed Practice (by Practice Assessor)
PW:	Project Work (i.e., poster displays, scrapbooks, group presentations, teaching packs)
S:	Simulation in Skills Laboratory
T:	Testimony of others (i.e., written materials, letters, consumer feedback)
WR:	Written Reflection

Index